**The book that empowers you with knowledge . . .**
**and puts *you* in charge!**

There's no time like the present to take control of your eating . . . make smart, healthful food choices . . . and keep track of those all-important calories. And there's no better guide through the nutritional maze than Corinne T. Netzer, America's #1 authority on the nutritional content of food. With this slim, handy reference you can make the right choices for yourself and your family as you plan daily meals . . . dine out in style . . . shop the supermarket aisles . . . grab a quick snack on the run . . . prepare a holiday feast, and more! You'll find the latest information about the newest foods, updated facts about old favorites, and much more, in this indispensable pocket companion—the perfect guide for people on the go!

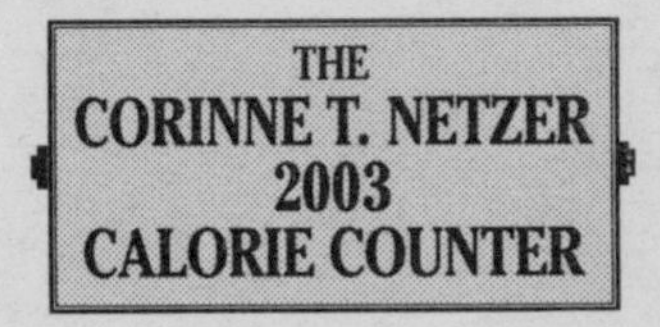

***Books by Corinne T. Netzer***

THE CORINNE T. NETZER ANNUAL CALORIE COUNTER
THE BRAND-NAME CALORIE COUNTER
THE BRAND-NAME CARBOHYDRATE GRAM COUNTER
THE CHOLESTEROL CONTENT OF FOOD
THE COMPLETE BOOK OF FOOD COUNTS
THE CORINNE T. NETZER CALORIE COUNTER
THE CORINNE T. NETZER CARBOHYDRATE GRAM COUNTER
THE CORINNE T. NETZER DIETER'S DIARY
THE CORINNE T. NETZER ENCYCLOPEDIA OF FOOD VALUES
THE CORINNE T. NETZER FAT GRAM COUNTER
THE CORINNE T. NETZER FIBER COUNTER
THE CORINNE T. NETZER LOW-FAT DIARY
THE DIETER'S CALORIE COUNTER
THE COMPLETE BOOK OF VITAMIN & MINERAL COUNTS

*THE COMPLETE BOOK OF FOOD COUNTS COOKBOOK SERIES:*
100 LOW FAT SMALL MEAL AND SALAD RECIPES
100 LOW FAT VEGETABLE AND LEGUME RECIPES
100 LOW FAT SOUP AND STEW RECIPES
100 LOW FAT PASTA AND GRAIN RECIPES
100 LOW FAT FISH AND SHELLFISH RECIPES
100 LOW FAT CHICKEN AND TURKEY RECIPES

# THE CORINNE T. NETZER 2003 CALORIE COUNTER

Corinne T. Netzer

A Dell Book

Published by
Dell Publishing
a division of
Random House, Inc.
1540 Broadway
New York, New York 10036




Cover design by Marietta Anastassatos



ISBN: 0-440-23679-7

Printed in the United States of America

Published simultaneously in Canada

September 2002

10 9 8 7 6 5 4 3 2
OPM

# Introduction

*The Corinne T. Netzer Calorie Counter* has been compiled with a twofold purpose: as an annual to keep you up-to-date on many of the changes made by the food industry, and to provide a handy source that you can carry in purse or pocket.

To keep this book concise yet comprehensive, I have grouped together listings of the same manufacturer whenever possible. Many brand-name yogurts, for example, are listed as "all fruit flavors." Therefore, instead of three pages filled with individual flavors of yogurt, all with identical calorie counts, I have been able to use the extra space for many other products. And for many basic foods and beverages (such as oil, milk, cream, and alcoholic beverages), I have used generic listings rather than include the numerous brands with the same or similar caloric values.

Finally, in the process of updating this edition, it was necessary to eliminate many previous listings and brands to accommodate new products and different brands. If you do not find a specific brand-name food that was listed in a previous edition of this book, this does not necessarily mean that the food product is no longer available. Also, since food producers are constantly revising and improving products, the caloric counts of your favorite foods may have changed even if the description of the product hasn't. Be sure to check for updated entries.

This book contains data from individual producers and manufacturers and from the United States government. It contains the most current information available as we go to press.

Good luck—and good eating.

*C.T.N.*

## ABBREVIATIONS

| | |
|---|---|
| approx. | approximately |
| cont. | container |
| diam. | diameter |
| fl. | fluid |
| lb. | pound |
| oz. | ounce |
| pc. | piece |
| pkg. | package |
| pkt. | packet |
| tbsp. | tablespoon |
| tsp. | teaspoon |
| w/ | with |

## SYMBOLS

| | |
|---|---|
| " | inch |
| * | prepared according to basic package directions |

***NOTE:*** *Brand-name foods and restaurants listed in italics denote registered trademarks.*

# THE CORINNE T. NETZER 2003 CALORIE COUNTER

# A

| FOOD AND MEASURE | CALORIES |
| --- | --- |
| **Abalone,** meat only, raw, 4 oz. | 119 |
| **Abruzzese sausage** (*Boar's Head*), 1 oz. | 100 |
| **Acerola,** fresh, trimmed, ½ cup | 16 |
| **Acorn squash:** | |
| raw (*Frieda's*), ¾ cup, 3 oz. | 35 |
| boiled, mashed, ½ cup | 41 |
| **Adobo sauce** (*Doña Maria*), 2 tbsp. | 230 |
| **Adzuki bean,** boiled, ½ cup | 147 |
| **Alfredo sauce** (see also "Cheese sauce, cooking") in jars: | |
| (*Five Brothers* Creamy), ¼ cup | 110 |
| (*Progresso* Authentic), ½ cup | 200 |
| garlic (*Five Brothers* Creamy), ¼ cup | 100 |
| mushroom (*Healthy Choice*), ¼ cup | 45 |
| **Alfredo sauce,** refrigerated, ¼ cup: | |
| (*Buitoni*) | 130 |
| (*Buitoni* Light) | 80 |
| **Alfredo sauce mix** (*Knorr* Pasta Sauces), 2 tbsp. | 60 |
| **Almond,** shelled: | |
| (*Fisher*), 1 oz. | 170 |
| whole, natural (*Blue Diamond*), 3 tbsp. | 180 |
| dry-roasted, 1 oz. | 167 |
| lightly salted (*Blue Diamond*), 3 tbsp. | 180 |
| oil-roasted (*Blue Diamond* 6 oz.), 3 tbsp. | 180 |
| sliced, blanched (*Blue Diamond*), ⅓ cup | 200 |
| slivered (*Planters*), 2-oz. pkg. | 340 |
| slivered, blanched (*Blue Diamond*), ¼ cup | 200 |
| honey-roasted (*Blue Diamond* 8 oz.), 3 tbsp. | 170 |
| smoke flavor (*Blue Diamond Smokehouse*), 3 tbsp. | 180 |
| smoked (*Planters*), 1 oz. | 170 |
| **Almond paste** (*Blue Diamond* Baker's), 2 tbsp. | 150 |
| **Anchovy,** fresh, meat only, European, raw, 1 oz. | 37 |
| **Anchovy, canned,** in olive oil (*Bumble Bee*), 6 pcs. | 25 |
| **Angel-hair pasta,** dry, see "Pasta" | |

**Angel-hair pasta entree,** frozen, 1 pkg.:
(*Lean Cuisine Everyday Favorites*), 10 oz. . . . . . . . . . . . . . .240
chunky tomatoes, meat sauce (*Budget Gourmet*), 8 oz. . . .240
**Angel-hair pasta mix,** 1 cup*:
garlic and butter (*Pasta Roni*) . . . . . . . . . . . . . . . . . . . . .260
w/herbs or Parmesan cheese (*Pasta Roni*) . . . . . . . . . . . . .320
primavera (*Pasta Roni*) . . . . . . . . . . . . . . . . . . . . . . . . . .330
tomato Parmesan (*Pasta Roni*) . . . . . . . . . . . . . . . . . . . . .280
**Anise seed,** 1 tsp. . . . . . . . . . . . . . . . . . . . . . . . . . . . . . .7
**Apple,** fresh:
w/peel (*Dole*), 1 medium . . . . . . . . . . . . . . . . . . . . . . . . .80
w/peel, 2¾" diam. . . . . . . . . . . . . . . . . . . . . . . . . . . . . . .81
w/peel, sliced, ½ cup . . . . . . . . . . . . . . . . . . . . . . . . . . . .32
peeled, 2¾" diam. . . . . . . . . . . . . . . . . . . . . . . . . . . . . . .72
peeled, sliced, ½ cup . . . . . . . . . . . . . . . . . . . . . . . . . . . .31
**Apple, coated,** candy or caramel (*Tastee*), 3-oz. apple . . . .160
**Apple, dried** (*Sunsweet*), 1.4 oz., ¼ cup . . . . . . . . . . . . . .110
**Apple, scalloped,** see "Apple dish"
**Apple butter,** 1 tbsp.:
(*Lucky Leaf/Musselman's*) . . . . . . . . . . . . . . . . . . . . . . . . .30
(*Smucker's* Cider) . . . . . . . . . . . . . . . . . . . . . . . . . . . . . . .45
**Apple chips** (*Tastee*), 1 oz. . . . . . . . . . . . . . . . . . . . . . . .130
**Apple cider,** see "Apple drink" and "Apple juice"
**Apple cider, alcoholic** (*Hard Core* Crisp), 12 fl. oz. . . . . . . .190
**Apple dip,** 2 tbsp.:
caramel (*Marzetti*) . . . . . . . . . . . . . . . . . . . . . . . . . . . . . .150
caramel (*Marzetti* Fat Free) . . . . . . . . . . . . . . . . . . . . . . . .120
peanut butter caramel (*Marzetti*) . . . . . . . . . . . . . . . . . . . .130
**Apple dish,** frozen:
cinnamon (*Boston Market*), ½ cup . . . . . . . . . . . . . . . . . . .260
scalloped (*Stouffer's* Side Dish), ½ of 12-oz. pkg. . . . . . . . .210
**Apple drink:**
(*Libby's* Nectar), 11.5-fl-oz. can . . . . . . . . . . . . . . . . . . . .200
(*Musselman's* Little Brown Jug Cider), 8 fl. oz. . . . . . . . . . .120
sparkling (*Lucky Leaf/Musselman's* Cider), 8 fl. oz. . . . . . . .150
**Apple drink blends,** 8 fl. oz., except as noted:
cranberry (*Tropicana*), 11.5 fl. oz. . . . . . . . . . . . . . . . . . . .200
herbal cider (*Turkey Hill*) . . . . . . . . . . . . . . . . . . . . . . . . . .100
raspberry blackberry (*Tropicana Twister*) . . . . . . . . . . . . . .120
raspberry blackberry (*Tropicana Twister*), 11.5 fl. oz. . . . . .180

**Apple dumpling,** frozen (*Pepperidge Farm*), 3-oz. pc. . . . . .250
**Apple fritters,** frozen (*Mrs. Paul's*), 2 pcs. . . . . . . . . . . . . . .240
**Apple juice,** 8 fl. oz.:
(*Dole*) . . . . . . . . . . . . . . . . . . . . . . . . . . . . . . .110
(*Lincoln*) . . . . . . . . . . . . . . . . . . . . . . . . . . . . . .120
(*Martinelli's* Juice/Cider) . . . . . . . . . . . . . . . . . . . . .140
(*Mott's* Natural) . . . . . . . . . . . . . . . . . . . . . . . . . .110
(*Mott's* From Concentrate) . . . . . . . . . . . . . . . . . . . .120
(*Nantucket Nectars* Cider/Pressed) . . . . . . . . . . . . . . .100
(*Season's Best*) . . . . . . . . . . . . . . . . . . . . . . . . . . .110
frozen* (*Cascadian Farm*) . . . . . . . . . . . . . . . . . . . . .120
**Apple juice blend,** 8 fl. oz.:
all blends (*Martinelli's*) . . . . . . . . . . . . . . . . . . . . . .110
grape (*Juicy Juice*) . . . . . . . . . . . . . . . . . . . . . . . . .120
**Apple pastry** (see also specific listings):
puffs (*Entenmann's*), 3-oz. pc. . . . . . . . . . . . . . . . . . . .270
strudel (*Entenmann's*), ¼ pastry . . . . . . . . . . . . . . . . . .340
**Applesauce,** ½ cup, except as noted:
(*Lucky Leaf/Lucky Leaf* Chunky) . . . . . . . . . . . . . . . . . .90
(*Mott's* Original) . . . . . . . . . . . . . . . . . . . . . . . . . .110
(*Mott's* Original), 4-oz. cont. . . . . . . . . . . . . . . . . . . . .90
(*Musselman's*) . . . . . . . . . . . . . . . . . . . . . . . . . . . .90
(*Musselman's* Chunky) . . . . . . . . . . . . . . . . . . . . . . .100
cinnamon (*Apple Time*) . . . . . . . . . . . . . . . . . . . . . . .100
cinnamon (*Lucky Leaf/Musselman's*) . . . . . . . . . . . . . . .100
cinnamon (*Mott's*), 4-oz. cont. . . . . . . . . . . . . . . . . . . .100
unsweetened/natural:
(*Apple Time* Original) . . . . . . . . . . . . . . . . . . . . . . .50
(*Langers*) . . . . . . . . . . . . . . . . . . . . . . . . . . . . . .50
(*Lucky Leaf* Old Fashioned/Musselman's) . . . . . . . . . . . .50
(*Mott's*), 3.9-oz. cont. . . . . . . . . . . . . . . . . . . . . . . .50
**Applesauce blends,** 4-oz. cont., except as noted:
all fruits (*Mott's Fruitsations*) . . . . . . . . . . . . . . . . . . .90
berry, mixed (*Mott's*) . . . . . . . . . . . . . . . . . . . . . . . .90
strawberry (*Mott's*) . . . . . . . . . . . . . . . . . . . . . . . . .80
**Apricot,** fresh:
(*Dole*), 3 medium, 4 oz. . . . . . . . . . . . . . . . . . . . . . . .60
pitted, halves, ½ cup . . . . . . . . . . . . . . . . . . . . . . . . .37
**Apricot, canned,** ½ cup, halves, except as noted:
(*Del Monte* Lite) . . . . . . . . . . . . . . . . . . . . . . . . . . .60

**Apricot, canned *(cont.)***
in juice (*Libby's*) . . . . . . . . . . . . . . . . . . . . . . . . . . . . . . .80
in light syrup (*Del Monte Orchard Select*) . . . . . . . . . . . . . . .80
in light syrup almond-flavor (*Del Monte*) . . . . . . . . . . . . . . .90
in heavy syrup (*Del Monte*) . . . . . . . . . . . . . . . . . . . . . . . . .100
in heavy syrup, whole, peeled (*S&W*) . . . . . . . . . . . . . . . . .120
**Apricot, dried:**
(*Sun•Maid Fast Fruit* California), 1.4 oz., ¼ cup . . . . . . . . .110
(*Sunsweet Fruitlings*), 1.4 oz., ⅓ cup . . . . . . . . . . . . . . . . .110
sun-dried (*Sunsweet* California), 1.4 oz., about 6 pcs. . . . . .100
**Apricot juice,** blend (*Ceres*), 5.25 fl. oz. . . . . . . . . . . . . . . .87
**Apricot nectar** (*Libby's*), 8 fl. oz. . . . . . . . . . . . . . . . . . . . .150
**Apricot syrup** (*Knott's Berry Farm*), ¼ cup . . . . . . . . . . . . .210
**Artichoke,** globe, fresh:
(*Dole*), 1 medium, 2 oz. edible . . . . . . . . . . . . . . . . . . . . . . .25
boiled, drained, 4.2 oz. . . . . . . . . . . . . . . . . . . . . . . . . . . . . .60
hearts, boiled, drained, ½ cup . . . . . . . . . . . . . . . . . . . . . . . .42
**Artichoke, can or jar** (see also "Artichoke appetizer"):
(*Progresso*), 1 pc., 2.9 oz. . . . . . . . . . . . . . . . . . . . . . . . . . .30
bottoms (*Gourmet Award*), 3 pcs. . . . . . . . . . . . . . . . . . . . . .18
hearts (*Pompeian*), ½ cup . . . . . . . . . . . . . . . . . . . . . . . . . . .35
hearts (*Reese*), 4.5 oz., 4 quarters . . . . . . . . . . . . . . . . . . . .50
**Artichoke, frozen:**
bottoms (*Bonduelle*), 3 oz. . . . . . . . . . . . . . . . . . . . . . . . . . .25
hearts (*Birds Eye* Deluxe), ½ cup . . . . . . . . . . . . . . . . . . . . .40
hearts, quartered (*Bonduelle*), 3 oz. . . . . . . . . . . . . . . . . . . .35
**Artichoke appetizer,** marinated:
(*Pompeian*), 1 oz. . . . . . . . . . . . . . . . . . . . . . . . . . . . . . . . .25
(*Progresso*), 2 pcs., 1.1 oz. . . . . . . . . . . . . . . . . . . . . . . . . .50
salad (*Reese*), ⅓ cup . . . . . . . . . . . . . . . . . . . . . . . . . . . . .150
**Artichoke dip** (*Victoria*), 2 tbsp. . . . . . . . . . . . . . . . . . . . . .30
**Arugula,** fresh:
trimmed, 1 oz. . . . . . . . . . . . . . . . . . . . . . . . . . . . . . . . . . . .7
½ cup . . . . . . . . . . . . . . . . . . . . . . . . . . . . . . . . . . . . . . . . .3
**Asparagus,** fresh, trimmed:
raw (*Dole*), 5 spears, 3.3 oz. . . . . . . . . . . . . . . . . . . . . . . . .25
raw, 4 spears, 2 oz. . . . . . . . . . . . . . . . . . . . . . . . . . . . . . . .14
raw, purple or white (*Frieda's*), 3 oz. . . . . . . . . . . . . . . . . . .20
boiled, 4 spears, ½"-diam. base . . . . . . . . . . . . . . . . . . . . . .14
boiled, drained, cuts, ½ cup . . . . . . . . . . . . . . . . . . . . . . . . .22

**Asparagus, can or jar:**
all styles (*Del Monte*), ½ cup .......................... 20
spears (*Green Giant*), 4.5 oz., about 5 pcs. ............... 20
spears (*Reese* White), ⅓ of 15-oz. can ................... 20
spears, pickled (*Hogue Farms*), 3 spears, 1.1 oz. ......... 10
cuts (*Bush's Best*), ½ cup ............................. 25
cuts (*Green Giant*), ½ cup ............................. 20
cuts (*Libby's*), ½ cup ................................. 20
**Asparagus, frozen:**
spears (*Birds Eye* Deluxe), 3 oz. ........................ 20
spears (*Seabrook Farms*), 7 pcs., 3 oz. .................. 20
spears, boiled, 4 pcs. ................................... 17
cuts (*Birds Eye* Deluxe), ½ cup ......................... 25
cuts (*Green Giant*), ⅔ cup .............................. 20
stir-fry blend (*Birds Eye*), 2 cups frozen ............... 90
**Au jus gravy** (*Franco-American*), ¼ cup ................. 10
**Au jus gravy mix** (*Lawry's*), 1 tsp. .................... 10
**Aubergine,** see "Eggplant"
**Australian blue squash** (*Frieda's*), ¾ cup, 3 oz. ........ 30
**Avocado,** fresh:
(*Frieda's Cocktail*), 1.4-oz. pc. ........................ 60
all varieties, cubed, ½ cup ............................. 203
California, 1 medium, 8 oz. ............................. 306
California, pureed, ½ cup ............................... 204
Florida, pureed, ½ cup .................................. 130

# B

| FOOD AND MEASURE | CALORIES |
|---|---|
| **Babaganoush,** see "Eggplant appetizer" | |
| **Bacon** (see also "Turkey bacon"), cooked: | |
| (*Armour*), 2 slices | 90 |
| (*Boar's Head*), 2 slices | 60 |
| (*Hormel* Fully Cooked), 2½ slices | 70 |
| (*Thorn Apple Valley*), 2 slices | 80 |
| (*Tobin's First Prize* Hardwood), 2 slices | 100 |
| thick cut (*Oscar Mayer*), 1 slice, ⅛" | 60 |
| **Bacon, Canadian** (*Boar's Head*), 2 oz. | 70 |
| **Bacon, Italian** (*Daniele* Pancetta), .5-oz. slice | 50 |
| **Bacon bits:** | |
| imitation (*Bac 'n Pieces*), 1½ tbsp. | 30 |
| real (*Oscar Mayer*), 1 tbsp. | 25 |
| **Bagel,** 1 pc., except as noted: | |
| plain (*Awrey's*), 4 oz. | 270 |
| plain or cinnamon raisin (*Awrey's*), 2 oz. | 150 |
| plain or cinnamon raisin (*Awrey's*), 2.6 oz. | 190 |
| plain, multigrain, onion, or whole wheat (*Thomas'*) | 280 |
| cranberry orange (*Thomas'* Gourmet), ½ pc. | 150 |
| sesame or blueberry (*Thomas'*) | 300 |
| wildberry blueberry (*Thomas'* Gourmet), ½ pc. | 170 |
| **Bagel, frozen** 1 pc., except as noted: | |
| all varieties, except cinnamon raisin (*Sara Lee*) | 210 |
| plain (*Lender's*) | 150 |
| plain (*Lender's* Bagelette), 2 pcs. | 140 |
| plain or blueberry (*Lender's Big 'n Crusty*) | 250 |
| blueberry or chocolate chip swirl (*Lender's*) | 160 |
| cinnamon raisin (*Lender's*) | 160 |
| cinnamon raisin (*Lender's Big 'n Crusty*) | 260 |
| cinnamon raisin (*Sara Lee*) | 220 |
| egg (*Lender's*) | 160 |
| egg (*Lender's Big 'n Crusty*) | 260 |
| garlic or onion (*Lender's*) | 150 |
| honey wheat (*Lender's Big 'n Crusty*) | 230 |

onion (*Lender's Big 'n Crusty*) . . . . . . . . . . . . . . . . . . . . .250
poppy, sesame seed, pumpernickel, or rye (*Lender's*) . . . . .150
soft (*Lender's* Original) . . . . . . . . . . . . . . . . . . . . . . . . . .210
**Baked beans,** canned, ½ cup:
(*Bush's Best* Bold & Spicy) . . . . . . . . . . . . . . . . . . . . . . .120
(*Bush's Best* Boston Recipe/Country Style) . . . . . . . . . . . . .170
(*Bush's Best* Original/Homestyle) . . . . . . . . . . . . . . . . . . .150
(*Campbell's* New England Style) . . . . . . . . . . . . . . . . . . . .160
(*Campbell's* Old Fashioned) . . . . . . . . . . . . . . . . . . . . . .180
w/bacon and onion (*B&M*) . . . . . . . . . . . . . . . . . . . . . . . .190
barbecue (*Bush's Best*) . . . . . . . . . . . . . . . . . . . . . . . . . .160
maple cured or w/onion (*Bush's Best*) . . . . . . . . . . . . . . . .150
w/pork (*Campbell's*) . . . . . . . . . . . . . . . . . . . . . . . . . . . .110
w/pork, peas (*East Texas Fair* Peas n' Pork) . . . . . . . . . . .110
w/pork, tomato sauce (*Campbell's*) . . . . . . . . . . . . . . . . . .130
sugar and bacon flavor (*Campbell's* Old Fashioned) . . . . . .160
vegetarian (*Bush's Best*) . . . . . . . . . . . . . . . . . . . . . . . . .130
vegetarian (*Heinz*) . . . . . . . . . . . . . . . . . . . . . . . . . . . . .140
**Baking mix,** ⅓ cup:
(*Bisquick*) . . . . . . . . . . . . . . . . . . . . . . . . . . . . . . . . . . .160
(*Bisquick* Reduced Fat) . . . . . . . . . . . . . . . . . . . . . . . . . .140
(*Hodgson Mill* InstaBake) . . . . . . . . . . . . . . . . . . . . . . . .150
sweet (*Bisquick*) . . . . . . . . . . . . . . . . . . . . . . . . . . . . . . .170
**Baking powder or soda,** ½ tsp. . . . . . . . . . . . . . . . . . . . . . .0
**Baklava,** frozen (*Apollo/Athens*), 4½ pcs., 4.4 oz. . . . . . . .540
**Balsam pear:**
leafy-tips, boiled, drained, ½ cup . . . . . . . . . . . . . . . . . . . .10
pods, ½" pcs., boiled, drained, ½ cup . . . . . . . . . . . . . . . . .12
**Bamboo shoots, canned** (*La Choy*), ½ cup . . . . . . . . . . . . .10
**Banana,** fresh:
(*Dole*), 1 medium, 4.4 oz. . . . . . . . . . . . . . . . . . . . . . . . .110
(*Frieda's* Baby Nino/Burro/Ice Cream), 3 oz. . . . . . . . . . . . .80
(*Frieda's* Red), 5 oz. . . . . . . . . . . . . . . . . . . . . . . . . . . . .130
common, 8¾" banana . . . . . . . . . . . . . . . . . . . . . . . . . . . .105
**Banana, baking,** see "Plantain"
**Banana, dried** (*Frieda's*), 1.2-oz. pc. . . . . . . . . . . . . . . . . .30
**Banana nectar** (*Libby's*), 11.5-fl.-oz. can . . . . . . . . . . . . .190
**Banana squash,** raw (*Frieda's*), ¾ cup, 3 oz. . . . . . . . . . . . .30
**Barbecue sauce** (see also "Grilling sauce"), 2 tbsp.:
(*Honeycup*) . . . . . . . . . . . . . . . . . . . . . . . . . . . . . . . . . . .50

**Barbecue sauce *(cont.)***
(*Hunt's* Original) .50
(*KC Masterpiece* Original) .60
(*Kraft* Original) .40
(*Lea & Perrins* Original) .50
(*Maull's*) .40
(*Maull's* Sweet-N-Mild/Smoky) .60
(*Silver Dollar City* Original) .40
(*Silver Dollar City* Ozark Recipe) .50
(*Sweet Baby Ray's*) .70
(*Sylvia's* Original) .40
(*Texas Best* Original Rib Style) .50
all varieties (*Muir Glen*) .40
beer (*Maull's*) .45
Cajun or mesquite (*Texas Best*) .50
hickory and brown sugar (*Hunt's*) .70
honey (*Sweet Baby Ray's*) .70
honey, honey teriyaki, or Dijon (*KC Masterpiece*) .60
hot (*D. L. Jardine's* Killer Hot) .35
jalapeño (*Maull's*) .50
Kansas City style (*Maull's*) .60
Korean style (*Sun Luck*) .45
mesquite (*D. L. Jardine's*) .35
mustard (*D. L. Jardine's* Chick'n-Lik'n) .40
onion bits (*Maull's*) .45
pecan, Texas (*D.L. Jardine's*) .35
smoky (*Maull's*) .40
spicy (*KC Masterpiece*) .60
tropical (*World Harbors Maui Mountain*) .50
**Barley,** pearled:
dry (*Quaker* Scotch Quick), ⅓ cup .170
dry (*Quaker* Scotch Regular), ¼ cup .170
cooked, 1 cup .193
**Barley flakes,** rolled (*Arrowhead Mills*), ⅓ cup .110
**Basil,** fresh, 5 medium leaves or 2 tbsp. chopped .1
**Basil, dried,** ground, 1 tbsp. .11
**Bass** (see also "Sea bass"), meat only, 4 oz.:
freshwater, raw .129
freshwater, baked, broiled, or microwaved .166

striped, raw . . . . . . . . . . . . . . . . . . . . . . . . . . . . . 110
striped, baked, broiled, or microwaved . . . . . . . . . . . . . . . 141
**Batter and seasoning mix,** all purpose (*Don's Chuck Wagon*), ¼ cup . . . . . . . . . . . . . . . . . . . . . . . . . . 100
**Bay leaf,** dried, crumbled, 1 tsp. . . . . . . . . . . . . . . . . . . . 5
**Bean dip,** 2 tbsp.:
(*Fritos*) . . . . . . . . . . . . . . . . . . . . . . . . . . . . . . . . 40
(*Marie's*) . . . . . . . . . . . . . . . . . . . . . . . . . . . . . . . 140
black bean, mild or spicy (*Guiltless Gourmet*) . . . . . . . . . . . 30
hot (*Fritos*) . . . . . . . . . . . . . . . . . . . . . . . . . . . . . . 40
**Bean dishes,** see specific bean listings
**Bean salad,** 3-bean, in jars (*Green Giant*), ½ cup . . . . . . . . 90
**Bean sprouts,** fresh, see specific listings
**Bean sprouts, canned** (*La Choy*), ⅔ cup . . . . . . . . . . . . . . 15
**Bean–carrot blend,** frozen, baby (*Birds Eye*), 3 oz. . . . . . . . . 30
**Beans,** see specific listings
**Beans, baked,** see "Baked beans"
**Beans, snap or string,** see "Green bean"
**Bearnaise sauce,** in jars (*Maille* Dipping), 2 tbsp. . . . . . . . 140
**Beef,** choice grade, meat only, trimmed to ¼" fat, except as noted, 4 oz.:
brisket, whole, braised, lean w/fat . . . . . . . . . . . . . . . . . 437
brisket, whole, braised, lean only . . . . . . . . . . . . . . . . . . 274
chuck, arm pot roast, braised, lean w/fat . . . . . . . . . . . . . . 395
chuck, arm pot roast, braised, lean only . . . . . . . . . . . . . . 255
chuck, blade roast, braised, lean w/fat . . . . . . . . . . . . . . . 412
chuck, blade roast, braised, lean only . . . . . . . . . . . . . . . 298
flank steak, trimmed to 0" fat, broiled, lean only . . . . . . . . . 256
ground, broiled, medium, extra lean . . . . . . . . . . . . . . . . 290
ground, broiled, medium, lean . . . . . . . . . . . . . . . . . . . . 308
ground, broiled, medium, regular . . . . . . . . . . . . . . . . . . 328
porterhouse steak, broiled, lean w/fat . . . . . . . . . . . . . . . 346
porterhouse steak, broiled, lean only . . . . . . . . . . . . . . . 247
rib, whole, roasted, lean w/fat . . . . . . . . . . . . . . . . . . . 426
rib, whole, roasted, lean only . . . . . . . . . . . . . . . . . . . . 276
rib, large end (ribs 6–9), roasted, lean w/fat . . . . . . . . . . . 434
rib, large end (ribs 6–9), roasted, lean only . . . . . . . . . . . . 284
rib, small end (ribs 10–12), broiled, lean w/fat . . . . . . . . . . 376
rib, small end (ribs 10–12), broiled, lean only . . . . . . . . . . . 264

**Beef** ***(cont.)***
round, bottom, braised, lean w/fat . . . . . . . . . . . . . . . . . . . .322
round, bottom, braised, lean only . . . . . . . . . . . . . . . . . . . . .249
round, eye of, roasted, lean w/fat . . . . . . . . . . . . . . . . . . . . .273
round, eye of, roasted, lean only . . . . . . . . . . . . . . . . . . . . . .198
round, full cut, broiled, lean w/fat . . . . . . . . . . . . . . . . . . . .272
round, full cut, broiled, lean only . . . . . . . . . . . . . . . . . . . .217
round, tip, roasted, lean w/fat . . . . . . . . . . . . . . . . . . . . . . .280
round tip, roasted, lean only . . . . . . . . . . . . . . . . . . . . . . . .213
round, top, broiled, lean w/fat . . . . . . . . . . . . . . . . . . . . . . .254
round, top, broiled, lean only . . . . . . . . . . . . . . . . . . . . . . .214
round, top, fried, lean w/fat . . . . . . . . . . . . . . . . . . . . . . . .314
round, top, fried, lean only . . . . . . . . . . . . . . . . . . . . . . . . .257
shank, crosscuts, braised, lean w/fat . . . . . . . . . . . . . . . . . .298
shank, crosscuts, braised, lean only . . . . . . . . . . . . . . . . . . .228
shortribs, braised, lean w/fat . . . . . . . . . . . . . . . . . . . . . . . .534
shortribs, braised, lean only . . . . . . . . . . . . . . . . . . . . . . . .335
sirloin, top, broiled, lean w/fat . . . . . . . . . . . . . . . . . . . . . .305
sirloin, top, broiled, lean only . . . . . . . . . . . . . . . . . . . . . . .229
sirloin, top, fried, lean w/fat . . . . . . . . . . . . . . . . . . . . . . . .370
sirloin, top, fried, lean only . . . . . . . . . . . . . . . . . . . . . . . . .270
T-bone steak, broiled, lean w/fat . . . . . . . . . . . . . . . . . . . . .338
T-bone steak, broiled, lean only . . . . . . . . . . . . . . . . . . . . . .243
tenderloin, broiled, lean w/fat . . . . . . . . . . . . . . . . . . . . . . .345
tenderloin, broiled, lean only . . . . . . . . . . . . . . . . . . . . . . . .252
top loin, broiled, lean w/fat . . . . . . . . . . . . . . . . . . . . . . . . .338
top loin, broiled, lean only . . . . . . . . . . . . . . . . . . . . . . . . . .243
**Beef, canned,** see specific listings
**Beef, corned** (see also "Beef lunch meat"):
brisket, cooked, 4 oz. . . . . . . . . . . . . . . . . . . . . . . . . . . . . .285
canned (*Libby's*), 2 oz. . . . . . . . . . . . . . . . . . . . . . . . . . . .120
**Beef, dried,** cured, 1 oz. . . . . . . . . . . . . . . . . . . . . . . . . . . .47
**"Beef," vegetarian,** frozen:
corned (*Worthington* Meatless), 2 oz. . . . . . . . . . . . . . . . . . .140
smoked (*Worthington* Meatless), 6 slices, 2 oz. . . . . . . . . . .120
**Beef dinner,** frozen, 1 pkg.:
chicken-fried steak (*Banquet Extra Helping*), 16 oz. . . . . . . .820
mesquite w/barbecue sauce (*Healthy Choice*), 11 oz. . . . . .320
oven roasted (*Healthy Choice*), 10.15 oz. . . . . . . . . . . . . . .280
patty, char-broiled (*Healthy Choice*), 11 oz. . . . . . . . . . . . . .310

pot roast (*Swanson Hungry-Man*), 18.5 oz. . . . . . . . . . . . .390
pot roast (*Swanson Traditional Favorites*), 14 oz. . . . . . . . .320
pot roast, Yankee (*Banquet Extra Helping*), 14.5 oz. . . . . . .410
pot roast, Yankee (*Healthy Choice*), 11 oz. . . . . . . . . . . . .330
pot roast, Yankee (*Stouffer's* HomeStyle), 16 oz. . . . . . . . . .360
roast, gravy (*Swanson Traditional Favorites*), 10.5 oz. . . . . .370
Salisbury steak (*Banquet Extra Helping*), 16.5 oz. . . . . . . . .740
Salisbury steak (*Healthy Choice*), 11.5 oz. . . . . . . . . . . . .330
Salisbury steak (*Stouffer's* HomeStyle), 16 oz. . . . . . . . . . .550
Salisbury steak (*Swanson Hungry-Man*), 16.25 oz. . . . . . . .610
sirloin, chopped (*Swanson Traditional Favorites*),
14.75 oz. . . . . . . . . . . . . . . . . . . . . . . . . . . . . . .490
sirloin tips (*Swanson Hungry-Man*), 15.75 oz. . . . . . . . . . .440
steak, country-fried (*Stouffer's* HomeStyle), 16 oz. . . . . . . .560
Stroganoff (*Healthy Choice*), 11 oz. . . . . . . . . . . . . . . . . .330
tips, portobello (*Healthy Choice*), 11.25 oz. . . . . . . . . . . . . .310
**Beef entree, can or pkg.**, 1 cont., except as noted:
hash, see "Beef hash"
pot roast (*Dinty Moore American Classics*) . . . . . . . . . . . .200
roast, w/gravy (*Hormel*), ½ cup . . . . . . . . . . . . . . . . . . . .150
roast, w/potato (*Dinty Moore American Classics*) . . . . . . . .240
Salisbury steak (*Dinty Moore American Classics*) . . . . . . . .320
stew (*Castleberry* Original), 1 cup . . . . . . . . . . . . . . . . . .340
stew (*Dinty Moore* Can), 1 cup . . . . . . . . . . . . . . . . . . . .180
stew (*Dinty Moore* Can), 7.5-oz. can . . . . . . . . . . . . . . . .190
stew (*Dinty Moore* Microwave Cup) . . . . . . . . . . . . . . . .160
stew (*Dinty Moore American Classics*) . . . . . . . . . . . . . . .250
stew (*Hormel* Microcup), 1 cup . . . . . . . . . . . . . . . . . . .150
stew, burger (*Dinty Moore* Microwave Cup) . . . . . . . . . . . .240
**Beef entree, frozen,** 1 pkg., except as noted:
barbecue sauce, rice, beans (*Healthy Choice* Duo),
8.5 oz. . . . . . . . . . . . . . . . . . . . . . . . . . . . . . . . .250
and broccoli (*Healthy Choice* Bowl), 10.5 oz. . . . . . . . . . .300
and broccoli, Hunan (*Lean Cuisine Everyday Favorites*),
8.5 oz. . . . . . . . . . . . . . . . . . . . . . . . . . . . . . . . .240
chipped, creamed (*Stouffer's*), ½ of 11-oz. pkg. . . . . . . . . .160
chunky, and tomato (*Stouffer's* HomeStyle), 10 oz. . . . . . . .280
cured, shaved, cream sauce w/ (*Michelina's*), 8 oz. . . . . . . .420
enchilada, see "Enchilada entree"
homestyle (*Lean Cuisine Hearty Portions*), 14.25 oz. . . . . . .350

**Beef entree, frozen *(cont.)***
homestyle (*Stouffer's Skillet Sensations*),
½ of 25-oz. pkg. . . . . . . . . . . . . . . . . . . . . . . . . . . . .350
macaroni and, see "Macaroni entree, frozen"
noodles w/, see "Noodle entree, frozen"
Oriental (*Budget Gourmet*), 8 oz. . . . . . . . . . . . . . . . . . . . .200
Oriental (*Lean Cuisine Cafe Classics*), 9.25 oz. . . . . . . . . . .210
patty, char-broiled:
gravy and (*Freezer Queen* Meal), 9.5 oz. . . . . . . . . . . . .270
gravy and (*Morton*), 9 oz. . . . . . . . . . . . . . . . . . . . . . . .310
mushroom gravy and (*Freezer Queen* Family), 1 patty
w/gravy . . . . . . . . . . . . . . . . . . . . . . . . . . . . . . . . . .180
patty, w/vegetables (*Banquet*), 9.5 oz. . . . . . . . . . . . . . . . .310
pepper steak (*Marie Callender's* Skillet Meal), ½ of
24-oz. pkg. . . . . . . . . . . . . . . . . . . . . . . . . . . . . . . . . .320
pepper steak (*Michelina's*), 8 oz. . . . . . . . . . . . . . . . . . . . .260
pepper steak w/rice (*Budget Gourmet*), 8.5 oz. . . . . . . . . . .230
peppercorn, sirloin (*Michelina's*), 8.5 oz. . . . . . . . . . . . . . .290
and peppers (*Freezer Queen* Deluxe Family), 1 cup . . . . . . .230
pie (*Marie Callender's*), 9.5 oz. . . . . . . . . . . . . . . . . . . . . .630
pie (*Swanson*), 7 oz. . . . . . . . . . . . . . . . . . . . . . . . . . . . .420
pie (*Swanson Potato-Topped*), 12 oz. . . . . . . . . . . . . . . . . .480
pot roast (*Country Skillet*), ¼ of 32-oz. pkg. . . . . . . . . . . . .200
pot roast (*Freezer Queen* Deluxe Family), 1 cup . . . . . . . . .170
pot roast (*Lean Cuisine Cafe Classics*), 9 oz. . . . . . . . . . . . .190
pot roast (*Michelina's*), 10 oz. . . . . . . . . . . . . . . . . . . . . .270
pot roast, country (*Marie Callender's* Bowl), 11.85 oz. . . . .250
pot roast, Yankee (*Banquet*), 9.4 oz. . . . . . . . . . . . . . . . . . .210
pot roast, Yankee (*Stouffer's Oven Sensations*),
½ of 24-oz. pkg. . . . . . . . . . . . . . . . . . . . . . . . . . . . . .320
w/roast potato and peppers (*Stouffer's Oven Sensations*),
½ of 24-oz. pkg. . . . . . . . . . . . . . . . . . . . . . . . . . . . . .300
roast, oven (*Lean Cuisine Cafe Classics*), 9.25 oz. . . . . . . . .260
roast, sirloin (*Michelina's* Supreme), 8 oz. . . . . . . . . . . . . .240
Salisbury steak:
(*Freezer Queen* Meal), 9.5 oz. . . . . . . . . . . . . . . . . . . . .280
(*Lean Cuisine Cafe Classics*), 9.5 oz. . . . . . . . . . . . . . . .290
(*Marie Callender's*), 10 oz. . . . . . . . . . . . . . . . . . . . . . .320
and gravy (*Marie Callender's*), 14 oz. . . . . . . . . . . . . . . .550

and gravy (*Michelina's* Family), ¼ of 32-oz. pkg. . . . . . .320
and gravy, w/mashed potato (*Michelina's*), 8 oz. . . . . . .330
and gravy, w/whipped potato (*Freezer Queen* Homestyle), 8.5 oz. . . . . . . . . . . . . . . . . . . . . . . .300
gravy and (*Freezer Queen* Family), 1 patty w/gravy . . . .160
and red skin potato (*Healthy Choice* Duo), 8 oz. . . . . . . . .210
w/shells and cheese (*Michelina's*), 10.5 oz. . . . . . . . . . .450
sandwich, see "Beef sandwich"
sliced, gravy and:
(*Freezer Queen* Cook-in-Pouch), 4 oz. . . . . . . . . . . . . . . .60
(*Freezer Queen* Deluxe Family), ⅔ cup . . . . . . . . . . . . . .80
w/mashed potato (*Freezer Queen Family Buffet*), ¼ pkg. . . . . . . . . . . . . . . . . . . . . . . . . . . . . . . . .220
w/mashed potato, carrots (*Freezer Queen*), 9 oz. . . . . . .140
steak, Philly (*Healthy Choice* Bread Stuffs), 6.1 oz. . . . . . . .310
steak, sirloin, and garlic potato (*Birds Eye Steak Voila!*), 1 cup cooked . . . . . . . . . . . . . . . . . . . . . . . . . . .240
stir-fry (*Contessa*), 1¾ cups . . . . . . . . . . . . . . . . . . . . . . .190
Stroganoff:
(*Budget Gourmet*), 8 oz. . . . . . . . . . . . . . . . . . . . . . . . . .240
(*Marie Callender's*), 13 oz. . . . . . . . . . . . . . . . . . . . . . . . .510
(*Marie Callender's* Skillet Meal), ½ of 22-oz. pkg. . . . . . .340
(*Marie Callender's* Skillet Meal), ¼ of 35-oz. pkg. . . . . . .270
(*Stouffer's* HomeStyle), 9.75 oz. . . . . . . . . . . . . . . . . . .370
teriyaki (*Healthy Choice* Medley), 9.5 oz. . . . . . . . . . . . . . . .330
teriyaki (*Lean Cuisine Skillet Sensations*), ½ of 24-oz. pkg. . . . . . . . . . . . . . . . . . . . . . . . . . . .320
teriyaki w/rice (*Yu Sing*), 8 oz. . . . . . . . . . . . . . . . . . . . . . .270
tips, sirloin, mushroom rice (*Healthy Choice* Duo), 8 oz. . . .270
tips, spiral pasta and (*Healthy Choice* Medley), 9.5 oz. . . . .300
w/vegetables (*Lean Cuisine Cafe Classics*), 9 oz. . . . . . . . . .200
w/vegetables (*Lean Cuisine Skillet Sensations*), ½ of 24-oz. pkg. . . . . . . . . . . . . . . . . . . . . . . . . . . .290

**Beef gravy,** ¼ cup:
(*Franco-American/Franco-American Slow Roast*) . . . . . . . . .25
(*Heinz* Savory Fat Free) . . . . . . . . . . . . . . . . . . . . . . . . . .20

**Beef hash,** canned, 1 cup, except as noted:
corned (*Broadcast*) . . . . . . . . . . . . . . . . . . . . . . . . . . . . .420
corned (*Libby's Morning Classics*) . . . . . . . . . . . . . . . . . . .360

**Beef hash *(cont.)***
corned (*Mary Kitchen*) .390
corned (*Mary Kitchen* 50% Less Fat) .280
roast (*Mary Kitchen*) .390
**Beef jerky,** see "Sausage stick"
**Beef lunch meat** (see also "Bologna," etc.):
corned (*Boar's Head* Brisket), 2 oz. .120
corned (*Boar's Head* Brisket First Cut), 2 oz. .80
corned (*Boar's Head Custom Cut* Round), 2 oz. .80
corned (*Sara Lee*), 2 slices, 1.6 oz. .45
eye round, pepper-seasoned (*Boar's Head*), 2 oz. .90
eye round, oven-roasted (*Boar's Head*), 2 oz. .80
flame-roasted, medium (*Sara Lee*), 2 oz. .70
flame-roasted, rare (*Sara Lee*), 2 oz. .80
peppered (*Sara Lee*), 2 oz. .70
roast (*Alpine Lace*), 2 oz. .70
roast (*Healthy Choice*), 2 oz. .60
roast (*Healthy Choice Deli Traditions*), 1-oz. slice .30
roast, Cajun (*Boar's Head*), 2 oz. .80
roast, Italian style (*Healthy Choice*), 2 oz. .60
roast, Italian style (*Healthy Deli*), 2 oz. .70
roast, medium (*Healthy Choice*), 2 oz. .70
top round (*Boar's Head* Cap Off No Salt), 2 oz. .70
top round, seasoned filet (*Boar's Head*), 2 oz. .80
**Beef pocket,** frozen, 4.5-oz. pc.:
barbecue (*Hot Pockets*) .340
and cheddar (*Hot Pockets*) .350
cheeseburger (*Hot Pockets*) .330
cheeseburger (*Lean Pockets*) .300
fajita (*Hot Pockets*) .330
jalapeño steak (*Hot Pockets*) .330
Philly steak/cheese (*Croissant Pockets*) .350
Philly steak/cheese (*Deli Stuffs*) .340
Philly steak/cheese (*Lean Pockets*) .280
**Beef sauce,** see "Steak sauce" and specific listings
**Beef stew seasoning mix** (*Lawry's*), 1 tsp. .10
**Beef Stroganoff seasoning mix** (*Lawry's*), 1 tbsp. .20
**Beer,** regular, 12 fl. oz. .146
**Beet,** fresh:
raw, trimmed, sliced, ½ cup .29

boiled, drained, 2 medium, 2" diam. . . . . . . . . . . . . . . . . . . . . .44
boiled, drained, sliced, ½ cup . . . . . . . . . . . . . . . . . . . . . . . .38
**Beet, can or jar,** ½ cup, except as noted:
whole or sliced (*Aunt Nellie's*) . . . . . . . . . . . . . . . . . . . . . .35
whole or sliced (*Libby's*) . . . . . . . . . . . . . . . . . . . . . . . . . .35
whole or sliced (*Veg-All*) . . . . . . . . . . . . . . . . . . . . . . . . . .40
sliced, w/ or w/out onion (*Aunt Nellie's/Lohmann/Libby's*),
4 slices, 1 oz. . . . . . . . . . . . . . . . . . . . . . . . . . . . . . . . .20
Harvard (*Aunt Nellie's/Lohmann*), ⅓ cup . . . . . . . . . . . . . . .60
Harvard (*Greenwood* Sweet & Tangy) . . . . . . . . . . . . . . . .100
Harvard (*Libby's*), ⅓ cup . . . . . . . . . . . . . . . . . . . . . . . . . .60
pickled (*Aunt Nellie's/Lohmann/Libby's*), 2 pcs. . . . . . . . . . .20
pickled (*Greenwood* Sweet & Tangy), 1 oz. . . . . . . . . . . . . . .25
**Berliner,** pork and beef, 1 oz. . . . . . . . . . . . . . . . . . . . . . . .65
**Berries, mixed,** frozen:
(*Cascadian Farm Harvest Berries*), 1 cup . . . . . . . . . . . . . . .65
in syrup (*Big Valley Burst O'Berries/Flavorland Berry
Bonanza*), ⅔ cup . . . . . . . . . . . . . . . . . . . . . . . . . . . . . .160
**Berry drink blends:**
black and blue (*WhipperSnapple*), 10 fl. oz. . . . . . . . . . . . .160
punch (*Tropicana*), 8 fl. oz. . . . . . . . . . . . . . . . . . . . . . . . .130
**Berry juice** (*Juicy Juice*), 8 fl. oz. . . . . . . . . . . . . . . . . . . .130
**Biscuit,** buttermilk, all varieties (*Awrey's*), 2 oz. . . . . . . . . .200
**Biscuit, frozen or refrigerated,** 1 pc., except
as noted:
(*Big Country Butter Tastin'*) . . . . . . . . . . . . . . . . . . . . . . . .100
(*Grands!* Extra Rich) . . . . . . . . . . . . . . . . . . . . . . . . . . . . .220
(*Grands!/Pillsbury Butter Tastin'*) . . . . . . . . . . . . . . . . . . .180
(*Pillsbury* Country), 3 pcs. . . . . . . . . . . . . . . . . . . . . . . . .150
buttermilk (*Big Country* Fluffy) . . . . . . . . . . . . . . . . . . . . .100
buttermilk (*Pillsbury*), 3 pcs. . . . . . . . . . . . . . . . . . . . . . . .150
buttermilk (*Hungry Jack*) . . . . . . . . . . . . . . . . . . . . . . . . . .100
buttermilk (*Pillsbury* Homestyle) . . . . . . . . . . . . . . . . . . . .190
buttermilk (*Pillsbury* Tender Layer), 3 pcs. . . . . . . . . . . . .160
buttermilk or corn (*Grands!*) . . . . . . . . . . . . . . . . . . . . . . .190
cheddar garlic (*Pillsbury Home Baked Classics*) . . . . . . . . .190
flaky (*Grands!*) . . . . . . . . . . . . . . . . . . . . . . . . . . . . . . . . .200
flaky (*Hungry Jack*) . . . . . . . . . . . . . . . . . . . . . . . . . . . . . .100
honey butter (*Hungry Jack*) . . . . . . . . . . . . . . . . . . . . . . . .110
Southern style (*Big Country*) . . . . . . . . . . . . . . . . . . . . . . .100

**Biscuit, frozen or refrigerated *(cont.)***
Southern style (*Pillsbury* Homestyle) . . . . . . . . . . . . . . . . . .180
wheat, golden (*Grands!* Reduced Fat) . . . . . . . . . . . . . . . . . . .190
**Black bean:**
dry (*Frieda's*), ⅓ cup, 3 oz. . . . . . . . . . . . . . . . . . . . . . . . . .120
boiled, ½ cup . . . . . . . . . . . . . . . . . . . . . . . . . . . . . . . . .113
**Black bean, canned** (see also "Refried beans"):
(*Bush's Best*), ½ cup . . . . . . . . . . . . . . . . . . . . . . . . . . . .100
(*S&W*), ½ cup . . . . . . . . . . . . . . . . . . . . . . . . . . . . . . . .70
w/ginger and lemon (*Eden* Organic), ½ cup . . . . . . . . . . . .120
turtle (*Hain* Organic), ½ cup . . . . . . . . . . . . . . . . . . . . . . .100
**Black bean sauce,** 1 tbsp.:
(*Ka•Me*) . . . . . . . . . . . . . . . . . . . . . . . . . . . . . . . . . . . . .20
chili (*Heaven and Earth*) . . . . . . . . . . . . . . . . . . . . . . . . . .30
garlic, spicy (*Annie Chun's*) . . . . . . . . . . . . . . . . . . . . . . .50
**Blackberry,** fresh, ½ cup . . . . . . . . . . . . . . . . . . . . . . . . .37
**Blackberry, canned** (*Allens*), ⅔ cup . . . . . . . . . . . . . . . . . .60
**Blackberry, frozen** (*Cascadian Farm*), 1 cup . . . . . . . . . . . .80
**Blackberry syrup** (*Smucker's*), ¼ cup . . . . . . . . . . . . . . . .210
**Black-eyed peas,** fresh, see "Cowpeas"
**Black-eyed peas, canned,** ½ cup:
fresh shell, w/ or w/out snaps (*Bush's Best*) . . . . . . . . . . . .110
mature (*Bush's Best*) . . . . . . . . . . . . . . . . . . . . . . . . . . . .100
mature, w/bacon (*Bush's Best*) . . . . . . . . . . . . . . . . . . . . . .110
mature, w/bacon and jalapeño (*Bush's Best*) . . . . . . . . . . .120
mature, seasoned (*Glory Foods*) . . . . . . . . . . . . . . . . . . . . .120
***Blimpie,*** 1 serving:
6" cold sub:
*Blimpie Best* . . . . . . . . . . . . . . . . . . . . . . . . . . . . . . . . .410
cheese trio/wheat . . . . . . . . . . . . . . . . . . . . . . . . . . . . . .490
cheese trio/white . . . . . . . . . . . . . . . . . . . . . . . . . . . . . . .490
club/wheat . . . . . . . . . . . . . . . . . . . . . . . . . . . . . . . . . . .370
club/white . . . . . . . . . . . . . . . . . . . . . . . . . . . . . . . . . . . .370
ham, salami, provolone/wheat . . . . . . . . . . . . . . . . . . . . . .450
ham, salami, provolone/white . . . . . . . . . . . . . . . . . . . . . . .480
ham and Swiss/wheat . . . . . . . . . . . . . . . . . . . . . . . . . . . .400
ham and Swiss/white . . . . . . . . . . . . . . . . . . . . . . . . . . . .410
roast beef/wheat or white . . . . . . . . . . . . . . . . . . . . . . . . .390
tuna/wheat . . . . . . . . . . . . . . . . . . . . . . . . . . . . . . . . . . .650

tuna/white . . . . . . . . . . . . . . . . . . . . . . . . . . .660
turkey/wheat . . . . . . . . . . . . . . . . . . . . . . . . . .330
turkey/white . . . . . . . . . . . . . . . . . . . . . . . . . .330

6" hot sub:
beef melt, smoky cheddar . . . . . . . . . . . . . . . . .380
Chik Max/wheat . . . . . . . . . . . . . . . . . . . . . . .495
Chik Max/white . . . . . . . . . . . . . . . . . . . . . . . .483
Grille Max/wheat . . . . . . . . . . . . . . . . . . . . . . .425
Grille Max/white . . . . . . . . . . . . . . . . . . . . . . .413
grilled chicken . . . . . . . . . . . . . . . . . . . . . . . .400
Italian meatball . . . . . . . . . . . . . . . . . . . . . . . .500
Mexi Max/wheat . . . . . . . . . . . . . . . . . . . . . . . .405
Mexi Max/white . . . . . . . . . . . . . . . . . . . . . . . .393
roast turkey Cordon Bleu . . . . . . . . . . . . . . . . . .430
steak and cheese . . . . . . . . . . . . . . . . . . . . . . .550
Vegi Max/wheat . . . . . . . . . . . . . . . . . . . . . . . .415
Vegi Max/white . . . . . . . . . . . . . . . . . . . . . . . . .403

wraps:
chicken Caesar . . . . . . . . . . . . . . . . . . . . . . . .610
Italian, zesty . . . . . . . . . . . . . . . . . . . . . . . . . .530
Southwestern . . . . . . . . . . . . . . . . . . . . . . . . . .590

salads/side, w/out dressing:
antipasto salad . . . . . . . . . . . . . . . . . . . . . . . .200
chef salad . . . . . . . . . . . . . . . . . . . . . . . . . . . .150
chili w/cheese and beef . . . . . . . . . . . . . . . . . .240
club salad . . . . . . . . . . . . . . . . . . . . . . . . . . . .130
coleslaw, ½ cup . . . . . . . . . . . . . . . . . . . . . . . .180
green salad, tossed . . . . . . . . . . . . . . . . . . . . . .35
ham and Swiss salad . . . . . . . . . . . . . . . . . . . . .170
macaroni salad, ⅔ cup . . . . . . . . . . . . . . . . . . .360
pasta, Italian, supreme salad . . . . . . . . . . . . . . .180
potato salad, ⅔ cup . . . . . . . . . . . . . . . . . . . . .270
potato salad, mustard, ⅔ cup . . . . . . . . . . . . . . .160
roast beef salad . . . . . . . . . . . . . . . . . . . . . . . .120
tuna salad . . . . . . . . . . . . . . . . . . . . . . . . . . . .130
turkey salad . . . . . . . . . . . . . . . . . . . . . . . . . . . .90

dressing, 1 fl. oz.:
*Blimpie* . . . . . . . . . . . . . . . . . . . . . . . . . . . . . .120
*Blimpie* Special Sub . . . . . . . . . . . . . . . . . . . . . .70

***Blimpie,* dressing *(cont.)***
blue cheese .......................................220
buttermilk ranch ..................................270
buttermilk ranch, light ............................90
honey French .......................................240
Italian, fat free or light ..........................20
Thousand Island ....................................210
sauces:
guacamole, 1 oz. ...................................194
mayonnaise, 1 tbsp. ................................100
soup, 1 cup:
chicken noodle .....................................140
chicken w/white and wild rice ......................230
potato, cream of ...................................190
*Blimpie* potato chips, all varieties ...............210
bread:
6" sub roll, marbled rye ...........................246
6" sub roll, wheat .................................235
6" sub roll, white .................................240
wrap, spinach herb .................................308
wrap, traditional ..................................301
wrap, veggie .......................................240
cookie:
chocolate chunk ....................................201
macadamia white chunk ..............................210
oatmeal raisin .....................................191
peanut butter ......................................221
sugar ..............................................330
baked goods:
brownie, fudge .....................................243
cinnamon roll ......................................631
muffin, banana nut .................................472
muffin, blueberry ..................................412
muffin, bran/raisin ................................442
**Blintz,** frozen, 1 pc.:
cheese (*Ratner's*) .................................90
potato (*Ratner's*) ................................110
**Blood sausage,** 1 oz. ..............................107
**Bloody Mary mixer,** 8 fl. oz., except as noted:
(*Mr & Mrs T*) ......................................40

spicy (*Mr & Mrs T* Rich & Spicy) . . . . . . . . . . . . . . . . . . . . .50
**Blueberry,** fresh, ½ cup . . . . . . . . . . . . . . . . . . . . . . . . . . .41
**Blueberry, dried** (*Sonoma*), ¼ cup, 1.4 oz. . . . . . . . . . . . .140
**Blueberry, frozen:**
(*Big Valley*), ⅔ cup . . . . . . . . . . . . . . . . . . . . . . . . . . . . .70
(*Cascadian Farm*), 1 cup . . . . . . . . . . . . . . . . . . . . . . . . . .90
**Blueberry syrup** (*Maple Grove Farms*), ¼ cup . . . . . . . . . .210
**Bluefish,** meat only:
raw, 4 oz. . . . . . . . . . . . . . . . . . . . . . . . . . . . . . . . . . . . . .141
baked, broiled, or microwaved, 4 oz. . . . . . . . . . . . . . . . . . .180
**Bocconcini pasta dish,** mix, four cheese Parmesano
(*Land O Lakes*), 2.5 oz. . . . . . . . . . . . . . . . . . . . . . . . . . .280
**Bockwurst,** raw, 1 oz. . . . . . . . . . . . . . . . . . . . . . . . . . . . .87
**Bok choy,** see "Cabbage, bok choy"
**Bologna** (see also "Ham bologna," etc.), 2 oz.:
(*Boar's Head*) . . . . . . . . . . . . . . . . . . . . . . . . . . . . . . . . .150
(*Boar's Head* Lebanon) . . . . . . . . . . . . . . . . . . . . . . . . . . .100
(*Johnsonville* Ring Original) . . . . . . . . . . . . . . . . . . . . . . .170
beef (*Hebrew National* Chub) . . . . . . . . . . . . . . . . . . . . . . .180
beef or garlic (*Boar's Head*) . . . . . . . . . . . . . . . . . . . . . . .150
**"Bologna," vegetarian,** frozen (*Yves* Deli Slices),
2.2 oz. . . . . . . . . . . . . . . . . . . . . . . . . . . . . . . . . . . . . . . .70
**Bonito,** meat only, raw, 4 oz. . . . . . . . . . . . . . . . . . . . . . .146
**Borage,** boiled, drained, 4 oz. . . . . . . . . . . . . . . . . . . . . . .28
***Boston Market,*** 1 serving:
entrees:
chicken, ½ w/skin . . . . . . . . . . . . . . . . . . . . . . . . . . . . . .590
chicken, dark, ¼ w/skin . . . . . . . . . . . . . . . . . . . . . . . . . .320
chicken, dark, ¼ w/out skin . . . . . . . . . . . . . . . . . . . . . . .190
chicken, white, ¼ w/skin, wing . . . . . . . . . . . . . . . . . . . .280
chicken, white, ¼ w/out skin, wing . . . . . . . . . . . . . . . . .170
chicken pot pie . . . . . . . . . . . . . . . . . . . . . . . . . . . . . . . .780
chicken salad, chunky, ¾ cup . . . . . . . . . . . . . . . . . . . . .370
ham, honey glaze, lean, 5 oz. . . . . . . . . . . . . . . . . . . . . .210
meat loaf, w/brown gravy, 7 oz. . . . . . . . . . . . . . . . . . . .390
meat loaf, w/tomato sauce, 8 oz. . . . . . . . . . . . . . . . . . . .370
turkey breast, rotisserie, 5 oz. . . . . . . . . . . . . . . . . . . . . .170
sandwiches:
chicken, w/cheese and sauce . . . . . . . . . . . . . . . . . . . . . .750
chicken, no cheese or sauce . . . . . . . . . . . . . . . . . . . . . .430

***Boston Market*, sandwiches *(cont.)***

chicken, BBQ .540
chicken salad .680
ham, w/cheese and sauce .750
ham, no cheese or sauce .440
meat loaf, w/cheese .860
meat loaf, no cheese .690
turkey, w/cheese and sauce .710
turkey, no cheese or sauce .400
turkey, open-face .500
turkey club .650

sides, hot, ¾ cup, except as noted:

apples, cinnamon .250
baked beans .270
black beans and rice, 1 cup .300
broccoli–rice casserole .240
butternut squash .160
carrots, glazed .280
chicken gravy, 1 oz. .15
corn, kernel .180
green-bean casserole .130
green beans .80
macaroni and cheese .280
potato, mashed, ⅔ cup .210
potato, mashed, and gravy .230
potatoes, new .130
red beans and rice, 1 cup .260
rice pilaf, ⅔ cup .180
spinach, creamed .260
squash casserole .330
stuffing, savory .310
sweet potato casserole .280
vegetables, steamed, ⅔ cup .35

sides, cold, ¾ cup, except as noted:

coleslaw .300
cranberry relish .370
cucumber salad .90
fruit salad .70
Jumpin Juice Squares, 3 oz. .60

potato salad .......................... 340
tortellini salad .......................... 380
salad, Caesar:
entree salad .......................... 670
w/out dressing .......................... 230
side salad .......................... 268
soup, 1 cup:
chicken noodle .......................... 130
chicken tortilla .......................... 220
baked goods:
apple pie, double crust .......................... 440
apple pie, Dutch .......................... 380
brownie, 1 pc. .......................... 450
chocolate chip cookie, 1 pc. .......................... 340
corn bread, 1 loaf .......................... 200
**Bouillon** (see also "Bouillon, liquid"):
beef (*Herb-Ox*), 1 cube .......................... 5
beef (*Herb-Ox* Instant Low Sodium), 1 pkt. .......................... 10
chicken (*Doña Maria*), 1 tsp. .......................... 10
chicken (*Herb-Ox/Herb-Ox* Instant), 1 cube, tsp., or pkt. ..... 5
chicken (*Herb-Ox* Instant Low Sodium), 1 pkt. .......................... 10
chicken tomato (*Doña Maria*), 1 tsp. .......................... 10
vegetable (*Maggi* Vegetarian), 1 cube .......................... 5
**Bouillon concentrate,** liquid, 2 tsp.:
beef (*Bovril*) .......................... 10
chicken (*Bovril*) .......................... 15
**Bow-tie pasta entree,** frozen, and chicken (*Lean Cuisine Cafe Classics*), 9.5-oz. pkg. .......................... 220
**Boysenberry,** fresh, see "Blackberry"
**Boysenberry, frozen,** unsweetened, ½ cup .......................... 33
**Boysenberry syrup** (*Maple Grove Farms*), ¼ cup .......................... 210
**Bran,** see "Cereal" and specific grains
**Bratwurst,** 1 link:
(*Johnsonville* Beef/Cooked/Stadium Style), 2.7 oz. .......................... 240
bites (*Johnsonville Brat Bites*), 6 links, 2 oz. .......................... 200
chicken, w/wild rice (*Bilinski's* Bratwurst), 2 oz. .......................... 70
fresh, grilled, 3 oz.:
(*Johnsonville/Johnsonville Beer'n Bratwurst*) .......................... 290
cheddar (*Johnsonville*) .......................... 300

**Bratwurst *(cont.)***
honey and garlic (*Johnsonville*) . . . . . . . . . . . . . . . . . . . .280
hot, roasted garlic, or savory onion (*Johnsonville*) . . . . .290
smoked (*Johnsonville* Light), 2.3 oz. . . . . . . . . . . . . . . . . . .140
**"Bratwurst," vegetarian,** frozen (*Boca*), 2.5-oz. link . . . . . .130
**Bratwurst burger,** grilled (*Johnsonville*), 2.5 oz. . . . . . . . . .240
**Braunschweiger** (see also "Liverwurst"):
chub (*Jones Dairy Farm* Light), 2 oz. . . . . . . . . . . . . . . . . .100
chub (*Jones Dairy Farm* Original 8 oz.), 2 oz. . . . . . . . . . . .160
chub (*Jones Dairy Farm* Original 16 oz.), 2 oz. . . . . . . . . . .150
chub, w/bacon, 20% (*Jones Dairy Farm*), 2 oz. . . . . . . . . . .150
chub, w/onion (*Jones Dairy Farm*), 2 oz. . . . . . . . . . . . . . .160
chunk (*Jones Dairy Farm* Original), 2 oz. . . . . . . . . . . . . . .180
sliced (*Oscar Mayer*), 1-oz. slice . . . . . . . . . . . . . . . . . . .100
**Brazil nuts,** shelled, 8 medium or 6 large, 1 oz. . . . . . . . . .186
**Bread,** 1 slice, except as noted:
(*Arnold Bran'nola/Health Nut*) . . . . . . . . . . . . . . . . . . . . . .110
banana swirl (*Pepperidge Farm*) . . . . . . . . . . . . . . . . . . . . . .90
bran (*Shiloh Farms*) . . . . . . . . . . . . . . . . . . . . . . . . . . . . . .80
buttermilk (*Pepperidge Farm Farmhouse* Sweet) . . . . . . . . .110
buttermilk (*Pillsbury*) . . . . . . . . . . . . . . . . . . . . . . . . . . . . .90
cheddar, white, garlic (*Great Harvest*) . . . . . . . . . . . . . . . .130
focaccia, sprouted 5 grain (*Shiloh Farms*), 4-oz. pc. . . . . . .360
French toast swirl:
brown sugar cinnamon (*Pepperidge Farm*) . . . . . . . . . .140
maple syrup cinnamon (*Pepperidge Farm*) . . . . . . . . . . .130
Italian (*Pepperidge Farm*) . . . . . . . . . . . . . . . . . . . . . . . . . .90
Italian (*Rhodes*) . . . . . . . . . . . . . . . . . . . . . . . . . . . . . . . .130
Italian (*Wonder* Seeded) . . . . . . . . . . . . . . . . . . . . . . . . . . .70
kamut (*Shiloh Farms* Egyptian Wheat) . . . . . . . . . . . . . . . . .90
mountain, see "Wraps"
multigrain:
(*LifeWorks*), 2 slices . . . . . . . . . . . . . . . . . . . . . . . . . . .170
5, sprouted (*Shiloh Farms* Hearth) . . . . . . . . . . . . . . . . . .130
5, sprouted (*Shiloh Farms*) . . . . . . . . . . . . . . . . . . . . . . . .90
5, sprouted, sourdough (*Shiloh Farms*) . . . . . . . . . . . . . .140
7 (*Healthy Choice*) . . . . . . . . . . . . . . . . . . . . . . . . . . . . . .80
7 (*Pepperidge Farm Farmhouse* Harvest) . . . . . . . . . . . . .110
7, sprouted (*Shiloh Farms*) . . . . . . . . . . . . . . . . . . . . . . . .90
9 (*Cobblestone Mill* Hearty) . . . . . . . . . . . . . . . . . . . . . . .120

9 (*Great Harvest*) . . . . . . . . . . . . . . . . . . . . . . . . . . .110
9 (*Pepperidge Farm* Natural Whole Grain) . . . . . . . . . . . .90
10, sprouted (*Shiloh Farms*), 2 slices . . . . . . . . . . . . . .140
12 (*Arnold*) . . . . . . . . . . . . . . . . . . . . . . . . . . . . . .110
soft (*Healthy Choice*) . . . . . . . . . . . . . . . . . . . . . . . .60
sprouted (*Shiloh Farms* Firehouse Unsliced), 2 oz. . . . . .160
sprouted (*Shiloh Farms* Sandwich) . . . . . . . . . . . . . . . . .80
oat, country (*Pepperidge Farm* Hearty Slices) . . . . . . . . . . .110
oat bran (*Arnold*), 2 slices . . . . . . . . . . . . . . . . . . . . . .170
oat bran (*Shiloh Farms*) . . . . . . . . . . . . . . . . . . . . . . . . .90
oatmeal (*Pepperidge Farm*) . . . . . . . . . . . . . . . . . . . . . . .60
oatmeal, soft (*Pepperidge Farm Farmhouse*) . . . . . . . . . . . .110
potato (*Home Pride*) . . . . . . . . . . . . . . . . . . . . . . . . . . .70
potato (*Martin's*) . . . . . . . . . . . . . . . . . . . . . . . . . . . .100
potato (*Stroehmann* Dutch Country) . . . . . . . . . . . . . . . . . .90
potato, golden (*Pepperidge Farm Farmhouse*) . . . . . . . . . . .110
pumpernickel (*Arnold*) . . . . . . . . . . . . . . . . . . . . . . . . . .80
pumpernickel (*Pepperidge Farm* Party), 5 slices . . . . . . . . .130
pumpernickel (*Rubschlager* Cocktail), 3 slices . . . . . . . . . . .80
pumpernickel (*Rubschlager* Danish/Westphalian) . . . . . . . . .70
raisin (*Monk's*) . . . . . . . . . . . . . . . . . . . . . . . . . . . . . .70
raisin whole wheat (*Shiloh Farms*), 2 slices . . . . . . . . . . .140
raisin cinnamon (*Great Harvest*) . . . . . . . . . . . . . . . . . . .100
raisin cinnamon swirl (*Pepperidge Farm*) . . . . . . . . . . . . . .80
raisin cinnamon swirl (*Sun•Maid*) . . . . . . . . . . . . . . . . . .80
rye (*Arnold* Real Jewish Melba Thin), 2 slices . . . . . . . . . . .110
rye (*Arnold* Real Jewish Seeds/Seedless) . . . . . . . . . . . . . . .80
rye (*Levy's* Real Jewish Seeds/Seedless) . . . . . . . . . . . . . . .90
rye (*Pepperidge Farm* Deli Seedless) . . . . . . . . . . . . . . . . .80
rye (*Pepperidge Farm* Jewish Party), 5 slices . . . . . . . . . . .120
rye, dill (*Arnold* Real Jewish) . . . . . . . . . . . . . . . . . . . . .80
rye, soft (*Beefsteak*) . . . . . . . . . . . . . . . . . . . . . . . . . . .70
rye, soft (*Beefsteak* Light), 2 slices . . . . . . . . . . . . . . . . .80
rye/pumpernickel, marble (*Arnold*) . . . . . . . . . . . . . . . . . .80
rye/pumpernickel swirl (*Pepperidge Farm* Deli Swirl) . . . . . .80
sesame wheat (*Pepperidge Farm* Hearty Slices) . . . . . . . . .110
sesame wheat (*Pepperidge Farm Farmhouse*) . . . . . . . . . . .110
sourdough (*Cobblestone Mill* San Francisco),
2 slices . . . . . . . . . . . . . . . . . . . . . . . . . . . . . . . . . .160
spelt (*Shiloh Farms*) . . . . . . . . . . . . . . . . . . . . . . . . . .100

**Bread *(cont.)***

stone-ground (*Home Pride*) .70
sunflower (*Great Harvest*) .110
sunflower and bran (*Monk's*) .60
sunflower whole wheat (*Shiloh Farms*), 2 slices .160
wheat (*Arnold* Country) .100
wheat (*Home Pride*) .80
wheat (*Nature's Own* Light), 2 slices .80
wheat (*Pan Wonder* De Trigo), 2 slices .110
wheat (*Pepperidge Farm* Very Thin), 3 slices .120
wheat (*Pillsbury*) .80
wheat (*Shiloh Farms* Butter Hearth) .150
wheat (*Shiloh Farms* Homestyle), 2 slices .160
wheat (*Wonder* Light), 2 slices .80
wheat, honey (*Nature's Own*) .60
wheat, honey (*Nature's Own* Light), 2 slices .80
wheat, honey, soft (*Healthy Choice*) .60
wheat, honey wheat berry (*Arnold*) .110
wheat, honey wheat berry (*Cobblestone Mill* Hearty) .110
wheat, honey wheat berry (*Home Pride*) .70
wheat, honey, whole (*Great Harvest*) .100
wheat, stone-ground (*Pepperidge Farm* 100%) .70
wheat, whole (*Arnold* 100%) .90
wheat, whole (*Arnold Brick Oven* 100%), 2 slices .130
wheat, whole (*Cobblestone Mill* 100% Hearty) .100
wheat, whole (*Monk's* 100%) .60
wheat, whole (*Nature's Own* 100%) .50
wheat, whole (*Nature's Own* 100% Sugar Free) .50
wheat, whole (*Shiloh Farms*), 2 slices .140
wheat, whole, stone-ground (*Wonder* 100%) .80
wheat, whole grain, dark (*Pepperidge Farm* German) .90
wheat and rye (*Shiloh Farms* Zesty), 2 slices .140
white (*Arnold* Country) .110
white (*Arnold Brick Oven*), 2 slices .130
white (*Arnold Brick Oven* Big Slice) .90
white (*Great Harvest*) .100
white (*Monk's*) .60
white (*Nature's Own* Butterbread) .60
white (*Nature's Own* Light Premium), 2 slices .80
white (*Pepperidge Farm* Original) .70

white (*Pepperidge Farm* Sandwich), 2 slices . . . . . . . . . . . . .130
white (*Pepperidge Farm Farmhouse* Hearty) . . . . . . . . . . . . .110
white (*Pillsbury*) . . . . . . . . . . . . . . . . . . . . . . . . . . . . . . . . .80
white (*Rhodes*) . . . . . . . . . . . . . . . . . . . . . . . . . . . . . . . . .140
white (*Wonder* Light), 2 slices . . . . . . . . . . . . . . . . . . . . . . .80
white (*Wonder* Giant), 2 slices . . . . . . . . . . . . . . . . . . . . . .120
white (*Wonder* Small), 2 slices . . . . . . . . . . . . . . . . . . . . . .110
white, honey (*Pillsbury*) . . . . . . . . . . . . . . . . . . . . . . . . . . .80
whole grain (*Healthy Choice* 100%) . . . . . . . . . . . . . . . . . . . .80
**Bread, frozen or refrigerated:**
buttermilk (*Pillsbury*), 1-oz. slice . . . . . . . . . . . . . . . . . . . . .90
corn bread (*Boston Market*), 2.25-oz. mini loaf . . . . . . . . .210
French, crusty (*Pillsbury* Tube), ⅕ loaf . . . . . . . . . . . . . . . . .150
garlic (*New York*), 2 slices, 1", 2 oz. . . . . . . . . . . . . . . . . . . .190
Texas toast:
 garlic (*New York*), 1" slice, 1.4 oz. . . . . . . . . . . . . . . . . .170
 garlic, w/cheese (*New York*), 1.7-oz. slice . . . . . . . . . . . .180
 garlic, Parmesan (*New York*), 1" slice, 1.7 oz. . . . . . . . . .190
 garlic, pizza (*New York*), 1.8-oz. slice . . . . . . . . . . . . . . .160
 Parmesan (*Pepperidge Farm*), 1.4-oz. slice . . . . . . . . . . .160
wheat or honey white (*Pillsbury*), 1-oz. slice . . . . . . . . . . . . .80
**Bread, mix** (see also "Bread mix, sweet"):
French or Italian (*Eagle Mills*), ⅑ loaf* . . . . . . . . . . . . . . . .160
multigrain or honey oat (*Eagle Mills*), 1/11 loaf* . . . . . . . . . .150
rye (*Eagle Mills* Old World), 1/11 loaf* . . . . . . . . . . . . . . . . .150
sourdough (*Eagle Mills* San Francisco), ⅑ loaf* . . . . . . . . .160
wheat, cracked (*Pillsbury* Bread Machine), 1/12 pkg. . . . . . . .130
wheat, whole (*Arrowhead Mills*), ⅓ cup . . . . . . . . . . . . . . .150
wheat, whole (*Eagle Mills* Harvest), 1/11 loaf* . . . . . . . . . . . .140
white (*Eagle Mills* Homestyle), ⅑ loaf* . . . . . . . . . . . . . . . . .160
white (*Hodgson Mill*), ¼ cup . . . . . . . . . . . . . . . . . . . . . . . .120
white (*Pillsbury* Bread Machine Country), 1/12 pkg. . . . . . . .130
**Bread mix, sweet,** dry, except as noted:
apple walnut, w/out icing (*Eagle Mills*), ¼ cup . . . . . . . . . .150
banana (*Betty Crocker* Quick), 1/12 loaf* . . . . . . . . . . . . . . . .170
chocolate, w/out icing (*Eagle Mills* Nugget), ¼ cup . . . . . . .150
cinnamon, w/out icing (*Eagle Mills* Sunrise), ¼ cup . . . . . .150
cinnamon streusel (*Betty Crocker* Quick), 1/14 loaf* . . . . . . .180
corn bread, see "Corn bread mix"
cranberry orange (*Betty Crocker* Quick), 1/12 loaf* . . . . . . . .180

**Bread mix, sweet *(cont.)***
date (*Pillsbury* Bread/Muffin), 1/14 pkg. . . . . . . . . . . . . . . . . . .130
gingerbread (*Hodgson Mill*), ¼ cup . . . . . . . . . . . . . . . . . . .110
lemon poppy (*Betty Crocker* Quick), 1/12 loaf* . . . . . . . . . . . .170
lemon poppy (*Pillsbury* Bread/Muffin), 1/14 pkg. . . . . . . . . . . .130
lemon poppy, w/out icing (*Eagle Mills*), ¼ cup . . . . . . . . . . .140
**Bread crumbs,** ¼ cup or 1 oz.:
all-purpose (*Golden Dipt* Fry Easy) . . . . . . . . . . . . . . . . . . .120
plain, Italian, or Parmesan (*Progresso*) . . . . . . . . . . . . . . . . .110
garlic and herb (*Progresso*) . . . . . . . . . . . . . . . . . . . . . . . .100
**Bread dough, sweet** (*Rhodes*), 1/9 loaf, 1.8 oz. . . . . . . . . . . .145
**Bread stick:**
(*Stella D'oro* Fat Free), 1 pc. . . . . . . . . . . . . . . . . . . . . . . . .70
(*Stella D'oro* Original/Onion), 1 pc. . . . . . . . . . . . . . . . . . . . .40
(*Stella D'oro* Sodium Free), 1 pc. . . . . . . . . . . . . . . . . . . . . .45
all varieties (*Stella D'oro* Snack Stix), 4 pcs. . . . . . . . . . . . . .70
garlic (*Stella D'oro* Traditional), 2 pcs. . . . . . . . . . . . . . . . . .70
onion or sesame (*Toufayan*), 2 pcs. . . . . . . . . . . . . . . . . . . . .55
sesame (*Stella D'oro*), 1 pc. . . . . . . . . . . . . . . . . . . . . . . . . .50
**Bread stick, frozen or refrigerated:**
corn bread twists (*Pillsbury*), 1 pc. . . . . . . . . . . . . . . . . . . .130
garlic (*Pepperidge Farm*), 1 pc. . . . . . . . . . . . . . . . . . . . . . .180
garlic w/herbs or Parmesan (*Pillsbury*), 2 pcs. . . . . . . . . . . .180
garlic Parmesan (*New York*), 1 pc. . . . . . . . . . . . . . . . . . . . .180
**Breakfast bar,** see "Granola and cereal bar"
**Breakfast sandwich** (see also "Burrito, breakfast" and "Toaster bagel, muffin, and pastry"), 1 pc.:
biscuit, sausage, egg (*Hormel Quick Meals*), 4.5 oz. . . . . . .390
biscuit, sausage, egg, cheese (*Great Starts*), 5.5 oz. . . . . . .460
croissant, sausage, egg, cheese (*Great Starts*), 5 oz. . . . . . .470
muffin, egg:
Canadian bacon, cheese (*Great Starts*), 4.1 oz. . . . . . . .290
Canadian bacon, cheese (*Great Starts* Lite), 4.2 oz. . . . .230
and cheese (*Hormel Quick Meals*), 4.5 oz. . . . . . . . . . . .260
pocket, egg, cheese, bacon (*Hot Pockets*) . . . . . . . . . . . . . .170
pocket, egg, cheese, sausage (*Croissant Pockets*) . . . . . . . . .340
pocket, egg, cheese, sausage (*Hot Pockets*) . . . . . . . . . . . . .180
**Broad bean,** raw (*Frieda's* Fava), ¾ cup, 3 oz. . . . . . . . . . .290
**Broad beans, mature** (see also "Habas"), boiled, ½ cup . . . . . . . . . . . . . . . . . . . . . . . . . . . . . . . . . . . .93

**Broccoli,** fresh:
raw (*Dole*), 5.2-oz. stalk . . . . . . . . . . . . . . . . . . . . . . . . .45
raw, chopped, ½ cup . . . . . . . . . . . . . . . . . . . . . . . . . . . . .12
raw, baby (*Mann's Broccolini*), 2.9 oz., about 8 stalks . . . . .35
boiled, drained, 1 stalk, 6.3 oz. . . . . . . . . . . . . . . . . . . . . .51
boiled, drained, chopped, ½ cup . . . . . . . . . . . . . . . . . . . . .22
**Broccoli, Chinese,** see "Kale, Chinese"
**Broccoli, frozen,** 1 cup, except as noted:
spears (*Birds Eye*), 3 oz. . . . . . . . . . . . . . . . . . . . . . . . . .25
florets (*Birds Eye* Deluxe), 3 oz. . . . . . . . . . . . . . . . . . . . .25
florets (*Green Giant*), 1⅓ cups . . . . . . . . . . . . . . . . . . . . .25
florets (*Seabrook Farms*) . . . . . . . . . . . . . . . . . . . . . . . . .25
florets, baby (*Birds Eye*), 3 oz. . . . . . . . . . . . . . . . . . . . .25
cuts (*Birds Eye*), ½ cup . . . . . . . . . . . . . . . . . . . . . . . . . .25
cuts (*Cascadian Farm*), ½ cup . . . . . . . . . . . . . . . . . . . . . .24
cuts (*Green Giant*) . . . . . . . . . . . . . . . . . . . . . . . . . . . . . .25
chopped (*Birds Eye*), ⅓ cup . . . . . . . . . . . . . . . . . . . . . . .25
chopped (*Green Giant*), ¾ cup . . . . . . . . . . . . . . . . . . . . . .25
in cheddar cheese sauce (*Cascadian Farm*), ½ cup . . . . . . . .60
in cheese sauce (*Birds Eye*), 4 oz. . . . . . . . . . . . . . . . . . . .70
in cheese sauce (*Green Giant*), ⅔ cup . . . . . . . . . . . . . . . .80
**Broccoli combinations,** fresh, 4 oz.:
carrots (*Mann's*) . . . . . . . . . . . . . . . . . . . . . . . . . . . . . . .35
carrots, red cabbage (*Mann's* Coleslaw) . . . . . . . . . . . . . . .35
carrots, snap peas, celery (*Mann's Broccoli Wokly*) . . . . . . .35
cauliflower, red cabbage (*Mann's* Rainbow Salad) . . . . . . . . .30
**Broccoli combinations, frozen** (see also "Broccoli dish"):
carrots, cauliflower (*Green Giant Select*), ⅔ cup . . . . . . . . .25
carrots, water chestnuts (*Birds Eye*), ½ cup . . . . . . . . . . . .30
carrots, water chestnuts (*Green Giant Select*),
⅔ cup . . . . . . . . . . . . . . . . . . . . . . . . . . . . . . . . . . . . . .25
cauliflower (*Birds Eye*), ½ cup . . . . . . . . . . . . . . . . . . . . . .20
cauliflower, carrots:
(*McKenzie's* Garden Fresh), ½ cup . . . . . . . . . . . . . . . . .25
in cheese sauce (*Birds Eye*), ½ cup . . . . . . . . . . . . . . . . .70
in cheese sauce (*Green Giant*), ⅔ cup . . . . . . . . . . . . . . .80
cauliflower, red pepper (*Birds Eye*), ½ cup . . . . . . . . . . . . .20
corn, red peppers (*Birds Eye*), ½ cup . . . . . . . . . . . . . . . . .50
red pepper, onion, mushrooms (*Birds Eye*), ½ cup . . . . . . . .25
stir-fry (*Birds Eye*), 1 cup . . . . . . . . . . . . . . . . . . . . . . . . .30

**Broccoli dish,** frozen:
in cheese sauce (*Freezer Queen* Family), ⅔ cup . . . . . . . . . . .80
and pasta, cauliflower, carrots, in cheese sauce
(*Freezer Queen* Family Side Dish), ⅔ cup . . . . . . . . . . .120
soufflé (*Melrose*), ⅓ cup . . . . . . . . . . . . . . . . . . . . . . . . . .80
**Broccoli rabe,** fresh (*Frieda's* Rapini), 3 oz. . . . . . . . . . . . . . .25
**Broccoli–cheese sandwich/pocket,** frozen, 1 pc.:
(*Amy's*), 4.5 oz. . . . . . . . . . . . . . . . . . . . . . . . . . . . . . . .270
croissant (*Sara Lee*), 3.7 oz. . . . . . . . . . . . . . . . . . . . . . . .280
**Brown gravy,** w/onions (*Franco-American*), ¼ cup . . . . . . . .25
**Brown gravy mix** (*Lawry's*), 2 tsp. . . . . . . . . . . . . . . . . . . .20
**Brownie:**
chocolate (*Awrey's* Decadent), 1 pc. . . . . . . . . . . . . . . . . . .220
chocolate chunk (*Entenmann's* Ultimate), 1 pc. . . . . . . . . . . .320
chocolate peanut (*Awrey's* Sensation), 1 pc. . . . . . . . . . . . . .230
fudge (*Entenmann's*), ½ pc., 1.5 oz. . . . . . . . . . . . . . . . . . .200
fudge nut (*Awrey's*), 1 pc. . . . . . . . . . . . . . . . . . . . . . . . .210
mini (*Entenmann's Little Bites*), 3 pcs., 2.2 oz. . . . . . . . . . .300
**Brownie mix,** 1 pc.*:
(*Duncan Hines Chocolate Lovers* Turtle) . . . . . . . . . . . . . . .150
chocolate, dark, fudge (*Betty Crocker* Supreme) . . . . . . . . . .170
chocolate, dark, fudge, w/chunks (*Duncan Hines*) . . . . . . . . .150
chocolate, German (*Betty Crocker* Supreme) . . . . . . . . . . . . .200
chocolate chunk (*Duncan Hines Chocolate Lovers*) . . . . . . .160
frosted (*Betty Crocker* Supreme) . . . . . . . . . . . . . . . . . . . .210
fudge (*Betty Crocker* Original Supreme) . . . . . . . . . . . . . . .160
fudge (*Betty Crocker* Pouch/Supreme) . . . . . . . . . . . . . . . .190
fudge (*Betty Crocker* Supreme Family No Cholesterol) . . . .140
fudge (*Sweet Rewards* Low Fat) . . . . . . . . . . . . . . . . . . . . .130
fudge (*Sweet Rewards* Reduced Fat) . . . . . . . . . . . . . . . . . .140
fudge, double (*Duncan Hines Chocolate Lovers*) . . . . . . . . . .170
peanut butter chunk (*Betty Crocker w/Reese's Pieces*) . . . .180
turtle (*Betty Crocker*) . . . . . . . . . . . . . . . . . . . . . . . . . . . .170
walnut (*Betty Crocker* Supreme) . . . . . . . . . . . . . . . . . . . .180
**Browning sauce** (*Gravy Master*), ¼ tsp. . . . . . . . . . . . . . . . . .0
**Brussels sprouts,** fresh:
raw (*Dole*), 4 sprouts, 3 oz. . . . . . . . . . . . . . . . . . . . . . . . .40
raw, ½ cup . . . . . . . . . . . . . . . . . . . . . . . . . . . . . . . . . . . .19
boiled, .7-oz. sprout . . . . . . . . . . . . . . . . . . . . . . . . . . . . . .8
boiled, drained, ½ cup . . . . . . . . . . . . . . . . . . . . . . . . . . . .30

**Brussels sprouts, frozen:**
(*Birds Eye* Deluxe), 11 pcs. . . . . . . . . . . . . . . . . . . . . . . . . .35
boiled, drained, ½ cup . . . . . . . . . . . . . . . . . . . . . . . . . .33
**Brussels sprouts combinations,** frozen, w/cauliflower
and carrots (*Birds Eye*), ½ cup . . . . . . . . . . . . . . . . . . . .30
**Buckwheat groats,** dry:
(*Wolff's* Kasha), ¼ cup . . . . . . . . . . . . . . . . . . . . . . . . . .170
brown (*Arrowhead Mills*), ¼ cup . . . . . . . . . . . . . . . . . . . .140
**Buffalo wing sauce,** 2 tbsp.:
hot (*Nance's* Chicken Wing) . . . . . . . . . . . . . . . . . . . . . . .15
hot (*World Harbors* After Glow) . . . . . . . . . . . . . . . . . . . .30
mild (*Nance's* Chicken Wing) . . . . . . . . . . . . . . . . . . . . . .20
**Bulgur** (see also "Tabouli"), cooked, 1 cup . . . . . . . . . . . .152
**Bun,** see "Roll"
**Bun, sweet,** 1 pc.:
cheese (*Entenmann's*) . . . . . . . . . . . . . . . . . . . . . . . . . . .300
cinnamon (*Entenmann's* Light) . . . . . . . . . . . . . . . . . . . . .170
cinnamon, iced (*Rhodes*) . . . . . . . . . . . . . . . . . . . . . . . . .265
cinnamon, w/out icing (*Rhodes*) . . . . . . . . . . . . . . . . . . . .220
cinnamon swirl (*Entenmann's*) . . . . . . . . . . . . . . . . . . . . .320
honey, iced (*Hostess*) . . . . . . . . . . . . . . . . . . . . . . . . . . .420
sticky (*Entenmann's*) . . . . . . . . . . . . . . . . . . . . . . . . . . .260
**Bun, sweet, frozen or refrigerated,** 1 pc.:
caramel, sticky (*Pillsbury*) . . . . . . . . . . . . . . . . . . . . . . .170
cinnamon, cream cheese iced (*Pillsbury*) . . . . . . . . . . . . . .150
cinnamon, iced (*Grands!*) . . . . . . . . . . . . . . . . . . . . . . . . .330
cinnamon, iced (*Pillsbury Home Baked Classics*) . . . . . . . .340
cinnamon, iced (*Pillsbury* Tube) . . . . . . . . . . . . . . . . . . . .150
orange flavor, w/icing (*Pillsbury*) . . . . . . . . . . . . . . . . . .170
**Burbot,** meat only:
raw, 4 oz. . . . . . . . . . . . . . . . . . . . . . . . . . . . . . . . . . . .102
baked, broiled, or microwaved, 4 oz. . . . . . . . . . . . . . . . . .130
**Burger, vegetarian, frozen,** 1 pc.:
(*Boca* Burger Vegan), 2.5 oz. . . . . . . . . . . . . . . . . . . . . . .90
(*Morningstar Farms* Quarter Prime), 3.4 oz. . . . . . . . . . . . .140
(*Morningstar Farms Better'n Burgers*), 2.75 oz. . . . . . . . . . .80
(*Morningstar Farms Garden Grille*), 2.5 oz. . . . . . . . . . . . .120
(*Natural Touch* Okara Patties), 2.25 oz. . . . . . . . . . . . . . . .110
(*Natural Touch Hard Rock Café*), 3 oz. . . . . . . . . . . . . . . . .170
(*Natural Touch Vegan Burger*), 2.75 oz. . . . . . . . . . . . . . . . .70

**Burger, vegetarian, frozen *(cont.)***
black bean, spicy (*Natural Touch*), 2.75 oz. . . . . . . . . . . . . . .110
black bean and mushroom (*Yves*), 3 oz. . . . . . . . . . . . . . . . .100
garden vegetable (*Morningstar Farms*), 2.4 oz. . . . . . . . . . . .100
garden vegetable (*Yves*), 3 oz. . . . . . . . . . . . . . . . . . . . . . . . .90
garlic, roasted (*Boca* Burger), 2.5 oz. . . . . . . . . . . . . . . . . .100
grilled vegetable (*Boca* Burger), 2.5 oz. . . . . . . . . . . . . . . . .80
Italian or Southwestern (*Morningstar Farms Harvest Burger*), 3.2 oz. . . . . . . . . . . . . . . . . . . . . . . . . . . . .140
onion, roasted, or salsa (*Boca* Burger), 2.5 oz. . . . . . . . . . . .90
***Burger King,*** 1 serving:
breakfast dishes:
biscuit . . . . . . . . . . . . . . . . . . . . . . . . . . . . . . . . . . . . .300
biscuit w/egg . . . . . . . . . . . . . . . . . . . . . . . . . . . . . . . .390
biscuit w/sausage . . . . . . . . . . . . . . . . . . . . . . . . . . . . .510
biscuit w/sausage, egg, and cheese . . . . . . . . . . . . . . . .650
cini-minis, w/out icing, 4 pcs. . . . . . . . . . . . . . . . . . . . .440
*Croissan'wich,* w/sausage, cheese . . . . . . . . . . . . . . . . .410
*Croissan'wich,* w/sausage, egg, cheese . . . . . . . . . . . . .500
french toast sticks, 5 pcs. . . . . . . . . . . . . . . . . . . . . . . .390
hash browns, large . . . . . . . . . . . . . . . . . . . . . . . . . . . .390
hash brown, small . . . . . . . . . . . . . . . . . . . . . . . . . . . . .240
breakfast components:
bacon, 3 pcs. . . . . . . . . . . . . . . . . . . . . . . . . . . . . . . . . .40
ham, 2 pcs. . . . . . . . . . . . . . . . . . . . . . . . . . . . . . . . . . .35
grape/strawberry jam . . . . . . . . . . . . . . . . . . . . . . . . . . .30
sausage patty . . . . . . . . . . . . . . . . . . . . . . . . . . . . . . . .210
syrup . . . . . . . . . . . . . . . . . . . . . . . . . . . . . . . . . . . . . . .80
vanilla icing, 1 oz. . . . . . . . . . . . . . . . . . . . . . . . . . . . .110
sandwiches:
bacon double cheeseburger . . . . . . . . . . . . . . . . . . . . . .610
*BK Big Fish* . . . . . . . . . . . . . . . . . . . . . . . . . . . . . . . . .710
*BK Broiler* chicken . . . . . . . . . . . . . . . . . . . . . . . . . . . .550
*BK Broiler* chicken, w/out mayo . . . . . . . . . . . . . . . . . .390
*Bull's-Eye* BBQ . . . . . . . . . . . . . . . . . . . . . . . . . . . . . .400
*Bull's-Eye* BBQ, w/out mayo . . . . . . . . . . . . . . . . . . . .310
cheeseburger . . . . . . . . . . . . . . . . . . . . . . . . . . . . . . . .370
cheeseburger, double . . . . . . . . . . . . . . . . . . . . . . . . . .570
chicken . . . . . . . . . . . . . . . . . . . . . . . . . . . . . . . . . . . .660
chicken, w/out mayo . . . . . . . . . . . . . . . . . . . . . . . . . . .460

chicken club . . . . . . . . . . . . . . . . . . . . . . . . . . . . .740
chicken club, w/out mayo . . . . . . . . . . . . . . . . . . . . .530
*Chicken Tenders* . . . . . . . . . . . . . . . . . . . . . . . . . . .450
*Chicken Tenders,* w/out mayo . . . . . . . . . . . . . . . . .290
*Double Whopper* . . . . . . . . . . . . . . . . . . . . . . . . . . .920
*Double Whopper,* w/out mayo . . . . . . . . . . . . . . . . . .760
*Double Whopper* w/cheese . . . . . . . . . . . . . . . . . . .1,020
*Double Whopper* w/cheese, w/out mayo . . . . . . . . . . . .860
hamburger . . . . . . . . . . . . . . . . . . . . . . . . . . . . . . .320
hamburger, double . . . . . . . . . . . . . . . . . . . . . . . . .480
*Whopper* . . . . . . . . . . . . . . . . . . . . . . . . . . . . . . . .680
*Whopper,* w/out mayo . . . . . . . . . . . . . . . . . . . . . . .530
*Whopper* w/cheese . . . . . . . . . . . . . . . . . . . . . . . . .780
*Whopper* w/cheese, w/out mayo . . . . . . . . . . . . . . . . .620
*Whopper Jr.* . . . . . . . . . . . . . . . . . . . . . . . . . . . . . .410
*Whopper Jr.,* w/out mayo . . . . . . . . . . . . . . . . . . . . .330
*Whopper Jr.* w/cheese . . . . . . . . . . . . . . . . . . . . . . .460
*Whopper Jr.* w/cheese, w/out mayo . . . . . . . . . . . . . . .370

sandwich condiments:

*Bull's-Eye* BBQ sauce, ½ oz. . . . . . . . . . . . . . . . . . . .20
ketchup, ½ oz. . . . . . . . . . . . . . . . . . . . . . . . . . . . . .15
tartar sauce, ½ oz. . . . . . . . . . . . . . . . . . . . . . . . . . .70

*Chicken Tenders:*

4 pcs. . . . . . . . . . . . . . . . . . . . . . . . . . . . . . . . . . .170
5 pcs. . . . . . . . . . . . . . . . . . . . . . . . . . . . . . . . . . .220
6 pcs. . . . . . . . . . . . . . . . . . . . . . . . . . . . . . . . . . .250
8 pcs. . . . . . . . . . . . . . . . . . . . . . . . . . . . . . . . . . .340

dipping sauce, 1 oz.:

barbecue . . . . . . . . . . . . . . . . . . . . . . . . . . . . . . . . .35
honey-flavored . . . . . . . . . . . . . . . . . . . . . . . . . . . . .90
honey mustard . . . . . . . . . . . . . . . . . . . . . . . . . . . . .90
marinara . . . . . . . . . . . . . . . . . . . . . . . . . . . . . . . . .20
ranch . . . . . . . . . . . . . . . . . . . . . . . . . . . . . . . . . . .120
sweet and sour . . . . . . . . . . . . . . . . . . . . . . . . . . . . .40

sides:

french fries, king size . . . . . . . . . . . . . . . . . . . . . . .600
french fries, large . . . . . . . . . . . . . . . . . . . . . . . . . .500
french fries, medium . . . . . . . . . . . . . . . . . . . . . . . .360
french fries, small . . . . . . . . . . . . . . . . . . . . . . . . . .230
*Jalapeño Poppers,* 4 pcs. . . . . . . . . . . . . . . . . . . . . .230

***Burger King*, sides *(cont.)***
mozzarella sticks, 4 pcs. . . . . . . . . . . . . . . . . . . . . . . . .290
onion rings, king size . . . . . . . . . . . . . . . . . . . . . . . .550
onion rings, large . . . . . . . . . . . . . . . . . . . . . . . . . .480
onion rings, medium . . . . . . . . . . . . . . . . . . . . . . . . .320
shakes:
chocolate, medium . . . . . . . . . . . . . . . . . . . . . . . . .440
chocolate, small . . . . . . . . . . . . . . . . . . . . . . . . . .340
vanilla, medium . . . . . . . . . . . . . . . . . . . . . . . . . .430
vanilla, small . . . . . . . . . . . . . . . . . . . . . . . . . . .330
syrup added, chocolate, medium . . . . . . . . . . . . . . . . .500
syrup added, chocolate, small . . . . . . . . . . . . . . . . . .400
syrup added, strawberry, medium . . . . . . . . . . . . . . . .500
syrup added, strawberry, small . . . . . . . . . . . . . . . . .390
dessert:
Dutch apple pie . . . . . . . . . . . . . . . . . . . . . . . . . . .340
*Hershey's* sundae pie . . . . . . . . . . . . . . . . . . . . . . .310
**Burrito,** frozen, 1 pc.:
(*El Monterey Family Classic* Supreme), 5 oz. . . . . . . . . . . . .290
bean, black, vegetable (*Amy's*), 6 oz. . . . . . . . . . . . . . . . . .320
bean/cheese (*Amy's*), 6 oz. . . . . . . . . . . . . . . . . . . . . . . .280
bean/cheese (*El Monterey*), 5 oz. . . . . . . . . . . . . . . . . . . .290
bean/rice (*Amy's*), 6 oz. . . . . . . . . . . . . . . . . . . . . . . . .270
bean/rice/cheese (*Cedarlane* Low Fat), 6 oz. . . . . . . . . . . . .260
beef/bean (*El Monterey*), 5 oz. . . . . . . . . . . . . . . . . . . . . .420
beef/bean, red hot or green chili (*El Monterey*), 5 oz. . . . . .370
beef/bean, red chili (*El Monterey*), 5 oz. . . . . . . . . . . . . . .350
chicken (*El Monterey*), 4 oz. . . . . . . . . . . . . . . . . . . . . . .210
chicken (*El Monterey Family Classic* Ultimate), 5 oz. . . . . . .290
chicken or steak fajita (*El Monterey Family Classic*),
5 oz. . . . . . . . . . . . . . . . . . . . . . . . . . . . . . . . . . .250
**Burrito, breakfast,** frozen, 1 pc.:
(*Amy's*), 6 oz. . . . . . . . . . . . . . . . . . . . . . . . . . . . . . .210
bacon (*Great Starts*), 3.5 oz. . . . . . . . . . . . . . . . . . . . . . .250
egg, bacon cheese (*El Monterey Family Classics*),
4.5 oz. . . . . . . . . . . . . . . . . . . . . . . . . . . . . . . . . . .270
sausage (*El Monterey Family Classics*), 4.5 oz. . . . . . . . . . .290
sausage (*Great Starts*), 3.5 oz. . . . . . . . . . . . . . . . . . . . .240
**Burrito dinner,** frozen, con queso (*Patio*),
10-oz. pkg. . . . . . . . . . . . . . . . . . . . . . . . . . . . . . . . .490

**Burrito entree,** frozen, 1 pkg.:
bean and cheese (*Michelina's*), 8.5 oz. . . . . . . . . . . . . . . . .400
spicy hot (*Patio*), 11 oz. . . . . . . . . . . . . . . . . . . . . . . . . . .390
**Butter,** 1 tbsp:
(*Land O Lakes*) . . . . . . . . . . . . . . . . . . . . . . . . . . . . . . . .100
(*Land O Lakes* Light) . . . . . . . . . . . . . . . . . . . . . . . . . . . .50
(*Land O Lakes Ultra Creamy*) . . . . . . . . . . . . . . . . . . . . . .110
whipped (*Land O Lakes*) . . . . . . . . . . . . . . . . . . . . . . . . . .70
whipped (*Land O Lakes* Light) . . . . . . . . . . . . . . . . . . . . . .35
**Butter, flavored,** 1 tbsp.:
garlic (*Land O Lakes*) . . . . . . . . . . . . . . . . . . . . . . . . . . .100
honey (*Land O Lakes*) . . . . . . . . . . . . . . . . . . . . . . . . . . . .90
**Butter beans,** see "Lima beans"
**Butter flavor seasoning** (*Molly McButter*), 1 tsp. . . . . . . . . . .5
**Butterbur,** fresh, boiled, drained, 4 oz. . . . . . . . . . . . . . . . . . .9
**Buttercup squash** (*Frieda's*), ¾ cup, 3 oz. . . . . . . . . . . . . . .30
**Butterfish,** meat only:
raw, 4 oz. . . . . . . . . . . . . . . . . . . . . . . . . . . . . . . . . . . . .166
baked, broiled, or microwaved, 4 oz. . . . . . . . . . . . . . . . . .212
**Butternut,** dried, shelled, 1 oz. . . . . . . . . . . . . . . . . . . . . . . .174
**Butternut squash,** fresh (*Frieda's*), ¾ cup, 3 oz. . . . . . . . . . .30
**Butterscotch baking chips** (*Nestlé*), 1 tbsp. . . . . . . . . . . . . .80
**Butterscotch syrup** (*Smucker's* Sundae), 2 tbsp. . . . . . . . . . .100
**Butterscotch topping,** 2 tbsp.:
(*Smucker's*) . . . . . . . . . . . . . . . . . . . . . . . . . . . . . . . . . . .130
regular or caramel (*Mrs. Richardson's*) . . . . . . . . . . . . . . . .130
caramel (*Smucker's* Special Recipe) . . . . . . . . . . . . . . . . . .130

# C

**FOOD AND MEASURE** | **CALORIES**

**Cabbage** (see also "Coleslaw blend"):
raw, shredded, ½ cup . . . . . . . . . . . . . . . . . . . . . . . . . . . .9
boiled, drained, shredded, ½ cup . . . . . . . . . . . . . . . . . . . . .17
**Cabbage, bok choy,** fresh:
(*Frieda's*), 1 cup, 3 oz. . . . . . . . . . . . . . . . . . . . . . . . . . . .10
boiled, drained, shredded . . . . . . . . . . . . . . . . . . . . . . . . . .10
**Cabbage, napa,** raw (*Frieda's*), 1 cup, 3 oz. . . . . . . . . . . . . .15
**Cabbage, red,** fresh:
raw, shredded (*Dole* Classic), 3 oz. . . . . . . . . . . . . . . . . . . . .25
boiled, drained, shredded, ½ cup . . . . . . . . . . . . . . . . . . . . .16
**Cabbage red, canned,** sweet/sour (*Greenwood*), ½ cup . . .100
**Cabbage, savoy,** raw (*Frieda's Salad Savoy*), 3 oz. . . . . . . . .25
**Cabbage entree,** frozen, stuffed (*Lean Cuisine Everyday Favorites*), 9.5-oz. pkg. . . . . . . . . . . . . . . . . . . . . . . . . .210
**Cactus,** see "Nopale"
**Cake,** ⅛ cake, except as noted:
almond-topped (*Entenmann's*) . . . . . . . . . . . . . . . . . . . . . . .180
apple crumb (*Entenmann's* Orchard Delight) . . . . . . . . . . . . .260
banana crunch (*Entenmann's*) . . . . . . . . . . . . . . . . . . . . . . .220
banana loaf (*Entenmann's* Light) . . . . . . . . . . . . . . . . . . . . .140
blueberry crumb (*Entenmann's* Orchard Delight) . . . . . . . . . .250
butter (*Entenmann's Deluxe Desserts* Sunshine), ⅙ cake . . .320
butter loaf (*Entenmann's*), ⅙ cake . . . . . . . . . . . . . . . . . . . .210
cheesecake, see "Cheesecake"
chocolate:
  blackout (*Entenmann's Deluxe Desserts*), ⅑ cake . . . . .240
  chip crumb (*Entenmann's Deluxe Desserts*), ⅑ cake . . .390
  creme-filled (*Entenmann's*) . . . . . . . . . . . . . . . . . . . . . .300
  crunch (*Entenmann's*), ⅑ cake . . . . . . . . . . . . . . . . . . . .300
  fudge (*Entenmann's*) . . . . . . . . . . . . . . . . . . . . . . . . . . . .260
coffee cake, butter (*Entenmann's* French) . . . . . . . . . . . . . .210
coffee cake, cheese (*Entenmann's*) . . . . . . . . . . . . . . . . . . . .160
coffee cake, cherry cheese (*Entenmann's* Light), ⅑ cake . . .140
crumb (*Entenmann's* Light Delight), ⅑ cake . . . . . . . . . . . . .210

crumb (*Entenmann's* Ultimate), 1/10 cake . . . . . . . . . . . . . . .250
Danish, pecan (*Entenmann's* Ultimate) . . . . . . . . . . . . . . . .250
Danish ring (*Entenmann's*), 1/5 cake . . . . . . . . . . . . . . . . . .250
Danish twist, cheese (*Entenmann's*) . . . . . . . . . . . . . . . . . .230
Danish twist, cinnamon apple (*Entenmann's* Light) . . . . . . .140
Danish twist, lemon (*Entenmann's* Light) . . . . . . . . . . . . . .130
devil's food, iced (*Entenmann's*) . . . . . . . . . . . . . . . . . . . . .280
fruit (*Claxton* Old Fashioned), 1/12 cake . . . . . . . . . . . . . . .420
golden, fudge-iced (*Entenmann's*), 1/6 cake . . . . . . . . . . . . .340
lemon coconut (*Entenmann's*), 1/6 cake . . . . . . . . . . . . . . . .380
lemon crunch (*Entenmann's*), 1/9 cake . . . . . . . . . . . . . . . . .320
marble loaf (*Entenmann's* All Butter) . . . . . . . . . . . . . . . . . .190
old-fashioned loaf (*Entenmann's*) . . . . . . . . . . . . . . . . . . . .200
pineapple, raisin, or sour cream loaf (*Entenmann's*) . . . . . .220
rocky road (*Entenmann's*) . . . . . . . . . . . . . . . . . . . . . . . . .260
**Cake, frozen,** 1/8 cake, except as noted:
cappuccino (*Manzoni*), 1/5 cake . . . . . . . . . . . . . . . . . . . . . .260
carrot (*Oregon Farms*), 1/6 cake . . . . . . . . . . . . . . . . . . . . . .300
cheesecake, see "Cheesecake, frozen"
chocolate layer, double (*Sara Lee*) . . . . . . . . . . . . . . . . . . .260
chocolate layer, fudge (*Pepperidge Farm*) . . . . . . . . . . . . . .250
chocolate layer, German (*Sara Lee*) . . . . . . . . . . . . . . . . . .280
chocolate mousse (*Manzoni*), 1/5 cake . . . . . . . . . . . . . . . . .270
coconut, layer (*Pepperidge Farm*) . . . . . . . . . . . . . . . . . . . .250
coconut layer (*Sara Lee*) . . . . . . . . . . . . . . . . . . . . . . . . . .260
coffee cake, butter streusel (*Sara Lee*), 1/6 cake . . . . . . . . . .220
coffee cake, cheese (*Sara Lee* Reduced Fat), 1/6 cake . . . . . .180
coffee cake, crumb (*Sara Lee*) . . . . . . . . . . . . . . . . . . . . . . .220
coffee cake, pecan (*Sara Lee*), 1/6 cake . . . . . . . . . . . . . . . .230
coffee cake, raspberry (*Sara Lee*), 1/6 cake . . . . . . . . . . . . .220
fudge stripe, three-layer (*Pepperidge Farm*) . . . . . . . . . . . .250
golden layer, fudge (*Sara Lee*) . . . . . . . . . . . . . . . . . . . . . .260
pound (*Sara Lee* Butter), 1/4 cake . . . . . . . . . . . . . . . . . . . .320
pound (*Sara Lee* Reduced Fat), 1/4 cake . . . . . . . . . . . . . . . .280
pound, chocolate swirl (*Sara Lee*), 1/4 cake . . . . . . . . . . . . .330
pound, strawberry swirl (*Sara Lee*), 1/4 cake . . . . . . . . . . . .290
strawberry layer, stripe (*Pepperidge Farm*) . . . . . . . . . . . . .250
strawberry shortcake layer (*Sara Lee*) . . . . . . . . . . . . . . . .180
tiramisu (*Manzoni*), 1/5 cake . . . . . . . . . . . . . . . . . . . . . . . .230
vanilla layer (*Sara Lee*) . . . . . . . . . . . . . . . . . . . . . . . . . . .260

**Cake, mix,** 1/12 cake*, except as noted:
angel food (*Duncan Hines* Moist Deluxe) . . . . . . . . . . . . . . .190
angel food (*SuperMoist* Traditional) . . . . . . . . . . . . . . . . . . . .130
angel food, chocolate swirl, or confetti (*SuperMoist*) . . . . .150
banana (*Duncan Hines* Moist Deluxe Supreme) . . . . . . . . . . .250
butter pecan (*SuperMoist*) . . . . . . . . . . . . . . . . . . . . . . . . . .240
butterscotch or caramel (*Duncan Hines* Moist Deluxe) . . . .250
carrot (*SuperMoist*), 1/10 cake* . . . . . . . . . . . . . . . . . . . . . .320
cheesecake, see "Cheesecake mix"
cherry chip (*SuperMoist*), 1/10 cake* . . . . . . . . . . . . . . . . . .300
cherry, wild, vanilla (*Duncan Hines* Moist Deluxe) . . . . . . . .250
chocolate:
chip or butter recipe (*SuperMoist*) . . . . . . . . . . . . . . . .250
dark, fudge (*Duncan Hines* Moist Deluxe) . . . . . . . . . . .290
fudge (*SuperMoist*) . . . . . . . . . . . . . . . . . . . . . . . . . . . .270
fudge, creamy swirls (*SuperMoist*), 1/9 cake* . . . . . . . .210
German (*Duncan Hines* Moist Deluxe) . . . . . . . . . . . . . .240
German or double swirl (*SuperMoist*) . . . . . . . . . . . . . .270
milk (*SuperMoist*) . . . . . . . . . . . . . . . . . . . . . . . . . . . . .240
mocha or Swiss (*Duncan Hines* Moist Deluxe) . . . . . . . .290
coffee cake, cinnamon (*Betty Crocker Stir 'n Bake*
Streusel), 1/6 pkg. . . . . . . . . . . . . . . . . . . . . . . . . . . . . . .200
devil's food (*Duncan Hines* Moist Deluxe) . . . . . . . . . . . . . .290
devil's food (*SuperMoist*) . . . . . . . . . . . . . . . . . . . . . . . . . .270
devil's food (*Sweet Rewards*) . . . . . . . . . . . . . . . . . . . . . . .200
fudge, butter (*Duncan Hines* Moist Deluxe), 1/10 cake* . . . . .320
fudge, marble (*Duncan Hines* Moist Deluxe) . . . . . . . . . . . .250
fudge, marble (*SuperMoist*), 1/10 cake* . . . . . . . . . . . . . . . .290
gingerbread (*Betty Crocker*), 1/8 cake* . . . . . . . . . . . . . . . .230
golden, butter recipe (*Duncan Hines* Moist Deluxe) . . . . . . .320
lemon (*Duncan Hines* Moist Deluxe Supreme) . . . . . . . . . . .250
lemon (*SuperMoist*) . . . . . . . . . . . . . . . . . . . . . . . . . . . . . .240
orange (*Duncan Hines* Moist Deluxe Supreme) . . . . . . . . . .250
pineapple (*Duncan Hines* Moist Deluxe Supreme) . . . . . . . .250
pineapple or party swirl (*SuperMoist*) . . . . . . . . . . . . . . . .250
pineapple upside down (*Betty Crocker*), 1/6 cake* . . . . . . . .400
pound (*Betty Crocker*), 1/8 cake . . . . . . . . . . . . . . . . . . . . . .260
rainbow chip (*SuperMoist*), 1/10 cake* . . . . . . . . . . . . . . . .300
red velvet (*Duncan Hines* Moist Deluxe) . . . . . . . . . . . . . . .240
sour cream white (*SuperMoist*), 1/10 cake* . . . . . . . . . . . . .280

spice (*Duncan Hines* Moist Deluxe) . . . . . . . . . . . . . . . . . .250
spice (*SuperMoist*) . . . . . . . . . . . . . . . . . . . . . . . . . . .240
strawberry (*SuperMoist*) . . . . . . . . . . . . . . . . . . . . . . . .250
vanilla, French (*Duncan Hines* Moist Deluxe) . . . . . . . . . . .250
vanilla, French or golden (*SuperMoist*) . . . . . . . . . . . . . . .240
white (*SuperMoist*) . . . . . . . . . . . . . . . . . . . . . . . . . . .230
white (*SuperMoist* Richer Recipe) . . . . . . . . . . . . . . . . . .250
white (*Sweet Rewards*) . . . . . . . . . . . . . . . . . . . . . . . . .190
yellow (*Duncan Hines* Moist Deluxe) . . . . . . . . . . . . . . . . .250
yellow (*SuperMoist*) . . . . . . . . . . . . . . . . . . . . . . . . . .250
yellow (*Sweet Rewards*) . . . . . . . . . . . . . . . . . . . . . . . .200
yellow, butter recipe (*SuperMoist*) . . . . . . . . . . . . . . . . . .260
yellow, w/fudge, creamy swirls (*SuperMoist*), 1/9 cake* . . . .210

**Cake, snack** (see also specific listings):
Boston creme (*Drake's*), 1.5 oz. . . . . . . . . . . . . . . . . . . . .180
butter loaf slice or cheese puffs (*Entenmann's*), 3 oz. . . . . .330
chocolate (*Devil Dogs*), 1.6 oz. . . . . . . . . . . . . . . . . . . . .180
chocolate (*Funny Bones*), 2 pcs., 2.5 oz. . . . . . . . . . . . . . .300
chocolate (*Hostess Ho-Ho's*), 2 pcs., 2 oz. . . . . . . . . . . . .250
chocolate (*Ring Dings*), 2 pcs., 2.7 oz. . . . . . . . . . . . . . . .340
chocolate (*Yodels*), 2 pcs., 2.2 oz. . . . . . . . . . . . . . . . . .290
coconut (*Drake's Mini Coco Bites*), 4 pcs., 2.5 oz. . . . . . . . .320
coffee cake (*Drake's*), 1.2-oz. pc. . . . . . . . . . . . . . . . . . .140
coffee cake (*Drake's*), 2.25-oz. pc. . . . . . . . . . . . . . . . . .270
coffee cake, crumb (*Hostess*), 1.1-oz. pc. . . . . . . . . . . . . .140
crumb cake (*Entenmann's*), 3 oz. . . . . . . . . . . . . . . . . . . .360
cupcake, creme-filled:
- (*Entenmann's* Light), 2 oz. . . . . . . . . . . . . . . . . . . . .160
- chocolate (*Entenmann's* Light), 2 oz. . . . . . . . . . . . . . .160
- chocolate (*Hostess*), 1.8-oz. pc. . . . . . . . . . . . . . . . . .180
- chocolate (*Yankee Doodles*), 3 pcs., 3 oz. . . . . . . . . . . .320
- chocolate mini (*Yankee Doodles*), 4 pcs., 1.8 oz. . . . . . .190
- golden (*Sunny Doodles*), 2 pcs., 2 oz. . . . . . . . . . . . . . .220
- orange (*Hostess*), 1.5-oz. pc. . . . . . . . . . . . . . . . . . . .160

devil's food, creme-filled (*Twinkies*), 1.6-oz. pc. . . . . . . . . .170
golden, creme-filled (*Twinkies*), 1.5-oz. pc. . . . . . . . . . . . . .150
golden, creme-filled (*Twinkies* Lowfat), 1.5-oz. pc. . . . . . . .130
marble (*Entenmann's*), 3 oz. . . . . . . . . . . . . . . . . . . . . . .320
pecan spinwheels (*Aunt Fanny's*), 1 oz. . . . . . . . . . . . . . . .100
pound (*Awrey's* Golden), 2.6 oz. . . . . . . . . . . . . . . . . . . . .250

**Cake, snack *(cont.)***
pound (*Drake's*), 2 pcs., 2.3 oz. . . . . . . . . . . . . . . . . . . . . . . .250
raspberry sponge (*Mr. Kipling*), 2 pcs., 2.3 oz. . . . . . . . . . . .260
**Cake, snack, mix** (see also specific listings), 1 pc.*:
chocolate bar (*Betty Crocker Hershey*) . . . . . . . . . . . . . . . .150
chocolate peanut butter bar (*Betty Crocker* Supreme) . . . . .190
date bar (*Betty Crocker*) . . . . . . . . . . . . . . . . . . . . . . . . . . .150
lemon bar (*Betty Crocker Sunkist*) . . . . . . . . . . . . . . . . . . .140
**Calamari dish,** frozen:
breaded (*Contessa*), 2 oz. or 13 pcs., w/2 tbsp. sauce . . . .170
crisps, breaded (*Acadian Gourmet*), 12 pcs., 3.1 oz. . . . . . .230
**Calves liver,** see "Liver"
**Candy:**
almond, candy-coated (*House of Bazzini* Jordan), 1 oz. . . . .180
almond, chocolate-coated (*Lindt*), 1.4 oz. . . . . . . . . . . . . . .220
almond bar (*Mars*), 1.8 oz. . . . . . . . . . . . . . . . . . . . . . . . . .240
(*Baby Ruth*), 2.1-oz. bar . . . . . . . . . . . . . . . . . . . . . . . . . . .270
(*Bittyfinger*), 2 bars . . . . . . . . . . . . . . . . . . . . . . . . . . . . . .170
butter rum (*LifeSavers*), 2 pcs. . . . . . . . . . . . . . . . . . . . . . . .20
(*Butterfinger*), 2.1-oz. bar . . . . . . . . . . . . . . . . . . . . . . . . .270
(*Butterfinger BB's*), 1.7-oz. bag . . . . . . . . . . . . . . . . . . . . .220
(*Butterfinger Treasures*), 3 pcs., 1.2 oz. . . . . . . . . . . . . . . .180
candy corn, 1 oz. . . . . . . . . . . . . . . . . . . . . . . . . . . . . . . . .110
caramel (*Nips*), 2 pcs. . . . . . . . . . . . . . . . . . . . . . . . . . . . . .60
caramel (*Treasures*), 3 pcs., 1.2 oz. . . . . . . . . . . . . . . . . . .170
caramel, chocolate-coated (*Pom Poms*), 1.6 oz. . . . . . . . . .200
cherries, chocolate-covered (*Cella*), 2 pcs. . . . . . . . . . . . . .110
cherry, chocolate thin (*Andes* Jubilee), 8 pcs. . . . . . . . . . . .200
chocolate, bittersweet (*Lindt Excellence*), 4 pcs., 1.4 oz. . . .220
chocolate, candy-coated (*M&M's*), 1.7 oz. . . . . . . . . . . . . .240
chocolate, candy-coated, almond (*M&M's*), 1.3 oz. . . . . . . .200
chocolate, candy-coated, peanut (*M&M's*), 1.7 oz. . . . . . . .250
chocolate, dark (*Ghirardelli*), 1.5 oz. . . . . . . . . . . . . . . . . .210
chocolate, dark (*Lindt* Thins), 15 pcs., 1.5 oz. . . . . . . . . . . .260
chocolate, milk:
(*Dove Promises*), 5 pcs., 1.4 oz. . . . . . . . . . . . . . . . . . . .220
(*Hershey's*), 1.5-oz. bar . . . . . . . . . . . . . . . . . . . . . . . . . .230
(*Hershey's Hugs and Kisses*), 9 pcs., 1.4 oz. . . . . . . . . . .220
(*Hershey's Nuggets*), 4 pcs., 1.4 oz. . . . . . . . . . . . . . . . .210
(*Lindt Excellence*), 12 pcs., 1.4 oz. . . . . . . . . . . . . . . . . .210

(*Lindt* Milk Truffle Bar), 5 pcs., 1.5 oz. . . . . . . . . . . . . . . .260
(*Lindt* Swiss Classic Milk), 12 pcs., 1.4 oz. . . . . . . . . . . .210
(*Lindt* Swiss Milk Gold), 5 pcs., 1.3 oz. . . . . . . . . . . . . .200
(*Nestlé*), 1.45-oz. bar . . . . . . . . . . . . . . . . . . . . . . .220
almond (*Ghirardelli*), 1.5 oz. . . . . . . . . . . . . . . . . . . . .230
almond (*Hershey's*), 1.4-oz. bar . . . . . . . . . . . . . . . . . . .230
almond (*Hershey's Kisses*), 9 pcs., 1.4 oz. . . . . . . . . . . . .230
almond (*Hershey's Nuggets*), 4 pcs., 1.3 oz. . . . . . . . . . .210
almond (*Lindt* Alba), 5 pcs., 1.5 oz. . . . . . . . . . . . . . . . .240
almond (*Lindt* Swiss), 12 pcs., 1.4 oz. . . . . . . . . . . . . . . .220
caramel (*Ghirardelli*), 3 pcs., 1.5 oz. . . . . . . . . . . . . . . .210
caramel (*Lindt*), 5 pcs., 1.5 oz. . . . . . . . . . . . . . . . . . .210
chocolate-filled (*Ghirardelli*), 3 pcs., 1.5 oz. . . . . . . . . . .210
crisps (*Cadbury's Krisp*), 9 blocks, 1.4 oz. . . . . . . . . . . . .200
crisps (*Krackel*), 1.4-oz. bar . . . . . . . . . . . . . . . . . . . .220
crisps (*Nestlé Crunch*), 1.55-oz. bar . . . . . . . . . . . . . .230
fruit, nuts (*Chunky*), 1.4-oz. bar . . . . . . . . . . . . . . . . .210
hazelnut (*Lindt* Swiss), 5 pcs., 1.3 oz. . . . . . . . . . . . . . .210
hazelnut (*Lindt* Swiss), 12 pcs., 1.4 oz. . . . . . . . . . . . . .230
hazelnut w/raisins (*Lindt*), 5 pcs., 1.3 oz. . . . . . . . . . . .210
peanut (*Mr. Goodbar*), 1.7-oz. bar . . . . . . . . . . . . . . . . .270
pistachio (*Lindt*), 5 pcs., 1.5 oz. . . . . . . . . . . . . . . . . . .250
raisins, hazelnuts, almonds (*Lindt*), 12 pcs., 1.4 oz. . . .200
chocolate, mint (*Ghirardelli*), 1.5 oz. . . . . . . . . . . . . . . . .220
chocolate, white:
(*Lindt* White Lindor Truffle), 7 pcs., 1.4 oz. . . . . . . . . .240
(*Lindt* Swiss), 4 pcs., 1.3 oz. . . . . . . . . . . . . . . . . . . . .220
(*Lindt* Swiss), 12 pcs., 1.4 oz. . . . . . . . . . . . . . . . . . . .230
w/cookie (*Hershey's Cookies n' Creme*), 1.5 oz. . . . . . . .230
w/crisps (*Nestlé White Crunch*), 1.4-oz. bar . . . . . . . . . .220
chocolate flavor (*Nips/Nips* Parfait), 2 pcs. . . . . . . . . . . . . . .60
chocolate truffles (*Godiva*), 1.5 oz. . . . . . . . . . . . . . . . . .220
chocolate twists (*Twizzlers*), 3 pcs., 1.5 oz. . . . . . . . . . . . .150
chocolate wafer bar (*Lindt*), 5 pcs., 1.5 oz. . . . . . . . . . . .220
coconut, chocolate-coated:
(*Mounds*), 1.9 oz. . . . . . . . . . . . . . . . . . . . . . . . . . . . .250
w/almonds (*Almond Joy*), 1.76 oz. . . . . . . . . . . . . . . . .240
white (*Lindt Excellence*), 4 pcs., 1.4 oz. . . . . . . . . . . . . .240
coffee (*Nips*), 2 pcs. . . . . . . . . . . . . . . . . . . . . . . . . . . . . .50
cotton candy (*Fluffy Stuff*), ½ bag, 1.6 oz. . . . . . . . . . . . .180

**Candy *(cont.)***

creme de menthe, chocolate thin (*Andes*), 8 pcs. . . . . . . . .200
fruit flavor:
(*Charms* Sour Balls), 1 pc. . . . . . . . . . . . . . . . . . . . . . . .20
(*LifeSavers*), 2 pcs. . . . . . . . . . . . . . . . . . . . . . . . . . . .20
(*LifeSavers* Large), 4 pcs. . . . . . . . . . . . . . . . . . . . . . . .60
(*LifeSavers Delites*), 5 pcs. . . . . . . . . . . . . . . . . . . . . . .30
(*Tootsie Flavor Roll*), 6 pcs., 1.4 oz. . . . . . . . . . . . . . . .170
chews (*Jolly Rancher*), 2-oz. pkg. . . . . . . . . . . . . . . . . . .210
chews (*LifeSavers Fruit Chews*), 11 pcs. . . . . . . . . . . . .150
chews (*Starburst*), 8 pcs., 1.4 oz. . . . . . . . . . . . . . . . . .160
and creme (*Creme Savers*), 3 pcs. . . . . . . . . . . . . . . . . . .60
gummed (*Dots*), 12 pcs., 1.5 oz. . . . . . . . . . . . . . . . . . .150
gummed (*Gummi Savers*), 10 pcs. . . . . . . . . . . . . . . . . .130
gummed (*Jolly Rancher* Jolly Jellies), 1.3-oz. pkg. . . . . .110
gummed (*Jolly Rancher Gummis*), 1.7-oz. pkg. . . . . . . .150
gummed (*Jujyfruits*), 2.1-oz. box . . . . . . . . . . . . . . . . .200
gum, chewing (*Doublemint/Juicy Fruit/Big Red/Winterfresh/Wrigley's Spearmint*), 1 pc. . . . . . . . . . .10
hard, see "fruit flavor," above, and specific flavors
hazelnuts, chocolate-coated (*Lindt*), 1.4 oz. . . . . . . . . . . .220
honey (*Bit-O-Honey*), 1.7-oz. bar . . . . . . . . . . . . . . . . . . .190
jelly beans (*Jolly Rancher* Jolly Beans), 25 pcs., 1.4 oz. . . .130
licorice (*Crows/Mason Dots*), 12 pcs., 1.5 oz. . . . . . . . . . .150
licorice (*Nibs*), 1.4 oz. . . . . . . . . . . . . . . . . . . . . . . . . .140
licorice (*Twizzlers* Twists), 2.5-oz. pkg. . . . . . . . . . . . . . .240
lollipop, all flavors, 1 pop, except as noted:
(*Charms Blow Pop/Sweet/Sour Pop* Regular) . . . . . . . . .70
(*Sugar Daddy* Large) . . . . . . . . . . . . . . . . . . . . . . . . . .200
(*Sugar Daddy* Junior), 3 pops . . . . . . . . . . . . . . . . . . .160
(*Tootsie Pops*) . . . . . . . . . . . . . . . . . . . . . . . . . . . . . . .60
malted milk balls (*Whoppers*), .75-oz. pouch . . . . . . . . . . .100
marshmallow (*Kraft Jet-Puffed*), 5 pcs. . . . . . . . . . . . . . . .110
marshmallow (*Spangler* Peanut), 6 pcs. . . . . . . . . . . . . . . .163
(*Milky Way*), 2-oz. bar . . . . . . . . . . . . . . . . . . . . . . . . . . .270
(*Milky Way* Dark), 1.75-oz. bar . . . . . . . . . . . . . . . . . . . .220
mint (*Junior* Chews), 26 pcs., 1.4 oz. . . . . . . . . . . . . . . . .150
mint (*LifeSavers*), 2 pcs. . . . . . . . . . . . . . . . . . . . . . . . . .20
mint (*LifeSavers* Large), 4 pcs. . . . . . . . . . . . . . . . . . . . . .60

mint w/chocolate (*Andes* Mint Parfait), 8 pcs. . . . . . . . . . . .210
mint w/chocolate (*Andes* Mint Patties), 3 pcs., 1.5 oz. . . . .180
mint w/chocolate (*Junior Mints*), 16 pcs., 1.4 oz. . . . . . . . .160
mint w/chocolate (*York* Peppermint Pattie), 1.4 oz. . . . . . . .160
(*Nestlé Mocha Crunch*), 1.3-oz. bar . . . . . . . . . . . . . . . . . .200
(*Nestlé Turtles*), 2 pcs. . . . . . . . . . . . . . . . . . . . . . . . . . .160
nonpareils (*Sno-Caps*), 2.3-oz. box . . . . . . . . . . . . . . . . . .300
nougat, chocolate-coated (*Charleston Chew*), 1.9 oz. . . . . .230
(*Oh Henry!*), .9-oz. bar . . . . . . . . . . . . . . . . . . . . . . . . . .120
(*100 Grand*), 1.5-oz. pkg. . . . . . . . . . . . . . . . . . . . . . . .190
peanut, butter toffee (*Fisher*), 1 oz. . . . . . . . . . . . . . . . . .130
peanut, chocolate-coated (*Goobers*), 1.38-oz. bag . . . . . . .210
peanut bar (*Planters*), 1.6 oz. . . . . . . . . . . . . . . . . . . . . . .230
peanut butter, chocolate (*Treasures*), 4 pcs., 1.5 oz. . . . . . .240
peanut butter, chocolate, candy (*Reese's Pieces*),
1.6 oz. . . . . . . . . . . . . . . . . . . . . . . . . . . . . . . . . . . . . .230
peanut butter cup (*Reese's*), 1.2-oz. pkg. . . . . . . . . . . . . . .180
peanut butter cookie (*Twix*), .9 oz. . . . . . . . . . . . . . . . . . . .130
peanut butter parfait (*Nips*), 2 pcs. . . . . . . . . . . . . . . . . . . .60
praline, chocolate (*Lindt*), 3 pcs., 1.3 oz. . . . . . . . . . . . . . .200
pretzel, chocolate, milk (*Flipz*), 1 oz. . . . . . . . . . . . . . . . . .130
pretzel, chocolate, white fudge (*Flipz*), 1 oz. . . . . . . . . . . .140
raisins, chocolate-coated (*Lindt*), 1.5 oz. . . . . . . . . . . . . . .190
raisins, chocolate-coated (*Raisinets*), 1.58-oz. bag . . . . . . .190
(*Snickers*), 2.1-oz. bar . . . . . . . . . . . . . . . . . . . . . . . . . .280
(*Spree/SweeTarts*), 8 pcs., .5 oz. . . . . . . . . . . . . . . . . . . . .60
(*Sugar Babies*), 30 pcs., 1.6 oz. . . . . . . . . . . . . . . . . . . . .180
(*3 Musketeers*), 2.1-oz. bar . . . . . . . . . . . . . . . . . . . . . . .260
strawberry twists (*Twizzlers*), 1.7-oz. pkg. . . . . . . . . . . . . .170
toffee (*Heath*), 1.4-oz. bar . . . . . . . . . . . . . . . . . . . . . . . .210
toffee crunch, chocolate thin (*Andes*), 8 pcs. . . . . . . . . . . .200
(*Tootsie Roll Midgees*), 6 pcs., 1.4 oz. . . . . . . . . . . . . . . .160
(*Tootsie Roll* Snack Bar), 2 bars, 1 oz. . . . . . . . . . . . . . . .110
truffle ball, .42-oz. pc.:
all varieties, except white chocolate (*Lindt Lindor*) . . . . . .70
white chocolate (*Lindt Lindor*) . . . . . . . . . . . . . . . . . . . .80
vanilla almond café (*Nips*), 2 pcs. . . . . . . . . . . . . . . . . . . .50
wafer, chocolate-coated (*Kit Kat*), 1.5-oz. bar . . . . . . . . . . .220
(*Wonderball*), 1-oz. pc. . . . . . . . . . . . . . . . . . . . . . . . . . .140

**Cannelloni entree,** frozen, 1 pkg.:
(*Lean Cuisine Everyday Favorites*), 9⅛ oz. . . . . . . . . . . . . .220
ricotta (*Wolfgang Puck's*), 12 oz. . . . . . . . . . . . . . . . . . . . . . .420
**Cantaloupe:**
½ of 5" melon . . . . . . . . . . . . . . . . . . . . . . . . . . . . . . . . . .94
pulp, cubed, ½ cup . . . . . . . . . . . . . . . . . . . . . . . . . . . . .28
**Capers** (*Italica*), 1 tbsp. . . . . . . . . . . . . . . . . . . . . . . . . . .0
**Capicola,** see "Ham lunch meat"
**Capon,** see "Chicken"
**Caponata,** see "Eggplant appetizer"
**Cappuccino,** see "Coffee, iced" and "Coffee, flavored, mix"
**Carambola,** fresh:
(*Frieda's* Starfruit), 5 oz. . . . . . . . . . . . . . . . . . . . . . . . . . .45
sliced, ½ cup . . . . . . . . . . . . . . . . . . . . . . . . . . . . . . . . . . .18
**Carambola, dried** (*Frieda's* Starfruit), ⅓ cup,
1.4 oz. . . . . . . . . . . . . . . . . . . . . . . . . . . . . . . . . . . . .120
**Caramel dip,** see "Apple dip"
**Caramel syrup** (*Smucker's* Sundae Syrup), 2 tbsp. . . . . . . .100
**Caramel topping** (see also "Butterscotch topping"):
(*Mrs. Richardson's*), 2 tbsp. . . . . . . . . . . . . . . . . . . . . . .130
(*Smucker's*), 2 tbsp. . . . . . . . . . . . . . . . . . . . . . . . . . . . .130
(*Smucker's Plate Scrapers*), 2 tbsp. . . . . . . . . . . . . . . . .100
hot (*Smucker's*), 2 tbsp. . . . . . . . . . . . . . . . . . . . . . . . . . .120
**Caraway seed,** 1 tsp. . . . . . . . . . . . . . . . . . . . . . . . . . . . . .7
**Carbonara sauce mix** (*Knorr* Pasta Sauces), 2 tbsp. . . . . . . .70
**Cardamom,** ground or seed, 1 tsp. . . . . . . . . . . . . . . . . . . . .6
**Cardoon,** boiled, drained, 4 oz. . . . . . . . . . . . . . . . . . . . . .25
***Carl's Jr.,*** 1 serving:
breakfast items:
bacon, 2 strips . . . . . . . . . . . . . . . . . . . . . . . . . . . . . . . .45
burrito . . . . . . . . . . . . . . . . . . . . . . . . . . . . . . . . . . . . .550
eggs, scrambled . . . . . . . . . . . . . . . . . . . . . . . . . . . . . . .180
English muffin w/margarine . . . . . . . . . . . . . . . . . . . . . .210
*French Toast Dips,* w/out syrup . . . . . . . . . . . . . . . . . . .370
sausage, 1 patty . . . . . . . . . . . . . . . . . . . . . . . . . . . . . . .190
sourdough . . . . . . . . . . . . . . . . . . . . . . . . . . . . . . . . . . .410
*Sunrise Sandwich,* w/out bacon or sausage . . . . . . . . . .360
quesadilla . . . . . . . . . . . . . . . . . . . . . . . . . . . . . . . . . . .370
sandwiches:
*Carl's* bacon Swiss crispy chicken . . . . . . . . . . . . . . . . . .760

*Carl's Catch Fish Sandwich* .530
*Carl's Famous Star* .590
*Carl's* ranch crispy chicken .660
*Carl's* western bacon crispy chicken .760
*Charbroiled BBQ Chicken Sandwich* .290
*Charbroiled BBQ Club Sandwich* .470
*Charbroiled Santa Fe Chicken Sandwich* .540
charbroiled sirloin steak .550
double sourdough bacon cheeseburger .880
*Double Western Bacon Cheeseburger* .920
*Famous Bacon Cheeseburger* .700
hamburger .280
sourdough bacon cheeseburger .640
sourdough ranch cheeseburger .720
Southwest spicy chicken .620
spicy chicken .480
*Super Star* .790
*Western Bacon Cheeseburger* .660
sandwich cheese, American, large .60
sandwich cheese, American, small, or Swiss style .50
side dishes:
chicken stars, 6 pcs. .260
*CrissCut Fries* .410
french fries, kids .250
french fries, large .620
french fries, medium .460
french fries, small .290
hash-brown nuggets .330
onion rings .430
zucchini .320
potato, plain, no margarine .290
potato, bacon/cheese .640
potato, broccoli/cheese .530
potato, sour cream/chives .430
salad, *Charbroiled Chicken Salad-to-Go* .200
salad, *Garden Salad-to-Go* .50
salad dressings, 2 oz.:
blue cheese .320
French, fat-free .60
house .220

***Carl's Jr.*, salad dressings *(cont.)***
Italian, fat-free .15
Thousand Island .230
breads/sauces:
bread sticks .35
croutons .30
BBQ, mustard, or sweet 'n sour sauce .50
grape jelly or strawberry jam .40
honey sauce or table syrup .90
salsa .10
bakery/desserts:
blueberry muffin .340
bran raisin muffin .370
cheese danish .400
chocolate cake .300
chocolate chip cookie .350
strawberry swirl cheesecake .290
shakes:
chocolate, regular .770
chocolate, small .530
strawberry, regular .750
strawberry, small .510
vanilla, regular .700
vanilla, small .470
**Carp,** meat only:
raw, 4 oz. .144
baked, broiled, or microwaved, 4 oz. .184
**Carrot,** fresh:
raw, whole, 7½" long, 2.8 oz. .31
raw, whole, baby, 1 medium, 2¾" long .4
raw, whole, baby, peeled mini (*Dole*), 3 oz. .40
raw, shredded (*Fresh Express*), 1 cup .45
raw, shredded, ½ cup .24
boiled, drained, sliced, ½ cup .35
**Carrot, can or jar,** ½ cup:
whole, baby (*Bonduelle*) .21
whole, baby (*Reese*) .15
whole, small, or julienne (*S&W*) .30
sliced (*Libby's*) .25
sliced (*Veg-All*) .30

**Carrot, frozen:**
baby (*Birds Eye*) ½ cup . . . . . . . . . . . . . . . . . . . . . . . . . .40
baby (*John Cope's*), 3 oz. . . . . . . . . . . . . . . . . . . . . . . . . .35
bell, small (*Bonduelle* Parisian), 3 oz. . . . . . . . . . . . . . . . .35
honey-glazed (*Green Giant*), 1 cup . . . . . . . . . . . . . . . . . . .90
honey-glazed, baby (*Cascadian Farm*), 1 cup . . . . . . . . . . . .60
sliced (*John Cope's*), ⅔ cup . . . . . . . . . . . . . . . . . . . . . . .35
**Carrot chips** (*Hain*), 22 pcs., 1.1 oz. . . . . . . . . . . . . . . . .160
**Carrot–fruit juice blend** (*AriZona* CrazyBerry/Cocktail), 8 fl. oz. . . . . . . . . . . . . . . . . . . . . . . . . . . . . . . . . . .110
**Casaba,** ⅒ of 7¾" melon . . . . . . . . . . . . . . . . . . . . . . . . .43
**Cashew,** 1 oz., except as noted:
(*Blue Diamond*) . . . . . . . . . . . . . . . . . . . . . . . . . . . . . . .190
(*Fisher* Jumbo) . . . . . . . . . . . . . . . . . . . . . . . . . . . . . . .170
(*Frito-Lay* Salted) . . . . . . . . . . . . . . . . . . . . . . . . . . . . .180
oil-roasted, whole (*Blue Diamond*), ¼ cup . . . . . . . . . . . . .210
roasted (*Setton Farms*), 1.2 oz. . . . . . . . . . . . . . . . . . . . . .200
**Catfish,** channel, meat only:
farmed, raw, 4 oz. . . . . . . . . . . . . . . . . . . . . . . . . . . . . . .153
farmed, baked, broiled, or microwaved, 4 oz. . . . . . . . . . . .172
wild, raw, 4 oz. . . . . . . . . . . . . . . . . . . . . . . . . . . . . . . . .108
wild, baked, broiled, or microwaved, 4 oz. . . . . . . . . . . . . .119
**Cauliflower,** fresh:
raw (*Dole*), ⅙ medium head, 3.5 oz. . . . . . . . . . . . . . . . . . .25
raw, florets, 3 pcs. . . . . . . . . . . . . . . . . . . . . . . . . . . . . . .14
raw, florets, 1" pcs., ½ cup . . . . . . . . . . . . . . . . . . . . . . . .13
boiled, drained, 1" pcs., ½ cup . . . . . . . . . . . . . . . . . . . . . .14
green, raw, 1" pcs., ½ cup . . . . . . . . . . . . . . . . . . . . . . . . .16
**Cauliflower, frozen:**
(*Birds Eye*), ½ cup . . . . . . . . . . . . . . . . . . . . . . . . . . . . . .20
florets (*Green Giant*), 1 cup . . . . . . . . . . . . . . . . . . . . . . .20
boiled, drained, 1" pcs., ½ cup . . . . . . . . . . . . . . . . . . . . . .17
**Cauliflower combinations,** frozen, nuggets, w/carrots and snow pea pods (*Birds Eye*), ½ cup . . . . . . . . . . . . . . . . .30
**Cavatelli pasta dish,** frozen, w/cheese (*Celentano*), 1 cup . . . . . . . . . . . . . . . . . . . . . . . . . . . . . . . . . . . .400
**Cavatappi pasta dish,** mix, sun-dried tomato basil pesto (*Land O Lakes*), 2.5 oz. . . . . . . . . . . . . . . . . . . . . . . . . .260
**Caviar** (see also "Roe"):
lumpfish, black, red, or gold (*Romanoff*), 1 tbsp. . . . . . . . . .15

**Caviar** ***(cont.)***
salmon (*Romanoff*), 1 tbsp. . . . . . . . . . . . . . . . . . . . . . . . .35
sturgeon (*Romanoff* Beluga/Osetra/Sevruga), 1 oz. . . . . . . . . .74
whitefish, black or gold (*Romanoff*), 1 tbsp. . . . . . . . . . . . . . .25
**Cayenne,** see "Pepper"
**Celeriac,** fresh, raw, trimmed, ½ cup . . . . . . . . . . . . . . . . . .31
**Celery:**
raw (*Dole*), 2 medium stalks . . . . . . . . . . . . . . . . . . . . . . . .20
raw, 7½" stalk, 1.6 oz. . . . . . . . . . . . . . . . . . . . . . . . . . . . . .6
raw, diced, ½ cup . . . . . . . . . . . . . . . . . . . . . . . . . . . . . . . .10
boiled, drained, diced, ½ cup . . . . . . . . . . . . . . . . . . . . . . . .13
**Celery, dried,** flake/seed, 1 tsp. . . . . . . . . . . . . . . . . . . . . . . .8
**Celery root,** see "Celeriac"
**Cellophane noodles,** see "Noodle, Chinese"
**Cereal, ready-to-eat** (see also specific grains), 1 cup, except as noted:
amaranth flakes (*Health Valley*), ¾ cup . . . . . . . . . . . . . . . . .100
bran (*Kellogg's All-Bran* Original), ½ cup . . . . . . . . . . . . . . . .80
bran (*Multi-Bran Chex*) . . . . . . . . . . . . . . . . . . . . . . . . . . . .200
bran, extra fiber (*Kellogg's All-Bran*), ½ cup . . . . . . . . . . . . .50
bran flakes (*Kellogg's Complete*), ¾ cup . . . . . . . . . . . . . . . .90
bran flakes, w/flax (*New Morning*) . . . . . . . . . . . . . . . . . . . .110
bran w/raisins (*Erewhon*) . . . . . . . . . . . . . . . . . . . . . . . . . .170
bran w/raisins (*Kellogg's*) . . . . . . . . . . . . . . . . . . . . . . . . . .190
bran w/raisins (*Malt-O-Meal*) . . . . . . . . . . . . . . . . . . . . . . .200
bran w/raisins and nuts (*General Mills*), ¾ cup . . . . . . . . . .200
corn (*Corn Bursts*) . . . . . . . . . . . . . . . . . . . . . . . . . . . . . . .120
corn (*Ginseng Crunch*), ¾ cup . . . . . . . . . . . . . . . . . . . . . . .110
corn (*Healthy Valley Crunch-Ems*), 1¼ cups . . . . . . . . . . . . .110
corn (*Kellogg's Corn Pops*) . . . . . . . . . . . . . . . . . . . . . . . . .120
corn flakes (*Country*) . . . . . . . . . . . . . . . . . . . . . . . . . . . . .110
corn flakes (*Kellogg's*) . . . . . . . . . . . . . . . . . . . . . . . . . . . .100
corn flakes (*Kellogg's Frosted/Honey Crunch*), ¾ cup . . . . .120
corn flakes (*Malt-O-Meal*) . . . . . . . . . . . . . . . . . . . . . . . . . .110
corn flakes, blue (*Health Valley* Organic), ¾ cup . . . . . . . . .100
corn flakes, w/flax (*New Morning*) . . . . . . . . . . . . . . . . . . . .120
corn, puffed (*Healthy Valley*) . . . . . . . . . . . . . . . . . . . . . . . .110
corn and amaranth (*Erewhon Aztec*) . . . . . . . . . . . . . . . . . .110
corn and rice (*Kellogg's Crispix*) . . . . . . . . . . . . . . . . . . . . .110
flax, golden (*Health Valley* Organic), ½ cup . . . . . . . . . . . .190

granola:
all varieties (*Health Valley* Low Fat), ⅔ cup . . . . . . . . . . .190
oats and honey (*Quaker* 100% Natural), ½ cup . . . . . . . .220
oats, honey, raisins (*Quaker* 100% Natural), ½ cup . . . .225
w/raisins (*Quaker* 100% Natural), ⅔ cup . . . . . . . . . . . . .210
kamut (*Kamutios*) . . . . . . . . . . . . . . . . . . . . . . . . . . . . .120
kamut flakes (*Erewhon*), ⅔ cup . . . . . . . . . . . . . . . . . . . .110
millet, puffed (*Arrowhead Mills*) . . . . . . . . . . . . . . . . . . . .60
multigrain (see also "granola," above):
(*Basic 4*) . . . . . . . . . . . . . . . . . . . . . . . . . . . . . . . . . . .200
(*Erewhon Apple Stroodles/Banana O's*), ¾ cup . . . . . . .110
(*Fiber One*), ½ cup . . . . . . . . . . . . . . . . . . . . . . . . . . . .60
(*General Mills* Cinnamon Grahams), ¾ cup . . . . . . . . . .120
(*GinkgOs*) . . . . . . . . . . . . . . . . . . . . . . . . . . . . . . . . . .120
(*Golden Puffs*), ¾ cup . . . . . . . . . . . . . . . . . . . . . . . . . .100
(*Grape-Nuts*), ½ cup . . . . . . . . . . . . . . . . . . . . . . . . . . .200
(*Honey Graham Crunch*), ¾ cup . . . . . . . . . . . . . . . . . .120
(*Honey Nut Chex*), ¾ cup . . . . . . . . . . . . . . . . . . . . . . .120
(*Kellogg's Apple Jacks/Fruit Loops*) . . . . . . . . . . . . . . . .120
(*Kellogg's Müeslix*), ⅔ cup . . . . . . . . . . . . . . . . . . . . . .200
(*Kellogg's Product 19*) . . . . . . . . . . . . . . . . . . . . . . . . .100
(*Kellogg's Special K Plus*) . . . . . . . . . . . . . . . . . . . . . . .210
(*Kix*), 1⅓ cups . . . . . . . . . . . . . . . . . . . . . . . . . . . . . .120
(*Multi-Grain Cheerios*) . . . . . . . . . . . . . . . . . . . . . . . . .110
(*Quaker Life*), ¾ cup . . . . . . . . . . . . . . . . . . . . . . . . . .120
(*Team Cheerios*) . . . . . . . . . . . . . . . . . . . . . . . . . . . . . .120
(*Total* Whole Grain), ¾ cup . . . . . . . . . . . . . . . . . . . . . .110
(*Trix*) . . . . . . . . . . . . . . . . . . . . . . . . . . . . . . . . . . . . .120
(*Wheaties Energy Crunch*) . . . . . . . . . . . . . . . . . . . . . . .210
brown sugar squares (*Kellogg's Healthy Choice*) . . . . . .190
w/fruit, nuts (*Kellogg's Just Right*) . . . . . . . . . . . . . . . .220
honey (*Health Valley* Fiber 7), ¾ cup . . . . . . . . . . . . . . .110
puffed (*Kashi*) . . . . . . . . . . . . . . . . . . . . . . . . . . . . . . . .70
oat bran (*Quaker*), 1¼ cups . . . . . . . . . . . . . . . . . . . . . . .210
oat bran flakes (*Kellogg's Complete*), ¾ cup . . . . . . . . . . . .110
oats/oatmeal:
(*Cheerios*) . . . . . . . . . . . . . . . . . . . . . . . . . . . . . . . . . .110
(*Frosted Cheerios/Honey Nut Cheerios*) . . . . . . . . . . . . .120
(*Frosted Toasty O's/Honey Nut Toasty O's*) . . . . . . . . . . .110
(*Kashi Heart to Heart*), ¾ cup . . . . . . . . . . . . . . . . . . . .110

**Cereal, ready-to-eat, oats/oatmeal *(cont.)***
(*Quaker* Oatmeal Squares) . . . . . . . . . . . . . . . . . . . . . .210
(*Quaker* Toasted) . . . . . . . . . . . . . . . . . . . . . . . . . . . . .110
(*Quaker* Toasted Oatmeal Original) . . . . . . . . . . . . . . . . . .190
(*Toasty O's*) . . . . . . . . . . . . . . . . . . . . . . . . . . . . . . .110
apple (*Health Valley* Crunch O's), ¾ cup . . . . . . . . . . . .120
apple cinnamon (*Toasty O's*), ¾ cup . . . . . . . . . . . . . . .120
cinnamon (*Quaker* Oatmeal Squares) . . . . . . . . . . . . . . .230
cinnamon (*Quaker Life*), ¾ cup . . . . . . . . . . . . . . . . . . . .120
flakes (*Mother's Harvest*), ¾ cup . . . . . . . . . . . . . . . . . .110
honey (*Health Valley* Crunch O's), ¾ cup . . . . . . . . . . . .120
honey nut (*Quaker* Toasted Oatmeal) . . . . . . . . . . . . . . .190
rice (*Kellogg's Rice Krispies*), 1¼ cups . . . . . . . . . . . . . . . .120
rice (*Kellogg's Special K*) . . . . . . . . . . . . . . . . . . . . . . . . . .110
rice (*Rice Chex*), 1¼ cups . . . . . . . . . . . . . . . . . . . . . . . . .120
rice, crispy (*Malt-O-Meal*), 1¼ cups . . . . . . . . . . . . . . . . . .130
rice, puffed (*Quaker*) . . . . . . . . . . . . . . . . . . . . . . . . . . . . .55
soy (*Health Valley*), ½ cup . . . . . . . . . . . . . . . . . . . . . . . . .180
spelt flakes (*Arrowhead Mills*) . . . . . . . . . . . . . . . . . . . . . .100
wheat (*Frosted Wheaties*), ¾ cup . . . . . . . . . . . . . . . . . . . .110
wheat (*Wheaties*) . . . . . . . . . . . . . . . . . . . . . . . . . . . . . . .110
wheat, puffed (*Kellogg's Smacks*), ¾ cup . . . . . . . . . . . . . .100
wheat, puffed (*Quaker*), 1¼ cups . . . . . . . . . . . . . . . . . . . . .55
wheat, shredded (*Nabisco*), 2 pcs. . . . . . . . . . . . . . . . . . . .160
wheat, shredded (*Nabisco Spoon Size*) . . . . . . . . . . . . . . . .170
wheat, shredded (*Quaker*), 3 pcs. . . . . . . . . . . . . . . . . . . . .220
wheat, shredded, w/bran (*Nabisco*), 1¼ cups . . . . . . . . . . .200
**Cereal, cooking/hot,** dry, 1 pkt., except as noted:
barley (*Erewhon Barley Plus*), ¼ cup . . . . . . . . . . . . . . . . .170
multigrain (*Country Choice Naturals*), ½ cup . . . . . . . . . . .130
multigrain (*Quaker*), ½ cup . . . . . . . . . . . . . . . . . . . . . . . .130
multigrain, apple cranberry cobbler (*Cream of Wheat*) . . . .140
oat bran (*Quaker*), ½ cup . . . . . . . . . . . . . . . . . . . . . . . . .150
oat bran w/toasted wheat germ (*Erewhon*), ⅓ cup . . . . . . .170
oats/oatmeal:
all varieties (*Quaker Express* Instant Oatmeal Cup) . . . . .200
(*Country Choice Naturals* Regular/Quick), ½ cup . . . . . .150
(*H-O* Instant/Quick), ½ cup . . . . . . . . . . . . . . . . . . . . . .150
(*H-O* Regular) . . . . . . . . . . . . . . . . . . . . . . . . . . . . . . . .110
(*Quaker* Instant Oatmeal) . . . . . . . . . . . . . . . . . . . . . . .100

(*Quaker* Old Fashioned/Quick Oats), ½ cup . . . . . . . . . .150
(*Quaker Sun Country* Fortified Quick Oats),
½ cup . . . . . . . . . . . . . . . . . . . . . . . . . . . . . . . .150
apple cinnamon (*H-O*) . . . . . . . . . . . . . . . . . . . . . . .130
apple cinnamon (*Quaker* Instant Oatmeal) . . . . . . . . . . .130
apple raisin (*Erewhon* Instant Oatmeal) . . . . . . . . . . . . .140
banana nut (*Health Valley Banana Gone Nuts!*, Cup) . . .240
brown sugar, golden (*Quaker* Instant Oatmeal) . . . . . . .165
cinnamon roll (*Quaker* Instant Oatmeal) . . . . . . . . . . . . .160
cinnamon spice (*Malt-O-Meal* Big Bowl) . . . . . . . . . . . .200
cinnamon spice (*Quaker* Instant Oatmeal) . . . . . . . . . . .170
honey nut (*Quaker* Instant Oatmeal) . . . . . . . . . . . . . . .170
maple (*Maypo* Vermont Style), ⅓ cup . . . . . . . . . . . . . .180
maple, apple, spice (*Arrowhead Mills* Instant) . . . . . . . .130
maple brown sugar (*H-O*) . . . . . . . . . . . . . . . . . . . . . .160
maple brown sugar (*Malt-O-Meal* Big Bowl) . . . . . . . . .230
maple brown sugar (*Quaker* Instant Oatmeal) . . . . . . . .160
maple spice (*Erewhon* Instant Oatmeal) . . . . . . . . . . . . .130
maple syrup (*Country Choice Naturals*) . . . . . . . . . . . . .170
peaches and cream (*Quaker* Instant Oatmeal) . . . . . . . .140
raisin, date, walnut (*Erewhon* Instant Oatmeal) . . . . . . .130
raisin, date, walnut (*Quaker* Instant Oatmeal) . . . . . . . . .140
raisin spice (*Quaker* Instant Oatmeal) . . . . . . . . . . . . . .150
strawberries and cream (*Quaker* Instant Oatmeal) . . . . .140
sweet and mellow (*H-O*) . . . . . . . . . . . . . . . . . . . . . . .150
vanilla, French (*Quaker* Instant Oatmeal) . . . . . . . . . . . .160
rice (*Cream of Rice*), ¼ cup . . . . . . . . . . . . . . . . . . . . .170
rice, brown (*Erewhon* Cream), ¼ cup . . . . . . . . . . . . . .170
wheat:
(*Arrowhead Mills Bear Mush*), ¼ cup . . . . . . . . . . . . . .160
(*Cream of Wheat* Instant Original) . . . . . . . . . . . . . . . .100
(*Cream of Wheat*) . . . . . . . . . . . . . . . . . . . . . . . . . . .120
(*Malt-O-Meal* Original), 3 tbsp. . . . . . . . . . . . . . . . . . .120
(*Wheatena*), ⅓ cup . . . . . . . . . . . . . . . . . . . . . . . . . .160
baked apple/brown sugar cinnamon (*Cream of Wheat*) . . . . . . . . . . . . . . . . . . . . . . . . . . . . . . .130
farina (*Cream of Wheat*), 3 tbsp. . . . . . . . . . . . . . . . . .120
farina (*Quaker* Creamy Wheat), ¼ cup . . . . . . . . . . . . .150
maple brown sugar (*Cream of Wheat*) . . . . . . . . . . . . . .130
maple brown sugar (*Malt-O-Meal*), 3 tbsp. . . . . . . . . . .120

**Cereal bar,** see "Granola and cereal bar"
**Cervelat,** see "Summer sausage"
**Chayote,** raw (*Frieda's*), ⅔ cup, 3 oz. . . . . . . . . . . . . . . . . . .20
**Cheese** (see also "Cheese Spread"), 1 oz., except as noted:
American (*Alpine Lace* Reduced Fat) . . . . . . . . . . . . . . . . . .80
American (*Kraft* Deluxe Loaf) . . . . . . . . . . . . . . . . . . . . . . .100
American (*Land O Lakes*), ¾-oz. slice . . . . . . . . . . . . . . . .70
American (*Sara Lee*) . . . . . . . . . . . . . . . . . . . . . . . . . . . .110
American (*Sargento* Deli), ⅔-oz. slice . . . . . . . . . . . . . . . .70
American, regular or sharp (*Land O Lakes*) . . . . . . . . . . . . .110
blue (*Flora Danica* Danish) . . . . . . . . . . . . . . . . . . . . . . . .110
brick (*Land O Lakes*) . . . . . . . . . . . . . . . . . . . . . . . . . . . .100
Brie . . . . . . . . . . . . . . . . . . . . . . . . . . . . . . . . . . . . . . . . .95
Camembert . . . . . . . . . . . . . . . . . . . . . . . . . . . . . . . . . . . .85
(*Chedarella*) . . . . . . . . . . . . . . . . . . . . . . . . . . . . . . . . . .100
cheddar (*Alpine Lace* Reduced Fat) . . . . . . . . . . . . . . . . . . .70
cheddar (*Sara Lee*) . . . . . . . . . . . . . . . . . . . . . . . . . . . . .110
cheddar, aged or medium (*Sargento* Deli), ¾-oz. slice . . . . .80
cheddar, extrasharp (*Cabot* Vermont) . . . . . . . . . . . . . . . . .110
cheddar, sharp or extrasharp (*Heluva* Good) . . . . . . . . . . . .110
cheddar, shredded (*Sargento* Chef Style), ¼ cup . . . . . . . . .110
Cheshire . . . . . . . . . . . . . . . . . . . . . . . . . . . . . . . . . . . . .110
Colby (*Sara Lee*) . . . . . . . . . . . . . . . . . . . . . . . . . . . . . . .110
Colby (*Sargento* Deli), ¾-oz. slice . . . . . . . . . . . . . . . . . . . .80
Colby jack (*Heluva* Good) . . . . . . . . . . . . . . . . . . . . . . . . . .110
Colby jack (*Land O Lakes*) . . . . . . . . . . . . . . . . . . . . . . . . .110
cottage, ½ cup:
  4% (*Friendship*) . . . . . . . . . . . . . . . . . . . . . . . . . . . . . .110
  2% (*Friendship* Pot Style) . . . . . . . . . . . . . . . . . . . . . . . .90
  1% (*Friendship* Lowfat) . . . . . . . . . . . . . . . . . . . . . . . . . .90
  1%, pineapple (*Friendship* Lowfat) . . . . . . . . . . . . . . . . . .120
  nonfat (*Crowley*) . . . . . . . . . . . . . . . . . . . . . . . . . . . . . .90
  nonfat (*Friendship*) . . . . . . . . . . . . . . . . . . . . . . . . . . . .80
  nonfat, peach or pineapple (*Friendship*) . . . . . . . . . . . . .110
cream cheese (*Friendship*), 2 tbsp. . . . . . . . . . . . . . . . . . .100
cream cheese (*Philadelphia*), 1 oz. . . . . . . . . . . . . . . . . . .100
cream cheese, whipped (*Breakstone's Temp-Tee*),
  3 tbsp. . . . . . . . . . . . . . . . . . . . . . . . . . . . . . . . . . . . .110
Edam . . . . . . . . . . . . . . . . . . . . . . . . . . . . . . . . . . . . . . . .90
farmer (*Friendship*) . . . . . . . . . . . . . . . . . . . . . . . . . . . . . .50

feta (*Athenos* Mild/Traditional) . . . . . . . . . . . . . . . . . . . . .80
feta, basil–tomato or garlic–herb (*Athenos*) . . . . . . . . . . . .80
fontina (*Denmark's Finest*) . . . . . . . . . . . . . . . . . . . . . . . . .90
goat (*Laura Chenel's Select* Chèvre) . . . . . . . . . . . . . . . . .80
goat, w/basil and roasted garlic (*Chavrie*), 1.1 oz. . . . . . . . . .50
goat, garlic herb (*Montchevré*) . . . . . . . . . . . . . . . . . . . . . .70
Gorgonzola (*Stella*) . . . . . . . . . . . . . . . . . . . . . . . . . . . . .100
Gouda (*Kraft*) . . . . . . . . . . . . . . . . . . . . . . . . . . . . . . . . .110
Gruyère . . . . . . . . . . . . . . . . . . . . . . . . . . . . . . . . . . . . . .117
Havarti (*Sara Lee*) . . . . . . . . . . . . . . . . . . . . . . . . . . . . . .120
Havarti, all varieties (*Boar's Head*) . . . . . . . . . . . . . . . . . .110
hoop (*Friendship*) . . . . . . . . . . . . . . . . . . . . . . . . . . . . . . .20
Italian blend, shredded, 6 cheese (*Sargento*), ¼ cup . . . . . . .90
jalapeño (*Alpine Lace* Reduced Fat) . . . . . . . . . . . . . . . . . . .80
jalapeño jack (*Land O Lakes*) . . . . . . . . . . . . . . . . . . . . . . .100
(*Jarlsberg*) . . . . . . . . . . . . . . . . . . . . . . . . . . . . . . . . . . .100
(*Jarlsberg Lite*) . . . . . . . . . . . . . . . . . . . . . . . . . . . . . . . .70
Limburger (*Kraft*) . . . . . . . . . . . . . . . . . . . . . . . . . . . . . . .90
mascarpone (*Bel Gioioso*) . . . . . . . . . . . . . . . . . . . . . . . . .124
Mexican, shredded, 4 cheese, (*Sargento*), ¼ cup . . . . . . . . .110
Monterey jack (*Land O Lakes*) . . . . . . . . . . . . . . . . . . . . . . .110
Monterey jack (*Sara Lee* Slice), ¾-oz. slice . . . . . . . . . . . . . .80
Monterey jack, hot pepper (*Land O Lakes*) . . . . . . . . . . . . . .110
Monterey jack, jalapeño (*Heluva* Good) . . . . . . . . . . . . . . . .100
mozzarella (*Alpine Lace* Reduced Fat) . . . . . . . . . . . . . . . . . .70
mozzarella (*Land O Lakes*) . . . . . . . . . . . . . . . . . . . . . . . . . .80
mozzarella (*Sargento* Deli), ¾-oz. slice . . . . . . . . . . . . . . . . .60
mozzarella, whole milk or part skim (*Maggio*) . . . . . . . . . . . .80
mozzarella, shredded, part skim (*Maggio*), ¼ cup . . . . . . . . . .80
Muenster (*Alpine Lace* Reduced Sodium) . . . . . . . . . . . . . . .110
Muenster (*Sara Lee* Slice), ¾-oz. slice . . . . . . . . . . . . . . . . .60
Muenster (*Sargento* Deli), ¾-oz. slice . . . . . . . . . . . . . . . . . .80
nacho/taco blend, shredded (*Sargento*), ¼ cup . . . . . . . . . . .110
Parmesan, grated (*Land O Lakes*), 1 tbsp. . . . . . . . . . . . . . . .20
Parmesan, grated (*Maggio*), 1 tbsp. . . . . . . . . . . . . . . . . . . . .25
Parmesan, grated or shredded (*Di Giorno*), 2 tsp. . . . . . . . . . .20
Parmesan, shredded (*Maggio*), 1 tbsp. . . . . . . . . . . . . . . . . . .20
Parmesan, shredded (*Sargento* Fancy), ¼ cup . . . . . . . . . . .110
Parmesan/mozzarella/Romano, shredded
(*Sargento Angel Hair* Blend), ¼ cup . . . . . . . . . . . . . . .100

**Cheese** ***(cont.)***
Parmesan/Romano shredded (*Sargento*), ¼ cup . . . . . . . . . .110
pepper-jack blend (*Sargento*), ¼ cup . . . . . . . . . . . . . . . . .110
pimiento, processed (*Kraft* Deluxe) . . . . . . . . . . . . . . . . . . .100
pizza blend, shredded (*Maggio* Fancy), ¼ cup . . . . . . . . . . .100
provolone (*Alpine Lace* Reduced Fat) . . . . . . . . . . . . . . . . . .70
provolone (*Land O Lakes*) . . . . . . . . . . . . . . . . . . . . . . . . .100
provolone (*Sara Lee*) . . . . . . . . . . . . . . . . . . . . . . . . . . . .100
provolone (*Sargento* Deli), ⅔-oz. slice . . . . . . . . . . . . . . . . .70
ricotta, whole milk (*Maggio*), ¼ cup . . . . . . . . . . . . . . . . . .100
ricotta, part skim (*Maggio*), ¼ cup . . . . . . . . . . . . . . . . . . . .80
ricotta, nonfat (*Maggio*), ¼ cup . . . . . . . . . . . . . . . . . . . . . .50
Romano, grated (*Di Giorno*), 2 tsp. . . . . . . . . . . . . . . . . . . . .20
Romano, grated (*Maggio*), 1 tbsp. . . . . . . . . . . . . . . . . . . . . .25
Romano, shredded (*Maggio*), 1 tbsp. . . . . . . . . . . . . . . . . . . .20
Roquefort . . . . . . . . . . . . . . . . . . . . . . . . . . . . . . . . . . . . .105
string (*Maggio*), 1-oz. pc. . . . . . . . . . . . . . . . . . . . . . . . . . .80
Swiss (*Alpine Lace* Reduced Fat) . . . . . . . . . . . . . . . . . . . . .90
Swiss (*Sara Lee*) . . . . . . . . . . . . . . . . . . . . . . . . . . . . . . .110
Swiss (*Sargento* Deli) . . . . . . . . . . . . . . . . . . . . . . . . . . . .110
Swiss, aged (*Sargento* Deli), ⅔-oz. slice . . . . . . . . . . . . . . . .70
Swiss, baby (*Land O Lakes*) . . . . . . . . . . . . . . . . . . . . . . . .110
Swiss, baby (*Sara Lee* Slice), ¾-oz. slice . . . . . . . . . . . . . . . .90
Swiss, shredded (*Sargento*), ¼ cup or 1 oz. . . . . . . . . . . . . .110
Swiss/American, processed (*Land O Lakes*) . . . . . . . . . . . .100
taco blend, shredded (*Sargento*), ¼ cup or 1 oz. . . . . . . . . . .110
**"Cheese," substitute and nondairy:**
(*Smart Beat* Lactose Free), ⅔-oz. slice . . . . . . . . . . . . . . . . .25
American (*Smart Beat*), ⅔-oz. slice . . . . . . . . . . . . . . . . . . . .25
American or cheddar (*Yves* The Good Slice), .7 oz. . . . . . . . .35
cheddar, mellow or sharp (*Smart Beat*), ⅔-oz. slice . . . . . . .25
jalapeño jack or Swiss (*Yves* The Good Slice), .7 oz. . . . . . . .35
mozzarella (*Yves* The Good Slice), .7-oz. slice . . . . . . . . . . .30
**Cheese dip,** 2 tbsp., except as noted:
blue (*Marzetti* Veggie Dip) . . . . . . . . . . . . . . . . . . . . . . . .180
cheddar, mild (*Fritos*) . . . . . . . . . . . . . . . . . . . . . . . . . . . . .60
cheddar, mild (*Snyder's*), 1 oz. . . . . . . . . . . . . . . . . . . . . . . .80
cheddar, jalapeño (*Fritos*) . . . . . . . . . . . . . . . . . . . . . . . . . .50
chili (*Fritos*) . . . . . . . . . . . . . . . . . . . . . . . . . . . . . . . . . . .45
nacho, beef (*Ortega*) . . . . . . . . . . . . . . . . . . . . . . . . . . . . .60

nacho, chicken (*Ortega*) . . . . . . . . . . . . . . . . . . . . . . . . . .45
salsa (*Chi-Chi's*) . . . . . . . . . . . . . . . . . . . . . . . . . . . . . . . .90
salsa (*Old El Paso*) . . . . . . . . . . . . . . . . . . . . . . . . . . . . . .40
salsa (*Tostitos*), 4 tbsp. . . . . . . . . . . . . . . . . . . . . . . . . . .80
**Cheese sauce, cooking,** in jars, ¼ cup:
Alfredo (*Ragú Cheese Creations!* Classic) . . . . . . . . . . . . . .110
Alfredo, 4 cheese (*Five Brothers*) . . . . . . . . . . . . . . . . . . . .120
Alfredo, 4 cheese (*Healthy Choice*) . . . . . . . . . . . . . . . . . . . .45
Alfredo, Parmesan, light (*Ragú Cheese Creations!*) . . . . . . . .80
cheddar, double (*Ragú Cheese Creations!*) . . . . . . . . . . . . . .100
garlic, roasted, Parmesan (*Ragú Cheese Creations!*) . . . . . .110
Parmesan and Romano (*Ragú Cheese Creations!*) . . . . . . . . .60
**Cheese sauce mix,** cheddar (*Knorr* Pasta Sauce), 2 tbsp. . . .60
**Cheese spread** (see also "Cheese," and "Cheese Product"),
2 tbsp., except as noted:
(*Cheez Whiz*) . . . . . . . . . . . . . . . . . . . . . . . . . . . . . . . . . . .90
(*Squeez-A-Snak*) . . . . . . . . . . . . . . . . . . . . . . . . . . . . . . . .90
(*Velveeta*), 1 oz. . . . . . . . . . . . . . . . . . . . . . . . . . . . . . . . .80
American (*Easy Cheese*) . . . . . . . . . . . . . . . . . . . . . . . . . . .100
cheddar (*Easy Cheese* Baseball) . . . . . . . . . . . . . . . . . . . . . .90
cheddar, sharp or and bacon (*Easy Cheese*) . . . . . . . . . . . .100
feta, w/garlic and chives (*Cypress*), 1 oz. . . . . . . . . . . . . . .110
feta, sun-dried tomato-basil (*Athenos*) . . . . . . . . . . . . . . . . .80
**Cheese sticks,** frozen, breaded, w/sauce:
mozzarella (*Farm Rich Dippers*), 2 pcs. . . . . . . . . . . . . . . . .180
mozzarella (*Giorgio*), 2 pcs. . . . . . . . . . . . . . . . . . . . . . . . .120
**Cheese topping,** see "Nacho topping"
**Cheese turnover,** see "Cheese appetizer"
**Cheeseburger,** see "Beef sandwich"
**Cheesecake,** pineapple (*Entenmann's*), ⅕ cake . . . . . . . . .350
**Cheesecake, frozen,** ¼ cake, except as noted:
(*Baby Watson* New York's), ⅙ cake . . . . . . . . . . . . . . . . . .260
(*Mrs. Smith's* Original), ⅙ cake . . . . . . . . . . . . . . . . . . . . .520
(*Mrs. Smith's Nestlé Butterfinger*), ⅙ cake . . . . . . . . . . . . .550
(*Sara Lee* Original) . . . . . . . . . . . . . . . . . . . . . . . . . . . . . .350
(*Sara Lee* 25% Reduced Fat) . . . . . . . . . . . . . . . . . . . . . . .310
cherry cream (*Sara Lee*) . . . . . . . . . . . . . . . . . . . . . . . . . . .350
chocolate (*Mrs. Smith's*), ⅙ cake . . . . . . . . . . . . . . . . . . . . .550
chocolate chip (*Sara Lee*) . . . . . . . . . . . . . . . . . . . . . . . . . .410
chocolate mousse (*Sara Lee*), ⅕ cake . . . . . . . . . . . . . . . . .400

**Cheesecake, frozen** ***(cont.)***
French (*Sara Lee*), ⅙ cake . . . . . . . . . . . . . . . . . . . . . . . .350
strawberry, cream (*Sara Lee*) . . . . . . . . . . . . . . . . . . . . . .330
strawberry, French (*Sara Lee*), ⅙ cake . . . . . . . . . . . . . . .320
strawberry, streusel (*Mrs. Smith's*), ⅙ cake . . . . . . . . . . . .530
**Cheesecake mix,** ⅛ cake*:
(*Betty Crocker* Original) . . . . . . . . . . . . . . . . . . . . . . . . .400
chocolate chip (*Betty Crocker*) . . . . . . . . . . . . . . . . . . . .410
strawberry swirl (*Betty Crocker*) . . . . . . . . . . . . . . . . . . .380
**Cherimoya** (*Frieda's*), 5 oz. . . . . . . . . . . . . . . . . . . . . . . .120
**Cherry,** fresh, ½ cup, except as noted:
(*Dole*), 1 cup, 21 cherries . . . . . . . . . . . . . . . . . . . . . . . . .90
sour, red, w/pits . . . . . . . . . . . . . . . . . . . . . . . . . . . . . . . . .26
sour, red, pitted . . . . . . . . . . . . . . . . . . . . . . . . . . . . . . . . .39
sweet, w/pits . . . . . . . . . . . . . . . . . . . . . . . . . . . . . . . . . . . .52
sweet, 10 medium, 2.6 oz. . . . . . . . . . . . . . . . . . . . . . . . . . .49
**Cherry, can or jar,** ½ cup:
sour, pitted, in heavy syrup . . . . . . . . . . . . . . . . . . . . . . . .116
sweet, w/pits, dark, in heavy syrup (*Oregon*) . . . . . . . . . . .100
sweet, pitted, dark, in heavy syrup (*Del Monte*) . . . . . . . . . .100
sweet, pitted, Royal Anne, in heavy syrup (*Oregon*) . . . . . .110
**Cherry, dried:**
Bing (*Frieda's*), ¼ cup, 1.4 oz. . . . . . . . . . . . . . . . . . . . . . .120
Bing or sweet-tart (*Sonoma*), ¼ cup, 1.4 oz. . . . . . . . . . . . .140
tart (*Frieda's*), ⅓ cup, 1.4 oz. . . . . . . . . . . . . . . . . . . . . . .150
**Cherry, frozen:**
dark, sweet (*Big Valley*), ¾ cup . . . . . . . . . . . . . . . . . . . . .90
dark, sweet (*Cascadian Farm*), 1 cup . . . . . . . . . . . . . . . . . .72
**Cherry, maraschino** (*Aunt Nellie's*), 1 pc. . . . . . . . . . . . . . . .10
**Cherry juice,** 8 fl. oz.:
(*Eden* Organic) . . . . . . . . . . . . . . . . . . . . . . . . . . . . . . . . .140
(*Juicy Juice*) . . . . . . . . . . . . . . . . . . . . . . . . . . . . . . . . . .130
**Cherry juice blend,** frozen* (*Cascadian Farm*), 8 fl. oz. . . .120
**Cherry–berry, dried** (*Sunsweet Fruitlings*), ⅓ cup . . . . . . .130
**Chervil,** dried, 1 tsp. . . . . . . . . . . . . . . . . . . . . . . . . . . . . . .1
**Chestnut, Chinese,** dried, 1 oz. . . . . . . . . . . . . . . . . . . . . . .103
**Chestnut, European:**
roasted, peeled, 1 cup, 17 kernels . . . . . . . . . . . . . . . . . . . .350
roasted, in jars (*Minerve*), 4 whole, 1.1 oz. . . . . . . . . . . . . . .50
**Chestnut, Japanese,** dried, 1 oz. . . . . . . . . . . . . . . . . . . . . .102

**Chicken,** fresh, 4 oz., except as noted:
broiler–fryer, roasted:
w/skin, ½ chicken, 10.5 oz. (15.8 oz. w/bone) . . . . . . . . 715
w/skin . . . . . . . . . . . . . . . . . . . . . . . . . . . . . . . . 271
meat only . . . . . . . . . . . . . . . . . . . . . . . . . . . . . . 215
meat only, chopped or diced, 1 cup . . . . . . . . . . . . . . . . 266
skin only, 1 oz. . . . . . . . . . . . . . . . . . . . . . . . . . . 129
dark meat only . . . . . . . . . . . . . . . . . . . . . . . . . . 232
light meat only . . . . . . . . . . . . . . . . . . . . . . . . . . 196
breast, w/skin, ½ breast, 3½ oz. (8½ oz. w/bone) . . . . . 193
drumstick, w/skin, 1.8 oz. (2.9 oz. w/bone) . . . . . . . . . . 112
leg, w/skin (5.7 oz. w/bone) . . . . . . . . . . . . . . . . . . . 265
thigh, w/skin, 2.2 oz. (2.9 oz. w/bone) . . . . . . . . . . . . . 153
wing, w/skin, 1.2 oz. (2.3 oz. w/bone) . . . . . . . . . . . . . . 99
capon, roasted, w/skin . . . . . . . . . . . . . . . . . . . . . . . 260
Cornish hen, see "Cornish hen"
ground, see "Chicken, ground"
roaster, roasted, meat w/skin . . . . . . . . . . . . . . . . . . . 253
stewing, stewed, meat w/skin . . . . . . . . . . . . . . . . . . . 323
stewing, stewed, meat only . . . . . . . . . . . . . . . . . . . . . 269
stewing, stewed, meat only, chopped or diced, 1 cup . . . . . 332
**Chicken, canned,** chunk, 2 oz.:
(*Hormel*) . . . . . . . . . . . . . . . . . . . . . . . . . . . . . . . . 70
breast (*Hormel*) . . . . . . . . . . . . . . . . . . . . . . . . . . . . 60
**Chicken, frozen or refrigerated,** cooked (see also "Chicken entree, frozen"), 3 oz., except as noted:
whole (*Tyson*) . . . . . . . . . . . . . . . . . . . . . . . . . . . . . 160
whole, garlic toasted, dark (*Perdue*) . . . . . . . . . . . . . . . 190
whole, garlic toasted, white (*Perdue*) . . . . . . . . . . . . . . 160
whole, rotisserie:
all flavors, except honey, dark (*Perdue*) . . . . . . . . . . . . 180
all flavors, except honey, white (*Perdue*) . . . . . . . . . . . 140
honey, dark (*Perdue*) . . . . . . . . . . . . . . . . . . . . . . . . 200
honey, white (*Perdue*) . . . . . . . . . . . . . . . . . . . . . . . 140
barbecue, smoky (*Wampler*), 1 cup . . . . . . . . . . . . . . . . 430
bites (*Country Skillet*), 10 pcs. . . . . . . . . . . . . . . . . . . 280
bites (*Country Skillet* Value Pack), 5 pcs. . . . . . . . . . . . . 270
breast, whole (*Perdue Oven Stuffer*) . . . . . . . . . . . . . . . 150
breast, split (*Tyson*), 5.1-oz. pc. . . . . . . . . . . . . . . . . . 260
breast, quarters (*Perdue*) . . . . . . . . . . . . . . . . . . . . . 170

**Chicken, frozen or refrigerated *(cont.)***

breast, boneless, skinless:
(*Perdue* Individually Frozen), 4.2 oz. . . . . . . . . . . . . . . . .140
(*Perdue Fit 'n Easy*) . . . . . . . . . . . . . . . . . . . . . . . .110
(*Perdue Oven Stuffer*) . . . . . . . . . . . . . . . . . . . . . . .120
(*Tyson*), 3.7-oz. pc. . . . . . . . . . . . . . . . . . . . . . . . .130
diced (*Tyson Time Trimmers*) . . . . . . . . . . . . . . . . . . .90
shredded (*Tyson*) . . . . . . . . . . . . . . . . . . . . . . . . . .110
tenderloin (*Perdue Fit 'n Easy*) . . . . . . . . . . . . . . . . . .100

breast, boneless, seasoned:
all flavors (*Perdue*) . . . . . . . . . . . . . . . . . . . . . . . . .90
all flavors, except roasted (*Perdue Short Cuts*), ½ cup . . . . . . . . . . . . . . . . . . . . . . . . . . . . . .100
roasted (*Perdue Short Cuts* Original), ½ cup . . . . . . . . . .90

breast fillet, breaded (*Tyson*), 2.8-oz. pc. . . . . . . . . . . . . .150
cacciatore (*Wampler*), 1 cup . . . . . . . . . . . . . . . . . . . . .260
cutlets, breaded (*Perdue*), 3.5 oz. . . . . . . . . . . . . . . . . . .220

drumstick:
barbecue, honey (*Tyson* Family Pack), 3.1-oz. pc. . . . . .150
barbecue, hot (*Tyson*), 2 pcs., 3.5 oz. . . . . . . . . . . . . .160
roasted (*Perdue*), 2.2 oz. . . . . . . . . . . . . . . . . . . . . . .110
roasted (*Perdue Oven Stuffer*), 3.6 oz. . . . . . . . . . . . . .190
roasted (*Tyson* Multi-Serve), 2 pcs., 3.8 oz. . . . . . . . . . .220
roasted (*Tyson* Single Serve), 3 pcs., 5.8 oz. . . . . . . . . .330

fajita (*Wampler*), 1 cup . . . . . . . . . . . . . . . . . . . . . . . .210
fried, bone-in (*Banquet* Original/Southern) . . . . . . . . . . . .280
fried, bone-in (*Country Skillet*) . . . . . . . . . . . . . . . . . . .270
fried, bone-in, honey barbecue, skinless (*Banquet*) . . . . . . .230
fried, bone-in, hot and spicy (*Banquet*) . . . . . . . . . . . . . .260
fried, bone-in, skinless (*Banquet*) . . . . . . . . . . . . . . . . . .220
leg, whole, roasted (*Perdue*), 5.6 oz. . . . . . . . . . . . . . . . .370

nuggets:
(*Country Skillet*), 5 pcs. . . . . . . . . . . . . . . . . . . . . . .270
(*Perdue*), 5 pcs. . . . . . . . . . . . . . . . . . . . . . . . . . . .210
(*Perdue* Individually Frozen), 5 pcs. . . . . . . . . . . . . . . .250
(*Tyson*), 6 pcs. . . . . . . . . . . . . . . . . . . . . . . . . . . . .280
(*Tyson* Family Pack), 6 pcs. . . . . . . . . . . . . . . . . . . . .240
breast (*Banquet*), 7 pcs. . . . . . . . . . . . . . . . . . . . . . .280
breast (*Perdue* Golden Brown), 5 pcs. . . . . . . . . . . . . . .240
breast (*Tyson*), 6 pcs. . . . . . . . . . . . . . . . . . . . . . . .220

w/cheese (*Perdue*), 5 pcs. . . . . . . . . . . . . . . . . . . . . . . .230
mozzarella (*Banquet*), 6 pcs. . . . . . . . . . . . . . . . . . . . . .280
Southern (*Tyson*), 6 pcs. . . . . . . . . . . . . . . . . . . . . . . . .260
Southern-fried (*Country Skillet*), 5 pcs. . . . . . . . . . . . . .270
patty (*Country Skillet*), 1 pc. . . . . . . . . . . . . . . . . . . . . . . .190
patty (*Tyson*), 2.6-oz. pc. . . . . . . . . . . . . . . . . . . . . . . . .180
patty (*Tyson* Family Pack), 1 pc. . . . . . . . . . . . . . . . . . . . .210
patty (*Tyson Thick'n Crispy*), 1 pc. . . . . . . . . . . . . . . . . . .220
popcorn (*Banquet*), 11 pcs. . . . . . . . . . . . . . . . . . . . . . . .190
popcorn (*Tyson Bites* Family Pack), 6 pcs. . . . . . . . . . . . . .210
shredded, barbecue (*Tyson*), ¼ cup . . . . . . . . . . . . . . . . . . .90
strips, breaded (*Perdue Kick 'N Chicken* Original) . . . . . . . . .120
strips, breast (*Tyson Time Trimmers*) . . . . . . . . . . . . . . . . . .90
strips, breast, Southwestern (*Tyson Time Trimmers*) . . . . . .110
strips, Buffalo style (*Tyson* Family Pack), 2 pcs., 3 oz. . . . . .190
strips, crispy (*Tyson* Family Pack), 2 pcs., 2.5 oz. . . . . . . . .160
strips, Parmesan garlic (*Perdue Simply Sauté*) . . . . . . . . . .100
strips, savory (*Perdue Simply Sauté* Classic) . . . . . . . . . . . .90
strips, spicy (*Perdue Simply Sauté* Fiesta) . . . . . . . . . . . .140
sweet and sour (*Wampler*), 1 cup . . . . . . . . . . . . . . . . . . .250
taco filling (*Tyson*), ¼ cup . . . . . . . . . . . . . . . . . . . . . . . . .90
tenderloin, breaded (*Perdue*) . . . . . . . . . . . . . . . . . . . . . .140
tenderloin, breaded (*Perdue* Individually Frozen) . . . . . . . . .200
tenderloin, breaded (*Tyson*), 2 pcs., 3 oz. . . . . . . . . . . . . . .180
tenderloin, breaded, spicy (*Tyson*), 2 pcs. . . . . . . . . . . . . . .200
tenders (*Tyson* Family Pack), 5 pcs., 3 oz. . . . . . . . . . . . . .240
tenders, breast (*Banquet* Fat Free), 3 pcs. . . . . . . . . . . . . . .120
tenders, breast (*Country Skillet*), 3 pcs. . . . . . . . . . . . . . . .240
tenders, breast, baked (*Butterball*), 3 pcs. . . . . . . . . . . . . .170
tenders, breast, breaded (*Tyson*), 5 pcs., 3 oz. . . . . . . . . . .230
tenders, breast, honey-battered (*Tyson*), 5 pcs., 3 oz. . . . . .220
tenders, Southern (*Banquet*), 3 pcs. . . . . . . . . . . . . . . . . .260
thigh, roasted (*Perdue*), 3.2-oz. pc. . . . . . . . . . . . . . . . . .240
thigh, roasted (*Tyson* Single Serve), 3.6-oz. pc. . . . . . . . . .270
wings:
(*Tyson Tabasco*), 3 pcs., 2.7 oz. . . . . . . . . . . . . . . . . . . . .170
barbecue (*Tyson*), 3 pcs., 3.2 oz. . . . . . . . . . . . . . . . . . . .200
barbecue, honey (*Tyson*), 5 pcs., 3 oz. . . . . . . . . . . . . . . .210
hot and spicy (*Banquet*), 4 pcs. . . . . . . . . . . . . . . . . . . .220
hot and spicy (*Perdue* Individually Frozen) . . . . . . . . . . . .180

**Chicken, frozen or refrigerated, wings *(cont.)***
hot and spicy (*Tyson*), 4 pcs., 3.4 oz. . . . . . . . . . . . . . .220
hot and spicy (*Tyson* Party Pack), 4 pcs., 3.2 oz. . . . . . .190
roasted (*Perdue*), 2 pcs., 3.2 oz. . . . . . . . . . . . . . . . . .210
teriyaki (*Tyson*), 4 pcs., 3.4 oz. . . . . . . . . . . . . . . . . . .190
wingettes, roasted (*Perdue*) 3 pcs. . . . . . . . . . . . . . . . . . . .210
**Chicken, ground**
raw (*Shady Brook Farms*), 4 oz. . . . . . . . . . . . . . . . . . . . .180
raw (*Tyson*), 4 oz. . . . . . . . . . . . . . . . . . . . . . . . . . . . . .150
cooked (*Tyson Crumbles*), 3 oz. . . . . . . . . . . . . . . . . . . . .110
cooked, breast (*Perdue Fit 'n Easy*), 3 oz. . . . . . . . . . . . . . .80
**Chicken dinner, frozen,** 1 pkg.:
baked (*Stouffer's* HomeStyle), 14 oz. . . . . . . . . . . . . . . . . .410
boneless, w/herb gravy (*Swanson Traditional Favorites*),
11 oz. . . . . . . . . . . . . . . . . . . . . . . . . . . . . . . . . . . . . . . .320
boneless, white (*Swanson Hungry-Man*), 13.75 oz. . . . . . . .660
breaded, country (*Healthy Choice*), 10.25 oz. . . . . . . . . . . .350
breast, stir-fry (*Healthy Choice*), 11.9 oz. . . . . . . . . . . . . . .360
broccoli Alfredo (*Healthy Choice*), 11.5 oz. . . . . . . . . . . . . .300
Dijon (*Healthy Choice*), 11 oz. . . . . . . . . . . . . . . . . . . . . . . .310
fettuccine (*Stouffer's* HomeStyle), 16.75 oz. . . . . . . . . . . .640
fried (*Banquet Extra Helping*), 14.7 oz. . . . . . . . . . . . . . . . .910
fried (*Swanson*), 11.5 oz. . . . . . . . . . . . . . . . . . . . . . . . . . .600
fried, boneless, white meat (*Banquet Extra Helping*), 13 oz. .720
herb, country (*Healthy Choice*), 11.35 oz. . . . . . . . . . . . . . .280
honey-glazed (*Healthy Choice*), 11 oz. . . . . . . . . . . . . . . . .320
mesquite, barbecue (*Healthy Choice*), 10.5 oz. . . . . . . . . . .320
nuggets (*Swanson Traditional Favorites*), 11 oz. . . . . . . . . .670
parmigiana (*Healthy Choice*), 11 oz. . . . . . . . . . . . . . . . . . .320
roast, w/herb gravy (*Swanson Hungry-Man*), 15.25 oz. . . . .540
roast, breast (*Healthy Choice*), 11 oz. . . . . . . . . . . . . . . . . .230
sesame, breast (*Healthy Choice*), 10.8 oz. . . . . . . . . . . . . . .360
sweet and sour (*Healthy Choice*), 11 oz. . . . . . . . . . . . . . . .350
teriyaki (*Healthy Choice*), 11 oz. . . . . . . . . . . . . . . . . . . . . .270
**Chicken entree, can or pkg.,** 1 cup, except as noted:
chow mein (*La Choy*) . . . . . . . . . . . . . . . . . . . . . . . . . . . . .80
and dumplings (*Dinty Moore*), 7.5-oz. can . . . . . . . . . . . . .200
and dumplings (*Dinty Moore* Microwave Cup) . . . . . . . . . .200
and dumplings, stew (*Dinty Moore* Can) . . . . . . . . . . . . . . .260
and noodles (*Dinty Moore American Classics*), 1 bowl . . . .270

noodles and, see "Noodle entree, can or pkg."
w/potatoes (*Dinty Moore American Classics*), 1 bowl .....240
stew (*Dinty Moore* Can) ..........................220

**Chicken entree, frozen** (see also "Chicken, frozen or refrigerated"), 1 pkg., except as noted:
à la king (*Stouffer's*), 11.5 oz. ......................370
à l'orange (*Lean Cuisine Cafe Classics*), 9 oz. ...........230
Alfredo:
(*Birds Eye Chicken Voila!*), 1 cup cooked ...........230
(*Lean Cuisine Skillet Sensations*), ¼ of 40-oz. pkg. ....280
(*Marie Callender's* Skillet Meal), ½ of 23-oz. pkg. .....500
and almonds, w/rice (*Yu Sing*), 9 oz. ..................300
bake, country (*Healthy Choice* Bowl), 11 oz. ............260
baked, and cheddar rice (*Stouffer's Oven Sensations*), ½ of 24-oz. pkg. ..............................390
baked, w/mashed potato (*Healthy Choice* Duo), 8.5 oz. ....210
barbecue (*Banquet*), 9.9 oz. ........................330
barbecue, honey, w/rice (*Michelina's*), 8.5 oz. ...........290
barbecue sauce (*Lean Cuisine Hearty Portions*), 13⅞ oz. ..370
basil cream sauce (*Lean Cuisine Cafe Classics*), 8.5 oz. ...290
breast, baked (*Stouffer's* HomeStyle), 8⅞ oz. ...........260
breast, barbecue sauce (*Stouffer's* HomeStyle), 10 oz. ....500
breast, cheesy rice and (*Marie Callender's*), 10 oz.........370
breast, mushroom gravy (*Stouffer's* HomeStyle), 10 oz. ...350
breast, oven-roasted (*Boston Market* Home Style), 6 oz. ...180
breast strips, breaded (*Marie Callender's*), 8.75 oz. .......500
breast strips, breaded, w/macaroni and cheese (*Healthy Choice* Duo), 8 oz. .....................270
breast and vegetables (*Healthy Choice* Medley), 11.5 oz. ....................................230
and broccoli (*Healthy Choice* Bread Stuffs), 6.1 oz. .......310
and broccoli bake (*Stouffer's Family-Style Favorites*), ⅕ of 40-oz. pkg. ..............................330
and broccoli w/cheese and rice (*Banquet* Family), 1 cup ....................................280
carbonara (*Healthy Choice* Medley), 9 oz. ..............310
carbonara (*Lean Cuisine Cafe Classics*), 9 oz. ...........280
cheddar cheese and, bake (*Stouffer's*), 11.5 oz. .........450
chow mein (*Contessa*), 1¾ cups ....................320
chow mein (*Yu Sing*), 8.75 oz. ......................270

**Chicken entree, frozen** ***(cont.)***
creamed (*Stouffer's*), 6.5 oz. . . . . . . . . . . . . . . . . . . . . . . .250
and dumplings (*Marie Callender's*), 14 oz. . . . . . . . . . . . . . .390
and dumplings (*Stouffer's* HomeStyle), 10 oz. . . . . . . . . . . .340
and dumplings, country style (*Banquet* Family), 1 cup . . . .290
enchilada, see "Enchilada"
fettuccine (*Lean Cuisine Everyday Favorites*), 9.25 oz. . . . . .270
fettuccine (*Lean Cuisine Hearty Portions*), 13⅝ oz. . . . . . .400
fettuccine (*Stouffer's* HomeStyle), 10.5 oz. . . . . . . . . . . . . .350
Florentine (*Lean Cuisine Everyday Favorites*), 8 oz. . . . . . . .220
Florentine (*Lean Cuisine Hearty Portions*), 13.25 oz. . . . . . .380
fingers (*Banquet* Meal), 7.1 oz. . . . . . . . . . . . . . . . . . . . . . .570
fingers BBQ sauce (*Freezer Queen* Meal), 9 oz. . . . . . . . . . .350
fried (*Banquet* Original), 9 oz. . . . . . . . . . . . . . . . . . . . . . . .470
fried (*Morton*), 9 oz. . . . . . . . . . . . . . . . . . . . . . . . . . . . . .470
fried, boneless white meat (*Banquet*), 8.25 oz. . . . . . . . . . .490
fried, breast (*Stouffer's* HomeStyle), 8⅞ oz. . . . . . . . . . . . .350
fried, country, and gravy (*Marie Callender's*), 16 oz. . . . . . .620
glazed (*Lean Cuisine Hearty Portions*), 13 oz. . . . . . . . . . . .360
glazed (*Michelina's*), 8 oz. . . . . . . . . . . . . . . . . . . . . . . . . .250
glazed, breast (*Marie Callender's*), 10 oz. . . . . . . . . . . . . . .340
glazed, orange (*Budget Gourmet*), 8 oz. . . . . . . . . . . . . . . . .270
glazed, w/rice (*Michelina's*), 9.5 oz. . . . . . . . . . . . . . . . . . .310
grilled:
(*Lean Cuisine Cafe Classics*), 9⅜ oz. . . . . . . . . . . . . . . . .250
Alfredo, w/broccoli (*Michelina's*), 10 oz. . . . . . . . . . . . .410
breast (*Marie Callender's*), 10 oz. . . . . . . . . . . . . . . . . . .300
breast, and pasta (*Healthy Choice* Duo), 9 oz. . . . . . . . .240
fiesta (*Lean Cuisine Cafe Classics*), 8.5 oz. . . . . . . . . . .260
w/mashed potato (*Healthy Choice* Duo/Medley),
8.5 oz. . . . . . . . . . . . . . . . . . . . . . . . . . . . . . . . . . . . . .200
and mashed potato (*Marie Callender's*), 10 oz. . . . . . . . .340
in mushroom sauce (*Marie Callender's*), 14 oz. . . . . . . .480
Southwestern style (*Marie Callender's*), 14 oz. . . . . . . . .410
herb (*Marie Callender's* Skillet Meal), ½ of 24-oz. pkg. . . . .290
herb, and roast potato (*Lean Cuisine Skillet Sensations*),
½ of 24-oz. pkg. . . . . . . . . . . . . . . . . . . . . . . . . . . . . . . .260
herb-roasted (*Lean Cuisine Cafe Classics*), 8 oz. . . . . . . . . .200
homestyle (*Country Skillet*), ¼ of 32-oz. pkg. . . . . . . . . . . .170
homestyle, and pasta (*Healthy Choice* Solo), 9 oz. . . . . . .270

honey mustard (*Lean Cuisine Cafe Classics*), 8 oz. . . . . . . .270
honey-roasted (*Lean Cuisine Cafe Classics*), 8.5 oz. . . . . . .270
honey-roasted (*Marie Callender's*), 14 oz. . . . . . . . . . . . . . .440
lemon herb (*Marie Callender's* Bowl), 12.4 oz. . . . . . . . . . .420
lo mein (*Yu Sing*), 8.5 oz. . . . . . . . . . . . . . . . . . . . . . .220
mandarin (*Budget Gourmet*), 8.5 oz. . . . . . . . . . . . . . . . .240
mandarin (*Lean Cuisine Everyday Favorites*), 9 oz. . . . . . . .240
Monterey, creamy (*Ortega* Skillet), ½ of 23-oz. pkg. . . . . . .430
nacho (*Ortega* Skillet Supreme), ½ of 23-oz. pkg. . . . . . . . .380
and noodles (*Budget Gourmet*), 8.5 oz. . . . . . . . . . . . . . . .370
and noodles, chunky (*Marie Callender's*), 10 oz. . . . . . . . . .430
and noodles, escalloped (*Stouffer's*), 10 oz. . . . . . . . . . . .460
noodles and, see "Noodle entree, frozen"
nuggets (see also "Chicken, frozen, and refrigerated"):
(*Freezer Queen* Meal), 6 oz. . . . . . . . . . . . . . . . . . . . . .250
(*Morton*), 7 oz. . . . . . . . . . . . . . . . . . . . . . . . . . . . .340
olé (*Healthy Choice* Solo), 9 oz. . . . . . . . . . . . . . . . . . . .270
Oriental:
(*Healthy Choice* Medley), 8.5 oz. . . . . . . . . . . . . . . . . .240
(*Lean Cuisine Skillet Sensations*), ½ of 24-oz. pkg. . . . .270
(*Stouffer's*), 10⅝ oz. . . . . . . . . . . . . . . . . . . . . . . . . .250
glazed (*Lean Cuisine Hearty Portions*), 14 oz. . . . . . . . .370
pappardelle (*Wolfgang Puck's*), 12 oz. . . . . . . . . . . . . . . .430
Parmesan (*Lean Cuisine Cafe Classics*), 10⅞ oz. . . . . . . . .300
Parmesan, breast (*Master Choice*), 1 pc. . . . . . . . . . . . . .240
parmigiana (*Marie Callender's*), 16 oz. . . . . . . . . . . . . . . .660
parmigiana (*Michelina's* Parmigiano), 10 oz. . . . . . . . . . . .410
parmigiana (*Stouffer's* HomeStyle), 12 oz. . . . . . . . . . . . .460
parmigiana (*Wolfgang Puck's*), 12 oz. . . . . . . . . . . . . . . . .540
pasta, vegetable and, bake (*Stouffer's*), 12 oz. . . . . . . . . .380
pasta primavera (*Banquet*), 9.5 oz. . . . . . . . . . . . . . . . . .320
patty (*Freezer Queen* Meal), 7.5 oz. . . . . . . . . . . . . . . . . .360
patty, breaded (*Morton*), 6.75 oz. . . . . . . . . . . . . . . . . . .340
penne and, bake (*Stouffer's*), 11.5 oz. . . . . . . . . . . . . . . .350
pesto, w/penne (*Michelina's*), 8 oz. . . . . . . . . . . . . . . . . .250
piccata (*Healthy Choice* Medley), 9 oz. . . . . . . . . . . . . . . .270
piccata (*Lean Cuisine Cafe Classics*), 9 oz. . . . . . . . . . . . .300
piccata (*Michelina's*), 9 oz. . . . . . . . . . . . . . . . . . . . . . .340
pie (*Lean Cuisine Everyday Favorites*), 9.5 oz. . . . . . . . . . .300
pie (*Marie Callender's*), 9.5 oz. . . . . . . . . . . . . . . . . . . . .680

**Chicken entree, frozen *(cont.)***
pie (*Stouffer's*), 10 oz. .730
pie (*Stouffer's*), ½ of 16-oz. pie .590
pie (*Swanson*), 7 oz. .410
pie (*Swanson Potato-Topped*), 12 oz. .440
pie, au gratin (*Marie Callender's* 16.5 oz.), 1 cup .580
pie, and broccoli (*Marie Callender's*), 9.5 oz. .670
pie, and broccoli, w/cheddar–potato top (*Swanson Potato-Topped*), 12 oz. .450
and potato casserole (*Marie Callender's* Bowl), 12.05 oz. .310
primavera (*Lean Cuisine Skillet Sensations*), ½ of 24-oz. pkg. .300
primavera, w/spirals (*Michelina's*), 8 oz. .250
and rice, w/broccoli and cheese (*Marie Callender's* Skillet Meal), ½ of 25-oz. pkg. .410
rice, fried (*Contessa*), 1¾ cups .260
rice, fried (*Michelina's* Family), 1 cup .270
rice, fried (*Yu Sing*), 8 oz. .360
rice, fried, and egg rolls (*Banquet*), 8.5 oz. .330
roast/roasted:
(*Lean Cuisine Everyday Favorites*), 8⅛ oz. .250
(*Lean Cuisine Hearty Portions*), 12.5 oz. .330
garlic (*Stouffer's Oven Sensations*), ½ of 24-oz. pkg. .320
herb (*Michelina's*), 10 oz. .270
red pepper (*Healthy Choice* Bowl), 9.5 oz. .340
and vegetables (*Marie Callender's* Skillet Meal), ½ of 25-oz. pkg. .300
sesame (*Healthy Choice* Medley), 9 oz. .240
Sorrentino, w/linguine (*Michelina's*), 8.5 oz. .320
stir-fry (*Contessa*), 1¾ cups .180
w/stuffing and gravy (*Stouffer's Oven Sensations*), ½ of 21-oz. pkg. .380
sweet and sour (*Healthy Choice* Bowl), 12 oz. .380
sweet and sour (*Freezer Queen* Homestyle), 8.5 oz. .280
sweet and sour (*Michelina's* Family), 1 cup .280
teriyaki:
(*Marie Callender's*), 10 oz. .310
(*Marie Callender's* Bowl), 12 oz. .400
(*Marie Callender's* Skillet Meal), ½ of 24-oz. pkg. .270

(*Stouffer's Skillet Sensations*), ½ of 25-oz. pkg. . . . . . .320
w/rice (*Healthy Choice* Bowl), 10.5 oz. . . . . . . . . . . . . . .300
tetrazzini (*Michelina's*), 8 oz. . . . . . . . . . . . . . . . . . . . . .320
and tomatoes, fire-roasted (*Michelina's*), 8 oz. . . . . . . . . . .240
and vegetables:
(*Lean Cuisine Cafe Classics*), 10.5 oz. . . . . . . . . . . . . . .250
grilled (*Stouffer's Skillet Sensations*),
½ of 25-oz. pkg. . . . . . . . . . . . . . . . . . . . . . . . . . . .400
herb, country (*Cascadian Farm*), 8.5 oz. . . . . . . . . . . . .240
w/noodles (*Freezer Queen* Homestyle), 8 oz. . . . . . . . . .170
orange Dijon or teriyaki (*Cascadian Farm*), 8.5 oz. . . . . .240
stir-fry (*Michelina's*), 8 oz. . . . . . . . . . . . . . . . . . . . . . .200
Thai (*Cascadian Farm*), 8.5 oz. . . . . . . . . . . . . . . . . . . . .260
in wine sauce (*Lean Cuisine Cafe Classics*), 8⅛ oz. . . . . . .220
**Chicken entree mix,** ⅙ pkg.*:
garlic, w/pasta (*Campbell's Supper Bakes*) . . . . . . . . . . . . .370
herb, w/rice (*Campbell's Supper Bakes*) . . . . . . . . . . . . . . . .330
lemon, w/herb rice (*Campbell's Supper Bakes*) . . . . . . . . . .340
**Chicken giblets,** simmered, chopped, 1 cup . . . . . . . . . . . .228
**Chicken gravy,** can or jar, ¼ cup:
(*Boston Market* Roasted) . . . . . . . . . . . . . . . . . . . . . . . . . . .30
(*Franco-American*) . . . . . . . . . . . . . . . . . . . . . . . . . . . . . . . .25
giblet (*Franco-American*) . . . . . . . . . . . . . . . . . . . . . . . . . . .20
**Chicken gravy mix** (*Lawry's*), 2 tsp. . . . . . . . . . . . . . . . . . . .25
**Chicken lunch meat,** breast, 2 oz., except as noted:
(*Healthy Choice* Skinless) . . . . . . . . . . . . . . . . . . . . . . . . . .50
(*Wampler* Gourmet) . . . . . . . . . . . . . . . . . . . . . . . . . . . . . . .60
(*Wampler* Premium) . . . . . . . . . . . . . . . . . . . . . . . . . . . . . . .90
barbecue (*Black Bear*) . . . . . . . . . . . . . . . . . . . . . . . . . . . . .70
barbecue (*Boar's Head* Bar B Q Sauce Basted) . . . . . . . . . . .60
browned (*Healthy Choice*) . . . . . . . . . . . . . . . . . . . . . . . . . .60
grilled (*Louis Rich Carving Board*), 6 slices, 1.6 oz. . . . . . .45
oil-browned (*Wampler*) . . . . . . . . . . . . . . . . . . . . . . . . . . . .60
oven-roasted:
(*Boar's Head* Golden Oven) . . . . . . . . . . . . . . . . . . . . . . . .50
(*Butterball*), 5 slices, 1.9 oz. . . . . . . . . . . . . . . . . . . . . . .50
(*Healthy Choice*), 1-oz. slice . . . . . . . . . . . . . . . . . . . . . . .25
(*Healthy Choice* 10 oz.), 1-oz. slice . . . . . . . . . . . . . . . . .35
(*Healthy Choice* Deli), 1-oz. slice . . . . . . . . . . . . . . . . . . .30
(*Healthy Choice Deli Traditions*), 6 slices, 1.8 oz. . . . . . . .60

**Chicken lunch meat *(cont.)***
(*Louis Rich*), 1-oz. slice .35
(*Sara Lee*) .50
(*Sara Lee*), 3 slices, 1.8 oz. .50
(*The Turkey Store*) .50
rotisserie flavor (*Sara Lee*) .50
slow-roasted (*Shady Brook Farms*) .60
smoked (*Healthy Choice*), 1-oz. slice .30
smoked (*Healthy Choice Deli Traditions*), 6 slices, 1.9 oz. .60
smoked, mesquite (*Healthy Choice*) .60
**Chicken pie,** see "Chicken entree, frozen"
**Chicken pocket,** frozen, 4.5-oz. pc., except as noted:
(*Mrs. Paterson's Aussie Pie*), 5.5 oz. 460
(*Mrs. Paterson's Aussie Pie* Low Fat), 5.5 oz. 380
broccoli (*Lean Pockets* Supreme) 280
broccoli and (*Hot Pockets*) 310
broccoli and cheddar (*Croissant Pockets*) 320
fajita (*Lean Pockets*) 260
fajita, potato top (*Mrs. Paterson's Aussie Pie*), 5.5 oz. 350
Italian melt (*Croissant Pockets*) 380
Parmesan (*Lean Pockets*) 300
**Chicken salad,** ⅓ cup:
(*Wampler*) 200
(*Wampler* Low Fat) 90
**Chicken sandwich,** 1 pc.:
breaded (*Hormel Quick Meal*) 340
grilled (*Hormel Quick Meal*) 310
**Chicken sauce, cooking,** ½ cup, except as noted:
cacciatore (*Chicken Tonight*) 70
Dijon (*Lawry's* Weekday Gourmet), 2 tbsp. 40
French, country (*Chicken Tonight*) 120
honey mustard, light (*Chicken Tonight*) 60
mushroom, creamy (*Chicken Tonight*) 80
orange (*Lawry's* Weekday Gourmet), 2 tbsp. 30
wing, see "Buffalo wing sauce"
**Chicken sausage,** see "Sausage"
**Chicken spread** (*Underwood*), ¼ cup 140
**Chickpeas,** see "Garbanzo beans"

**Chicory, witloof:**
(*Frieda's* Belgium Endive), 2 cups, 3 oz. . . . . . . . . . . . . . . . .15
5–7" head, 1.9 oz. . . . . . . . . . . . . . . . . . . . . . . . . . . . . .9
**Chili,** can or pkg., 1 cup:
w/beans (*Broadcast*) . . . . . . . . . . . . . . . . . . . . . . . . .350
w/beans (*Castleberry*) . . . . . . . . . . . . . . . . . . . . . . . .350
w/beans (*Hormel/Hormel* Chunky/Hot) . . . . . . . . . . . . . . . . .270
w/beans (*Hormel* Microcup) . . . . . . . . . . . . . . . . . . . . . .220
w/out bean (*Hormel/Hormel* Hot) . . . . . . . . . . . . . . . . . . .210
w/macaroni (*Hormel* Microcup Chili Mac) . . . . . . . . . . . . . .200
turkey, w/beans (*Health Valley* 99% Fat Free) . . . . . . . . . . .220
turkey, w/beans (*Hormel*) . . . . . . . . . . . . . . . . . . . . . . .210
turkey, w/out beans (*Hormel*) . . . . . . . . . . . . . . . . . . . .190
vegetarian (*Bearitos* Lowfat Premium Original) . . . . . . . . . .200
vegetarian (*Hormel*) . . . . . . . . . . . . . . . . . . . . . . . . . .200
vegetarian (*Natural Touch*) . . . . . . . . . . . . . . . . . . . . . .170
vegetarian, lentil, mild or spicy (*Health Valley*) . . . . . . . . . .160
**Chili beans** (see also "Mexican beans"), canned, ½ cup:
(*Eden* Organic) . . . . . . . . . . . . . . . . . . . . . . . . . . . . .130
regular or hot (*Bush's Best*) . . . . . . . . . . . . . . . . . . . . .120
spicy (*Eden* Organic Pintos) . . . . . . . . . . . . . . . . . . . . .125
**Chili entree, frozen,** 1 pkg., except as noted:
bean, 3 (*Lean Cuisine Everyday Favorites*), 10 oz. . . . . . . . .250
w/beans (*Stouffer's*), 8.75 oz. . . . . . . . . . . . . . . . . . . . .290
w/beans, rice (*Healthy Choice* Bowl Homestyle), 11 oz. . . . .380
black bean, w/rice (*Michelina's*), 10 oz. . . . . . . . . . . . . . . .400
and corn bread (*Marie Callender's*), 16 oz. . . . . . . . . . . . .560
w/macaroni (*Michelina's* Chili-Mac), 8 oz. . . . . . . . . . . . . .290
**Chili pepper,** see "Pepper, chili"
**Chili powder,** 1 tbsp. . . . . . . . . . . . . . . . . . . . . . . . . .24
**Chili relish,** hot, Indian (*Patak's* Chile), 1 tbsp. . . . . . . . . . .50
**Chili sauce,** tomato (see also "Hot sauce" and "Thai sauce"):
(*Bennetts*), 1 tbsp. . . . . . . . . . . . . . . . . . . . . . . . . . . .15
(*Heinz*), 1 tbsp. . . . . . . . . . . . . . . . . . . . . . . . . . . . . .15
(*Nance's*), 2 tbsp. . . . . . . . . . . . . . . . . . . . . . . . . . . .25
**Chili seasoning mix:**
(*Adolph's Meal Makers*), 1 tbsp. . . . . . . . . . . . . . . . . . . . .30
(*Lawry's*), 1 tbsp. . . . . . . . . . . . . . . . . . . . . . . . . . . . .25
(*Shotgun Willie's* Texas), 3 tbsp. . . . . . . . . . . . . . . . . . . .50

**Chimichanga,** frozen:
beef and bean (*El Monterey*), 4 oz. . . . . . . . . . . . . . . . . . . . .310
beef and cheese (*El Monterey Family Classic*), 5 oz. . . . . . . .310
chicken and cheese (*El Monterey Family Classic*), 5 oz. . . . . .320
**Chipotle sauce** (*La Morena* Homemade), 2 tbsp. . . . . . . . . . .25
**Chitterlings,** pork, simmered, 4 oz. . . . . . . . . . . . . . . . . . . . .344
**Chives,** fresh, chopped, 1 tbsp. . . . . . . . . . . . . . . . . . . . . . . . .1
**Chives, freeze-dried,** ¼ cup . . . . . . . . . . . . . . . . . . . . . . . . .2
**Chocolate,** see "Candy"
**Chocolate, baking,** ½ oz. or 1 tbsp., except as noted:
(*Nestlé Choco-Bake*) . . . . . . . . . . . . . . . . . . . . . . . . . . . . .80
bar, semisweet (*Nestlé*) . . . . . . . . . . . . . . . . . . . . . . . . . . . .70
bar, unsweetened (*Nestlé*) . . . . . . . . . . . . . . . . . . . . . . . . . .80
bar, white (*Nestlé* Premier) . . . . . . . . . . . . . . . . . . . . . . . . . .80
bits, milk (*M&M's*), 1 tbsp. . . . . . . . . . . . . . . . . . . . . . . . . . .70
chips or morsels:
  milk, mint, peanut butter, or semisweet (*Hershey's*) . . . . .80
  milk, mint, or semisweet (*Nestlé*) . . . . . . . . . . . . . . . . . .70
  white (*Nestlé* Premier) . . . . . . . . . . . . . . . . . . . . . . . . . .80
chunks (*Nestlé*) . . . . . . . . . . . . . . . . . . . . . . . . . . . . . . . . . .70
**Chocolate drink:**
(*Yoo-Hoo*), 9 fl. oz. . . . . . . . . . . . . . . . . . . . . . . . . . . . . .150
(*Yoo-Hoo* Lite), 9 fl. oz. . . . . . . . . . . . . . . . . . . . . . . . . . .70
**Chocolate drink mix,** 2 tbsp.:
(*Nesquik*) . . . . . . . . . . . . . . . . . . . . . . . . . . . . . . . . . . . . . .90
(*Nesquik* No Sugar) . . . . . . . . . . . . . . . . . . . . . . . . . . . . . . .40
**Chocolate fondue** (*Swiss Knight*), 1 oz. . . . . . . . . . . . . . . .160
**Chocolate milk,** see "Milk, flavored"
**Chocolate mousse mix,** see "Mousse Mix"
**Chocolate syrup,** 2 tbsp., except as noted:
(*Fox's U-Bet*) . . . . . . . . . . . . . . . . . . . . . . . . . . . . . . . . . .120
(*Hershey's*) . . . . . . . . . . . . . . . . . . . . . . . . . . . . . . . . . . .100
(*Nesquik*) . . . . . . . . . . . . . . . . . . . . . . . . . . . . . . . . . . . . .100
(*Smucker's* Sundae Syrup) . . . . . . . . . . . . . . . . . . . . . . . . .110
**Chocolate topping,** 2 tbsp.:
(*Smucker's Magic Shell*) . . . . . . . . . . . . . . . . . . . . . . . . . .210
(*Smucker's Plate Scrapers*) . . . . . . . . . . . . . . . . . . . . . . . .100
dark (*Dove*) . . . . . . . . . . . . . . . . . . . . . . . . . . . . . . . . . . . .140
fudge (*Mrs. Richardson's* Chocolate Lovers) . . . . . . . . . . . .130

fudge (*Smucker's*) . . . . . . . . . . . . . . . . . . . . . . . . . . . .130
fudge (*Smucker's Magic Shell*) . . . . . . . . . . . . . . . . . . . . .200
fudge, hot (*Mrs. Richardson's*) . . . . . . . . . . . . . . . . . . . . .140
fudge, hot (*Smucker's/Smucker's* Special Recipe) . . . . . . . .140
fudge, hot (*Smucker's* Microwave) . . . . . . . . . . . . . . . . . . .130
fudge, hot (*Smucker's* Microwave Fat Free) . . . . . . . . . . . . .110
milk (*Dove*) . . . . . . . . . . . . . . . . . . . . . . . . . . . . . . . . . .130
white (*Smucker's Plate Scrapers*) . . . . . . . . . . . . . . . . . . .110
**Chorizo,** see "Sausage"
**Chow chow pickle:**
hot or mild (*Mrs. Renfro's*), 1 tbsp. . . . . . . . . . . . . . . . . . . .10
relish (*Stubb's*), ¼ cup . . . . . . . . . . . . . . . . . . . . . . . . . . .70
***Church's Chicken:***
chicken, 1 pc.:
  breast, 2.8 oz. . . . . . . . . . . . . . . . . . . . . . . . . . . . . . .200
  leg, 2 oz. . . . . . . . . . . . . . . . . . . . . . . . . . . . . . . . . .140
  *Tender Strip,* 1.1 oz. . . . . . . . . . . . . . . . . . . . . . . . . . .80
  thigh, 2.8 oz. . . . . . . . . . . . . . . . . . . . . . . . . . . . . . .230
  wing, 3.1 oz. . . . . . . . . . . . . . . . . . . . . . . . . . . . . . .250
sides:
  biscuit, 2.1 oz. . . . . . . . . . . . . . . . . . . . . . . . . . . . . .250
  coleslaw, 3 oz. . . . . . . . . . . . . . . . . . . . . . . . . . . . . . .92
  corn on cob, 5.7 oz. . . . . . . . . . . . . . . . . . . . . . . . . . .139
  french fries, 2.7 oz. . . . . . . . . . . . . . . . . . . . . . . . . . .210
  jalapeño bombers, 5 oz. . . . . . . . . . . . . . . . . . . . . . . .300
  macaroni and cheese, 3.6 oz. . . . . . . . . . . . . . . . . . . . .140
  okra, fried, 2.8 oz. . . . . . . . . . . . . . . . . . . . . . . . . . . .210
  potatoes w/gravy, 3.7 oz. . . . . . . . . . . . . . . . . . . . . . . .90
  rice, Cajun, 3.1 oz. . . . . . . . . . . . . . . . . . . . . . . . . . .130
apple pie, 3.1 oz. . . . . . . . . . . . . . . . . . . . . . . . . . . . . . .280
**Churro,** cinnamon (*Bearitos*), ½ cup . . . . . . . . . . . . . . .150
**Chutney:**
(*Trader Vic's* Calcutta), 2 tbsp. . . . . . . . . . . . . . . . . . . . . .44
mango (*Bombay Brand* Major Grey's), 2 tbsp. . . . . . . . . . . .110
mango, ginger (*Bombay Brand*), 2 tbsp. . . . . . . . . . . . . . . . .90
tomato, dried (*Sonoma*), 1 tbsp. . . . . . . . . . . . . . . . . . . . . .35
**Cilantro,** see "Coriander"
**Cinnamon,** ground, 1 tsp. . . . . . . . . . . . . . . . . . . . . . . . . . .6
**Citron, candied,** diced (*Seneca* Glacé), 2 tbsp. . . . . . . . . . . .70

**Citrus drink blend,** 8 fl. oz.:
punch (*Tropicana*) . . . . . . . . . . . . . . . . . . . . . . . . . .140
tangy (*Sunny Delight*) . . . . . . . . . . . . . . . . . . . . . . . .120
**Clam,** meat only:
raw, 4 oz. . . . . . . . . . . . . . . . . . . . . . . . . . . . . . . . . .84
raw, 9 large or 20 small, 6.3 oz. . . . . . . . . . . . . . . . . . . .133
boiled, poached or steamed, 4 oz. . . . . . . . . . . . . . . . . . .168
**Clam, canned,** 2 oz. or ¼ cup, except as noted:
whole, baby (*Bumble Bee*) . . . . . . . . . . . . . . . . . . . . . . .50
whole, baby (*Chicken of the Sea*) . . . . . . . . . . . . . . . . . .30
whole, small (*3 Diamonds*) . . . . . . . . . . . . . . . . . . . . . . .45
chopped or minced (*Chicken of the Sea*) . . . . . . . . . . . . . .30
chopped or minced (*Doxsee*) . . . . . . . . . . . . . . . . . . . . .25
smoked, baby (*Reese*), ⅓ cup . . . . . . . . . . . . . . . . . . . .120
**Clam chowder,** see "Soup"
**Clam dish, frozen:**
casino (*Matlaw's*), 2 pcs., 1.3 oz. . . . . . . . . . . . . . . . . . .60
fried (*Chincoteague*), 3 oz. . . . . . . . . . . . . . . . . . . . . . .265
fried (*Gorton's*), 3 oz. . . . . . . . . . . . . . . . . . . . . . . . . .250
fried (*Mrs. Paul's/Van de Kamp's*), 18 pcs., 3 oz. . . . . . . .250
fried, crisps (*Acadian Gourmet*), 22 pcs., 3.1 oz. . . . . . . .310
on half shell (*Chincoteague*), 2 pcs. . . . . . . . . . . . . . . . .20
oreganata (*Matlaw's*), 2 pcs., 1.2 oz. . . . . . . . . . . . . . . . .90
stuffed (*Chincoteague*), 1 pc. . . . . . . . . . . . . . . . . . . . .130
stuffed (*Morning Catch*), 2 pcs. . . . . . . . . . . . . . . . . . . .180
stuffed (*Matlaw's* Box), 2 pcs., 3.7 oz. . . . . . . . . . . . . . .180
stuffed (*Matlaw's* Tray), 2.7-oz. pc. . . . . . . . . . . . . . . . .130
**Clam juice** (*Crown Prince*), 1 tbsp. . . . . . . . . . . . . . . . . . .5
**Clam sauce,** canned, ½ cup:
red (*Crown Prince*) . . . . . . . . . . . . . . . . . . . . . . . . . . . .60
red (*Rienzi*) . . . . . . . . . . . . . . . . . . . . . . . . . . . . . . . . .70
white (*Bookbinder's*) . . . . . . . . . . . . . . . . . . . . . . . . . .300
white (*Chincoteague*) . . . . . . . . . . . . . . . . . . . . . . . . . .120
white (*Crown Prince*) . . . . . . . . . . . . . . . . . . . . . . . . . . .90
white (*Olde Cape Cod*) . . . . . . . . . . . . . . . . . . . . . . . . .100
white, creamy (*Progresso*) . . . . . . . . . . . . . . . . . . . . . .110
**Clover sprouts,** fresh (*Jonathan's*), 1 cup . . . . . . . . . . . . .25
**Cloves,** ground, 1 tbsp. . . . . . . . . . . . . . . . . . . . . . . . . . .21
**Cocktail sauce,** see "Seafood sauce"

**Cocoa,** baking (*Nestlé*), 1 tbsp. . . . . . . . . . . . . . . . . . . . . . .15
**Cocoa mix,** hot, 1 pkt., except as noted:
chocolate:
(*Country Choice Naturals* Royal) . . . . . . . . . . . . . . . . . .100
all flavors, except black cherry (*Land O Lakes*) . . . . . . .160
cherry, black (*Land O Lakes*) . . . . . . . . . . . . . . . . . . . .150
dark (*Carnation* Homemade Classics), 1⅔ tbsp. . . . . . . .90
double (*Carnation* Meltdown) . . . . . . . . . . . . . . . . . . .150
double or hazelnut (*Ghirardelli*) . . . . . . . . . . . . . . . . . .90
milk (*Carnation* Homemade Classics), 1⅔ tbsp. . . . . . . .90
milk or rich (*Carnation*) . . . . . . . . . . . . . . . . . . . . . . .120
rich (*Carnation* Fat Free) . . . . . . . . . . . . . . . . . . . . . . .25
rich (*Carnation* No Sugar) . . . . . . . . . . . . . . . . . . . . . .50
w/marshmallows:
(*Carnation* Fat Free) . . . . . . . . . . . . . . . . . . . . . . . . . .40
(*Carnation Marshmallow Madness*) . . . . . . . . . . . . . . .180
chocolate, rich (*Carnation*) . . . . . . . . . . . . . . . . . . . . .120
chocolate, rich (*Carnation* No Sugar) . . . . . . . . . . . . . . .50
s'mores (*Carnation*) . . . . . . . . . . . . . . . . . . . . . . . . . .130
vanilla, French (*Carnation*) . . . . . . . . . . . . . . . . . . . . . .120
**Coconut,** fresh, shelled:
(*Frieda's* White/Young), ¼ cup, 1.4 oz. . . . . . . . . . . . . . . . .140
shredded or grated (*Dole*), 1 cup not packed . . . . . . . . . . .283
shredded or grated, 1 cup not packed . . . . . . . . . . . . . . . .283
**Coconut, dried,** flaked (*Baker's* Premium), 2 tbsp. . . . . . . . .60
**Coconut cream,** canned (*Goya* Coco Cream), 2 tbsp. . . . . .140
**Coconut milk, canned** (*Goya*), 1 tbsp. . . . . . . . . . . . . . . . .50
**Cod,** meat only:
Atlantic, raw, 4 oz. . . . . . . . . . . . . . . . . . . . . . . . . . . . . . .93
Atlantic, baked, broiled, or microwaved, 4 oz. . . . . . . . . . . .119
Pacific, raw, 4 oz. . . . . . . . . . . . . . . . . . . . . . . . . . . . . . . .93
Pacific, baked, broiled, or microwaved, 4 oz. . . . . . . . . . . .119
**Cod, canned,** in biscayan sauce (*Goya*), ¼ cup . . . . . . . . .100
**Cod, dried,** Atlantic, salted, 1 oz. . . . . . . . . . . . . . . . . . . . . .81
**Cod entree,** frozen:
au gratin (*Oven Poppers*), 5-oz. pc. . . . . . . . . . . . . . . . . . .220
fillets, breaded (*Mrs. Paul's* Premium), 1 pc. . . . . . . . . . . . .260
stuffed w/broccoli, cheese (*Oven Poppers*), 5-oz. pc. . . . . .150
**Coffee,** brewed, 6 fl. oz. . . . . . . . . . . . . . . . . . . . . . . . . . . .4

**Coffee, flavored, mix:**
cappuccino:
all flavors, except iced (*Land O Lakes*), 1 pkt. . . . . . . . .130
all flavors, iced (*Land O Lakes*), 1 pkt. . . . . . . . . . . . . . . .60
amaretto, caramel, or vanilla (*Nescafé Frothé*), 3 tbsp. . .80
latte (*Nescafé* Frothé), 3 tbsp. . . . . . . . . . . . . . . . . . . . .90
chocolate mocha, all varieties (*Nescafé Frothé*), 3 tbsp. . . . .80
**Coffee, iced:**
cappuccino, all flavors (*Starbucks Frappuccino*),
9.5 fl. oz. . . . . . . . . . . . . . . . . . . . . . . . . . . . . . .190
latte, supreme or mocha (*AriZona*), 8 fl. oz. . . . . . . . . . . . .110
**Coffee creamer,** see "Creamer, nondairy"
**Cold cuts,** see "Lunch meat" and specific listings
**Coleslaw blend,** see "Salad blend" and "Salad kit"
**Coleslaw dressing,** see "Salad dressing"
**Collard greens,** fresh:
raw, chopped, ½ cup . . . . . . . . . . . . . . . . . . . . . . . . . . . .6
boiled, drained, chopped, ½ cup . . . . . . . . . . . . . . . . . . . .17
**Collard greens, canned,** ½ cup:
chopped (*Bush's Best*) . . . . . . . . . . . . . . . . . . . . . . . . . .30
seasoned (*Glory Foods*) . . . . . . . . . . . . . . . . . . . . . . . . .50
seasoned (*Sylvia's*) . . . . . . . . . . . . . . . . . . . . . . . . . . . .45
**Collard greens, frozen,** chopped, boiled, drained, ½ cup . . .31
**Cookie** (see also "Cake, snack" and specific listings):
almond (*Frieda's*), 2 pcs., 1 oz. . . . . . . . . . . . . . . . . . . . .170
almond (*Grandma's Tiny Bites*), 11 pcs., 1 oz. . . . . . . . . . .260
almond, fudge-dipped (*Stella D'oro*), 1 pc. . . . . . . . . . . . . .120
almond toast (*Stella D'oro*), 2 pcs., 1 oz. . . . . . . . . . . . . .110
animal (*Nabisco Barnum's Animals*), 10 pcs., 1.1 oz. . . . . .140
animal, chocolate chip (*Keebler*), 7 pcs., 1 oz. . . . . . . . . . .130
animal, iced or sprinkled (*Keebler*), 6 pcs., 1.1 oz. . . . . . . .150
anisette (*Stella D'oro* Sponge), 2 pcs., 1 oz. . . . . . . . . . . . .90
anisette (*Stella D'oro* Toast), 3 pcs., 1.2 oz. . . . . . . . . . . .130
apple cinnamon (*Newtons Cobblers*), .75-oz. pc. . . . . . . . . .70
apple-filled (*Newtons* Fat Free), 2 pcs., 1 oz. . . . . . . . . . . . .90
apple raisin (*Health Valley* Fat Free Jumbo), .9-oz. pc. . . . . . .80
apricot raspberry (*Pepperidge Farm Verona*),
3 pcs., 1.1 oz. . . . . . . . . . . . . . . . . . . . . . . . . . . . . . .140
arrowroot (*Nabisco*), 1.2-oz. pc. . . . . . . . . . . . . . . . . . . . .20
biscotti (*Almondina* Choconut), 4 pcs., 1.1 oz. . . . . . . . . . .140

biscotti, almond or hazelnut (*Stella D'oro*), .8-oz. pc. . . . . .100
biscotti, chocolate chunk (*Stella D'oro*), .8-oz. pc. . . . . . . . .90
biscotti, chocolate-dipped (*Nonni's* Cioccolati),
  1.3-oz. pc. . . . . . . . . . . . . . . . . . . . . . . . . . . . . . . . .130
biscotti, vanilla, French, fudge-dipped (*Stella D'oro*),
  1 pc. . . . . . . . . . . . . . . . . . . . . . . . . . . . . . . . . . . . .120
butter (see also "shortbread," below):
  (*Demitasse* Minis Petit Buerre), 10 pcs., 1 oz. . . . . . . . .110
  (*Keebler*), 5 pcs., 1.1 oz. . . . . . . . . . . . . . . . . . . . . . . .150
  (*Pepperidge Farm* Chessman), 3 pcs., .9 oz. . . . . . . . . .120
  fudge-filled (*E.L. Fudge*), 2 pcs., .9 oz. . . . . . . . . . . . . .120
  waffle (*Jules Destrooper*), 2 pcs., .9 oz. . . . . . . . . . . . .130
cappuccino, crisp (*Murray* Sugar Free), 4 pcs., 1.1 oz. . . . .150
cappuccino sandwich (*Café Cremes*), 2 pcs. . . . . . . . . . . . .160
caramel (*SnackWell's* Delights), .6-oz. pc. . . . . . . . . . . . . . .70
chocolate:
  (*Stella D'oro*), 2 pcs., 1 oz. . . . . . . . . . . . . . . . . . . . . .130
  (*Stella D'oro* Breakfast Treat), .8-oz. pc. . . . . . . . . . . . . .100
  (*Stella D'oro Margherite*), 2 pcs., 1.1 oz. . . . . . . . . . . . .140
  crisps (*SnackWell's* Bite Size), 18 pcs., 1 oz. . . . . . . . . .130
  milk (*Carr's Imperials*), 2 pcs., 1 oz. . . . . . . . . . . . . . . .150
  top, w/nuts (*Pepperidge Farm Geneva*), 3 pcs., 1.1 oz. . .160
  wafer (*Nabisco Famous*), 5 pcs., 1.2 oz. . . . . . . . . . . . .140
  wafer (*Nilla*), 8 pcs., 1.1 oz. . . . . . . . . . . . . . . . . . . . . .110
chocolate almond (*Pepperidge Farm Dessert Bliss*),
  3 pcs., 1.1 oz. . . . . . . . . . . . . . . . . . . . . . . . . . . . . . . .170
chocolate chip/chunk:
  (*Chips Ahoy!*), 3 pcs., 1.1 oz. . . . . . . . . . . . . . . . . . . . .160
  (*Chips Ahoy!* Chewy), 3 pcs., 1.3 oz. . . . . . . . . . . . . . . .170
  (*Chips Ahoy!* Chunky), .6-oz. pc. . . . . . . . . . . . . . . . . . . .80
  (*Chips Ahoy!* Mini), 5 pcs., 1.1 oz. . . . . . . . . . . . . . . . . .150
  (*Chips Ahoy!* Reduced Fat), 3 pcs., 1.1 oz. . . . . . . . . . .140
  (*Entenmann's* Soft), 3 pcs., 1.1 oz. . . . . . . . . . . . . . . . .150
  (*Entenmann's* Soft Chocolatey), .7-oz. pc. . . . . . . . . . . .100
  (*Entenmann's* Soft Chunk), 1.8-oz. pc. . . . . . . . . . . . . . .240
  (*Famous Amos*), 4 pcs., 1 oz. . . . . . . . . . . . . . . . . . . . .130
  (*Famous Amos* Belgian Style), 4 pcs., 1 oz. . . . . . . . . . .150
  (*Famous Amos* Big Chunk), 1-oz. pc. . . . . . . . . . . . . . . .140
  (*Grandma's* Homestyle), 1.4-oz. pc. . . . . . . . . . . . . . . . .200
  (*Grandma's Tiny Bites*), 12 pcs., 1 oz. . . . . . . . . . . . . . .280

**Cookie, chocolate chip/chunk *(cont.)***

(*Health Valley Healthy Chips* Fat Free), 3 pcs., 1.2 oz. . . . . . . . . . . . . . . . . . . . . . . . . . . .100
(*Keebler Chips Deluxe*), .5-oz. pc. . . . . . . . . . . . . . . . . . . .80
(*Keebler Chips Deluxe* Chocolate Lovers'), .6-oz. pc. . . . .90
(*Keebler Chips Deluxe* Mini), 4 pcs., 1 oz. . . . . . . . . . . .150
(*Keebler Cookie Stix*), 4 pcs., 1 oz. . . . . . . . . . . . . . . . .130
(*Keebler Soft Batch*), .6-oz. pc. . . . . . . . . . . . . . . . . . . . .80
(*Pepperidge Farm Chesapeake/Tahoe*), .9-oz. pc. . . . . . .140
(*Pepperidge Farm Montauk*), .9-oz. pc. . . . . . . . . . . . . .130
(*Pepperidge Farm Nantucket*), 1-oz. pc. . . . . . . . . . . . . .140
(*SnackWell's* Bite Size), 13 pcs., 1 oz. . . . . . . . . . . . . . .130
w/cashews (*Famous Amos* Big Chunk), 1-oz. pc. . . . . . .140
coconut (*Keebler Chips Deluxe*), .6-oz. pc. . . . . . . . . . . . .80
crispy (*Entenmann's Little Bites*), 8 pcs., 1.8 oz. . . . . .240
double (*SnackWell's*), 13 pcs., 1.1 oz. . . . . . . . . . . . . . .130
fudge (*Chips Ahoy!*), 3 pcs., 1.1 oz. . . . . . . . . . . . . . . .160
fudge (*Grandma's* Homestyle/Mini), 1.4-oz. pc. . . . . . . .190
w/macadamias (*Famous Amos* Big Chunk), 1-oz. pc. . . .150
milk (*Entenmann's*), .7-oz. pc. . . . . . . . . . . . . . . . . . . . .100
w/pecans (*Chips Ahoy!* Mini), 5 pcs., 1.1 oz. . . . . . . . . .150
w/pecans (*Famous Amos*), 4 pcs., 1 oz. . . . . . . . . . . . .140
w/pecans or walnuts (*Westbrae Natural*), .9-oz. pc. . . . .110
w/peanut butter cup (*Keebler Chips Deluxe*), .6-oz. pc. . . . . . . . . . . . . . . . . . . . . . . . . . . . . .80
soft, chewy (*Keebler Chips Deluxe*), .6-oz. pc. . . . . . . . . .80
toffee (*Famous Amos*), 4 pcs., 1 oz. . . . . . . . . . . . . . . .130
walnut (*Country Choice Naturals*), .8-oz. pc. . . . . . . . . .100
walnut, crunch (*Keebler Chips Deluxe*), .6-oz. pc. . . . . . .90

chocolate mocha (*Pepperidge Farm Salzburg*), 2 pcs., 1 oz. . . . . . . . . . . . . . . . . . . . . . . . . . . . . . . . . .150

chocolate sandwich:
(*Hydrox*), 3 pcs., 1.1 oz. . . . . . . . . . . . . . . . . . . . . . . .150
(*Murray* Sugar Free), 3 pcs., 1 oz. . . . . . . . . . . . . . . . .120
(*Oreo*), 3 pcs., 1.2 oz. . . . . . . . . . . . . . . . . . . . . . . . . .160
(*Oreo* Mini), 9 pcs., 1 oz. . . . . . . . . . . . . . . . . . . . . . .140
(*Oreo* Reduced Fat), 3 pcs., 1.2 oz. . . . . . . . . . . . . . . .130
(*Oreo Double Stuff*), 2 pcs., 1 oz. . . . . . . . . . . . . . . . .140
(*Pepperidge Farm Bordeaux*), 4 pcs., 1 oz. . . . . . . . . . .130
(*Pepperidge Farm Brussels*), 3 pcs., 1.1 oz. . . . . . . . . . .150

(*Pepperidge Farm Milano*), 3 pcs., 1.2 oz. . . . . . . . . . . .180
(*SnackWell's*), 2 pcs., .9 oz. . . . . . . . . . . . . . . . . . . . . . .110
creme-filled (*Droxies*), 3 pcs., 1.1 oz. . . . . . . . . . . . . . .140
double (*Pepperidge Farm Milano*), 2 pcs., 1 oz. . . . . . . .140
fudge-covered (*Oreo*), .75-oz. pc. . . . . . . . . . . . . . . . . .110
milk (*Pepperidge Farm Milano*), 3 pcs., 1.2 oz. . . . . . . .170
mint or orange (*Pepperidge Farm Milano*), 2 pcs., .9 oz. . . . . . . . . . . . . . . . . . . . . . . . . . . . . . . . . .130
chocolate stick, wafer (*Lazzaroni* Cannoli), 4 pcs., 1.1 oz. . . . . . . . . . . . . . . . . . . . . . . . . . . . . . . . . . .150
cinnamon (*Stella D'oro* Viennese), 1-oz. pc. . . . . . . . . . . .100
coconut (*Lazzaroni* Samba), 5 pcs., 1.1 oz. . . . . . . . . . . . . .160
coconut creme (*SnackWell's*), 2 pcs., 1 oz. . . . . . . . . . . . . .110
coffee creme sandwich (*Peek Freans*), 2 pcs., 1.1 oz. . . . . .150
creme sandwich (*Peek Freans* Tropical Cremes), 2 pcs. . . . .130
creme sandwich (*SnackWell's*), 1.7-oz. pkg. . . . . . . . . . . . .210
Danish (*Keebler* Wedding), 4 pcs., 1 oz. . . . . . . . . . . . . . . .120
date (*Health Valley* Delight Fat Free), 3 pcs., 1.2 oz. . . . . . .100
(*Delicious Heath*), 3 pcs., 1.3 oz. . . . . . . . . . . . . . . . . . . .170
(*Delicious Nestlé Butterfinger*), 3 pcs., 1 oz. . . . . . . . . . . .130
devil's food (*SnackWell's*), 1.1-oz. pkg. . . . . . . . . . . . . . . . . .90
devil's food (*SnackWell's* Golden/Fat Free), .6-oz. pc. . . . . . .50
egg biscuit (*Stella D'oro* Jumbo), 2 pcs., .8 oz. . . . . . . . . . . .90
egg biscuit, vanilla (*Stella D'oro* Roman), 1.2-oz. pc. . . . . .140
fig bar (*Fig Newton*), 2 pcs., 1.1 oz. . . . . . . . . . . . . . . . . .110
fig bar (*Fig Newton* Fat Free), 2 pcs., 1 oz. . . . . . . . . . . . . . .90
fig-filled (*Health Valley Cobbler Bites*), 2 pcs., .9 oz. . . . . .100
fudge, double, caramel (*Fudge Shoppe*), 2 pcs., 1.1 oz. . . .140
fudge, mint (*Fudge Shoppe* Grasshoppers), 4 pcs., 1 oz. . . . . . . . . . . . . . . . . . . . . . . . . . . . . . . . . . . . .150
fudge brownie (*Country Choice Naturals*), .8-oz. pc. . . . . . . .80
fudge sandwich (*E.L. Fudge*), 2 pcs., .9 oz. . . . . . . . . . . . . .120
fudge-striped (*Fudge Shoppe*), 3 pcs., 1.1 oz. . . . . . . . . . . .160
ginger (*Country Choice Naturals*), .8-oz. pc. . . . . . . . . . . . . .90
ginger snaps (*Nabisco*), 4 pcs., 1 oz. . . . . . . . . . . . . . . . . .120
ginger snaps (*Sunshine*), 5 pcs., 1.2 oz. . . . . . . . . . . . . . . .150
graham (*Cinnamon Crisp*), 8 pcs., 1.1 oz. . . . . . . . . . . . . . .130
graham (*Graham Selects* Original), 8 pcs., 1 oz. . . . . . . . . .130
graham (*Honey Maid*), 8 pcs., 1 oz. . . . . . . . . . . . . . . . . . .120
graham (*Nabisco*), 4 pcs., 1 oz. . . . . . . . . . . . . . . . . . . . . .120

**Cookie *(cont.)***

graham, chocolate (*Dizzy Grizzlies*), 8 pcs., 1.1 oz. . . . . . . . .150
graham, chocolate (*Graham Selects*), 8 pcs., 1.1 oz. . . . . . . .130
graham, chocolate (*Honey Maid*), 8 pcs., 1 oz. . . . . . . . . . . .120
graham, chocolate (*New Morning*), 2 pcs., 1.1 oz. . . . . . . . .120
graham, cinnamon (*New Morning*), 2 pcs., 1.1 oz. . . . . . . . .100
graham, fudge-coated (*Fudge Shoppe Deluxe*),
  3 pcs., .9 oz. . . . . . . . . . . . . . . . . . . . . . . . . . . . . . . . . .140
graham, ginger (*New Morning*), 2 pcs., 1.1 oz. . . . . . . . . . . .140
graham, honey (*Blue's Clues*), 24 pcs., 1.1 oz. . . . . . . . . . .130
graham, honey (*Keebler*), 8 pcs., 1.1 oz. . . . . . . . . . . . . . .140
graham, honey (*New Morning*), 2 pcs., 1.1 oz. . . . . . . . . . . .110
graham, oat bran (*Health Valley*), 6 pcs., 1 oz. . . . . . . . . . .120
graham, oatmeal crunch (*Honey Maid*), 8 pcs., 1 oz. . . . . .130
graham, vanilla-frosted (*Dizzy Grizzlies*), 8 pcs., 1.1 oz. . . .150
honey almond (*Westbrae Natural*), .9-oz. pc. . . . . . . . . . . .110
lemon (*Country Choice Naturals*), .8-oz. pc. . . . . . . . . . . . . .90
lemon w/hazelnuts (*Lazzaroni* Limonelli), 5 pcs., 1 oz. . . . .140
lemon nut (*Pepperidge Farm*), 3 pcs., 1.1 oz. . . . . . . . . . . .170
lemon snaps (*Westbrae Natural*), 3 pcs., 1.1 oz. . . . . . . . . .140
lemon sandwich (*SnackWell's*), 3 pcs. . . . . . . . . . . . . . . . .140
lemon sandwich (*Vienna Fingers*), 2 pcs., 1 oz. . . . . . . . . .140
lime (*Peek Freans* Calypso), 2 pcs. . . . . . . . . . . . . . . . . . . .130
marshmallow, chocolate (*Mallomars*), 2 pcs., .9 oz. . . . . . .120
mint, fudge-coated (*Mystic Mint*), .6-oz. pc. . . . . . . . . . . . . .90
mint creme (*SnackWell's*), 2 pcs., .9 oz. . . . . . . . . . . . . . . .110
molasses (*Grandma's* Homestyle), 1.4-oz. pc. . . . . . . . . . . .160
molasses crisps (*Pepperidge Farm*), 5 pcs., 1.1 oz. . . . . . .150
oatmeal:
  (*Keebler* Country Style), 2 pcs., .8 oz. . . . . . . . . . . . . . .120
  (*Nabisco* Family Favorites), .6-oz. pc. . . . . . . . . . . . . . . .80
  chocolate chip (*Country Choice Naturals*), .8-oz. pc. . . .100
  chocolate chip (*Health Valley*), .8-oz. pc. . . . . . . . . . . . .100
  chocolate chip, walnut (*Famous Amos*),
    4 pcs., 1 oz. . . . . . . . . . . . . . . . . . . . . . . . . . . . . . . .140
  iced (*Nabisco* Family Favorites), .6-oz. pc. . . . . . . . . . . . .80
  peanut crunch (*Health Valley*), .8-oz. pc. . . . . . . . . . . . .100
oatmeal raisin (*Country Choice Naturals*), .8-oz. pc. . . . . . .100
oatmeal raisin (*Entenmann's* Soft Light), 2 pcs., 1.1 oz. . . .100
oatmeal raisin (*Famous Amos*), 4 pcs., 1 oz. . . . . . . . . . . . .130

oatmeal raisin (*Grandma's* Homestyle), 1.4-oz. pc. . . . . . . .180
oatmeal raisin (*Health Valley*), .8-oz. pc. . . . . . . . . . . . . . . . . .90
oatmeal raisin, soft (*Pepperidge Farm*), .9-oz. pc. . . . . . . . . .110
peach–apricot (*Newtons Cobblers*), .75-oz. pc. . . . . . . . . . . .70
peanut butter (*Country Choice Naturals*), .8-oz. pc. . . . . . . . .80
peanut butter (*Grandma's* Homestyle), 1.4-oz. pc. . . . . . . . . .200
peanut butter (*Murray* Sugar Free), 3 pcs., 1 oz. . . . . . . . . . .150
peanut butter fudge (*Fudge Shoppe* Sticks), 3 pcs.,
1 oz. . . . . . . . . . . . . . . . . . . . . . . . . . . . . . . . . . . . .150
peanut butter sandwich (*E.L. Fudge*), 2 pcs., .9 oz. . . . . . . .120
peanut butter sandwich (*Nutter Butter* Bite Size), 10 pcs. . . .150
peanut butter sandwich, chocolate (*Nutter Butter*),
2 pcs. . . . . . . . . . . . . . . . . . . . . . . . . . . . . . . . . . . . .130
peanut butter patties (*Nutter Butter*), 5 pcs. . . . . . . . . . . . .160
pecan, see "shortbread," below
(*Peek Freans* Nice), 4 pcs., 1.2 oz. . . . . . . . . . . . . . . . . . .160
pfeffernüsse (*Stella D'oro*), 3 pcs., 1 oz. . . . . . . . . . . . . . . .120
pralines and creme (*Pepperidge Farm Dessert Bliss*),
3 pcs., 1.1 oz. . . . . . . . . . . . . . . . . . . . . . . . . . . . . . . .160
rainbow (*Beigel's*), 1.2-oz. pc. . . . . . . . . . . . . . . . . . . . . .120
raspberry (*Health Valley* Fat Free Jumbo), .9-oz. pc. . . . . . . .80
raspberry-filled (*Barbara's* Fat/Wheat Free), .7-oz. pc. . . . . .60
raspberry vanilla (*Westbrae Natural*), .9-oz. pc. . . . . . . . . .110
rocky road (*Country Choice Naturals*), .8-oz. pc. . . . . . . . . . .90
sesame (*Stella D'oro Regina*), 3 pcs., 1.1 oz. . . . . . . . . . . .150
shortbread (*Lorna Doone*), 4 pcs., 1 oz. . . . . . . . . . . . . . . .140
shortbread (*Simply Sandies*), .6-oz. pc. . . . . . . . . . . . . . . . .80
shortbread (*SnackWell's*), 3 pcs. . . . . . . . . . . . . . . . . . . . .130
shortbread, almond (*Sandies*), .6-oz. pc. . . . . . . . . . . . . . . .80
shortbread, fudge (*Fudge Favorites*), 3 pcs., 1.1 oz. . . . . . .160
shortbread, pecan (*Pecanz*), .6-oz. pc. . . . . . . . . . . . . . . . . .90
shortbread, pecan (*Sandies*), .6-oz. pc. . . . . . . . . . . . . . . . . .80
(*Social Tea*), 6 pcs., 1 oz. . . . . . . . . . . . . . . . . . . . . . . . .120
(*Stella D'oro Angelica Goodies*), .8-oz. pc. . . . . . . . . . . . .100
(*Stella D'oro Margherite* Combination), 2 pcs., 1.1 oz. . . . .140
strawberry–kiwi (*Tropical Newtons*), 2 pcs., 1 oz. . . . . . . . . .90
sugar (*Grandma's Tiny Bites*), 12 pcs., 1 oz. . . . . . . . . . . . .280
sugar (*Pepperidge Farm*), 3 pcs., 1.1 oz. . . . . . . . . . . . . . .140
sugar wafer (*Biscos*), 8 pcs., 1 oz. . . . . . . . . . . . . . . . . . .140
sugar wafer (*Keebler*), 3 pcs., .9 oz. . . . . . . . . . . . . . . . . .130

**Cookie** ***(cont.)***
sugar wafer, chocolate (*Keebler*), 3 pcs., .9 oz. . . . . . . . . . .140
sugar wafer, lemon (*Keebler*), 3 pcs., .9 oz. . . . . . . . . . . . .130
sugar wafer, peanut butter (*Keebler*), 4 pcs., 1.1 oz. . . . . . .160
vanilla (*Grandma's* Mini), 9 pcs., 1 oz. . . . . . . . . . . . . . . . .150
vanilla fudge sandwich (*Café Cremes*), 2 pcs. . . . . . . . . . . .200
vanilla sandwich (*Café Cremes*), 2 pcs. . . . . . . . . . . . . . . . .160
vanilla sandwich (*Cameo*), 2 pcs., 1 oz. . . . . . . . . . . . . . . .130
vanilla sandwich (*Grandma's*), 5 pcs., 1 oz. . . . . . . . . . . . .210
vanilla sandwich (*Murray* Sugar Free), 3 pcs., 1 oz. . . . . . .120
vanilla sandwich (*Vienna Fingers*), 2 pcs., 1 oz. . . . . . . . . .140
vanilla wafer (*Keebler Golden*), 8 pcs., 1.1 oz. . . . . . . . . . . .150
vanilla wafer (*Murray* Sugar Free), 9 pcs., 1.1 oz. . . . . . . . .120
vanilla wafer (*Nilla*), 8 pcs., 1.1 oz. . . . . . . . . . . . . . . . . . . .140
vanilla wafer, rainbow (*Keebler*), 8 pcs., 1.1 oz. . . . . . . . . .130
**Cookie, mix,** 2 pcs.*:
chocolate chip (*Betty Crocker*) . . . . . . . . . . . . . . . . . . . . .160
chocolate chip (*Duncan Hines*) . . . . . . . . . . . . . . . . . . . . .170
chocolate chunk, double or peanut butter (*Betty Crocker*) . .150
oatmeal/oatmeal chocolate chip (*Betty Crocker*) . . . . . . . . .150
peanut butter (*Betty Crocker*) . . . . . . . . . . . . . . . . . . . . . .160
peanut butter (*Duncan Hines*) . . . . . . . . . . . . . . . . . . . . . .140
sugar, golden (*Duncan Hines*) . . . . . . . . . . . . . . . . . . . . . .150
sugar or white chunk (*Betty Crocker*) . . . . . . . . . . . . . . . .160
**Cookie, refrigerated,** 1 pc.*:
chocolate chip (*Nestlé Toll House/Toll House* Big Batch) . . .140
chocolate chip bar (*Nestlé Toll House*) . . . . . . . . . . . . . . . .110
chocolate chip peanut butter (*Nestlé Toll House*) . . . . . . . . .150
chocolate chip walnut (*Nestlé Toll House*) . . . . . . . . . . . . . .110
chocolate chip walnut (*Pillsbury* Ready to Bake!) . . . . . . . .120
chocolate chip and white fudge (*Nestlé Toll House*) . . . . . . .150
chocolate chunk (*Nestlé Toll House*) . . . . . . . . . . . . . . . . . .150
sugar (*Pillsbury* Ready to Bake!) . . . . . . . . . . . . . . . . . . . .110
sugar bar (*Nestlé Toll House*) . . . . . . . . . . . . . . . . . . . . . .110
**Cookie dough topping,** crunch (*Smucker's Magic Shell*),
2 tbsp. . . . . . . . . . . . . . . . . . . . . . . . . . . . . . . . . . . . . .210
**Coquito nuts** (*Frieda's*), 11 pcs., 1 oz. . . . . . . . . . . . . . . .110
**Coriander,** dried:
leaf, 1 tsp. . . . . . . . . . . . . . . . . . . . . . . . . . . . . . . . . . . . .2
seed, 1 tsp. . . . . . . . . . . . . . . . . . . . . . . . . . . . . . . . . . . .5

**Corkscrew pasta dish mix,** 1 cup*:
4-cheese sauce (*Pasta Roni*) . . . . . . . . . . . . . . . . . . . . . . .390
garlic sauce, creamy (*Pasta Roni*) . . . . . . . . . . . . . . . . . . .350
**Corn,** fresh:
raw, 1 large ear, 7¾–9" long . . . . . . . . . . . . . . . . . . . . . . .123
kernels, boiled, drained, ½ cup . . . . . . . . . . . . . . . . . . . . . .89
**Corn, canned,** ½ cup, except as noted:
kernel, gold (*Green Giant/Green Giant* Less Sodium) . . . . . . .80
kernel, gold (*Green Giant Niblets*), ⅓ cup . . . . . . . . . . . . . . .70
kernel, gold (*Green Giant Niblets* No Salt), ⅓ cup . . . . . . . . .60
kernel, gold (*Libby's*) . . . . . . . . . . . . . . . . . . . . . . . . . . . .90
kernel, gold (*Libby's* Sweet No Salt/Vac Pack) . . . . . . . . . . .80
kernel, gold (*Veg-All*) . . . . . . . . . . . . . . . . . . . . . . . . . . . .80
kernel, gold/white (*Green Giant* Super Sweet), ⅓ cup . . . . . .50
kernel, white (*Del Monte*) . . . . . . . . . . . . . . . . . . . . . . . . . .60
kernel, w/peppers (*Green Giant Mexicorn*), ⅓ cup . . . . . . . .60
kernel or cream style, gold (*Blue Boy*) . . . . . . . . . . . . . . . . .90
kernel or cream style, gold (*Del Monte*) . . . . . . . . . . . . . . . .90
cream style, gold (*Libby's*) . . . . . . . . . . . . . . . . . . . . . . . . .90
cream style, gold (*Veg-All*) . . . . . . . . . . . . . . . . . . . . . . . .100
**Corn, frozen:**
on cob, 1 ear, except as noted:
(*Birds Eye* 4 Pack) . . . . . . . . . . . . . . . . . . . . . . . . . . .140
(*Birds Eye* Little Ears 8 or 12 Pack) . . . . . . . . . . . . . . . .80
(*Cascadian Farm*), 2 ears . . . . . . . . . . . . . . . . . . . . . . .120
(*Green Giant Niblets*) . . . . . . . . . . . . . . . . . . . . . . . . . .150
(*John Cope's* 3"–5") . . . . . . . . . . . . . . . . . . . . . . . . . .140
(*John Cope's* Mini 2"–3") . . . . . . . . . . . . . . . . . . . . . . . .80
(*John Cope's* Super Sweet 5") . . . . . . . . . . . . . . . . . . . .120
white (*John Cope's* Silver Queen 5") . . . . . . . . . . . . . . .150
kernel, gold (*Birds Eye* Deluxe), ⅓ cup . . . . . . . . . . . . . . . . .60
kernel, gold (*Cascadian Farm*), ¾ cup . . . . . . . . . . . . . . . . .90
kernel, gold (*Green Giant Niblets* Extra Sweet), ⅔ cup . . . . .70
kernel, gold (*John Cope's/John Cope's* Shoepeg), ⅔ cup . . .80
kernel, gold (*Seabrook Farms*), ⅔ cup . . . . . . . . . . . . . . . . .80
kernel, gold (*Tree of Life* Organic), ⅔ cup . . . . . . . . . . . . . .80
kernel, gold/white (*Birds Eye*), ½ cup . . . . . . . . . . . . . . . . .60
kernel, gold/white (*Green Giant*), ¾ cup . . . . . . . . . . . . . . . .70
kernel, white (*Green Giant* Shoepeg), ¾ cup . . . . . . . . . . . .100
kernel, white (*John Cope's* Super Sweet), ⅓ cup . . . . . . . . .80

**Corn, frozen:**
kernel, white (*McKenzie's*), ½ cup . . . . . . . . . . . . . . . . . . . .80
kernel, white, baby (*Birds Eye*), ⅔ cup . . . . . . . . . . . . . . . .110
cream style, white (*John Cope's* Sweet 'n Creamy),
⅓ cup . . . . . . . . . . . . . . . . . . . . . . . . . . . . . . . . . . . . .100
in butter sauce (*Cascadian Farm*), ½ cup . . . . . . . . . . . . . .100
in butter sauce (*Green Giant Niblets*), ⅔ cup . . . . . . . . . . .110
**Corn, dried,** sweet (*John Cope's*), ¼ cup . . . . . . . . . . . . . . .130
**Corn blend,** frozen, baby, and bean (*Birds Eye*), 3 oz. . . . . . .60
**Corn bread,** see "Bread. frozen or refrigerated"
**Corn bread mix,** dry, ¼ cup, except as noted:
(*Aunt Jemima* Easy), ⅛ pkg. . . . . . . . . . . . . . . . . . . . . . . .145
(*Hodgson Mill* Corn bread/Muffin) . . . . . . . . . . . . . . . . . . . .130
(*Glory Foods*) . . . . . . . . . . . . . . . . . . . . . . . . . . . . . . . . . .140
jalapeño (*Hodgson Mill*) . . . . . . . . . . . . . . . . . . . . . . . . . . .100
sweet cake (*Chi-Chi's* Cake), ½ cup . . . . . . . . . . . . . . . . . .100
sweet cake (*El Torito*), ⅛ pkt. . . . . . . . . . . . . . . . . . . . . . .100
sweet cake (*Kentucky Kernel*) . . . . . . . . . . . . . . . . . . . . . .120
**Corn cake,** frozen (*El Torito*), ⅓ cup . . . . . . . . . . . . . . . . . .180
**Corn chips, puffs, and similar snacks** (see also
"Snack chips and crisps"), 1 oz., except as noted:
(*Bachman*), 1.1 oz. . . . . . . . . . . . . . . . . . . . . . . . . . . . . . .150
(*Bugles*), 1.1 oz. . . . . . . . . . . . . . . . . . . . . . . . . . . . . . . .160
(*Fritos/Fritos* King Size/Scoops) . . . . . . . . . . . . . . . . . . . .160
(*Snyder's*), 1.5 oz. . . . . . . . . . . . . . . . . . . . . . . . . . . . . . .240
(*Wahoos* Original) . . . . . . . . . . . . . . . . . . . . . . . . . . . . . . .140
barbecue (*Bachman*), 1.1 oz. . . . . . . . . . . . . . . . . . . . . . . .150
barbecue (*Utz*) . . . . . . . . . . . . . . . . . . . . . . . . . . . . . . . . .160
barbecue (*Wahoos*) . . . . . . . . . . . . . . . . . . . . . . . . . . . . . .140
barbecue, regular or honey (*Fritos*) . . . . . . . . . . . . . . . . . .150
cheese (*Chee•tos* Crunchy/Puffs/X's & O's) . . . . . . . . . . . . .160
cheese (*Chee•tos* Curls/Puffed Balls) . . . . . . . . . . . . . . . . .150
cheese (*Chee•tos* Zig Zags) . . . . . . . . . . . . . . . . . . . . . . . .170
cheese (*Jax* Baked) . . . . . . . . . . . . . . . . . . . . . . . . . . . . . .140
cheese (*Planters Cheez Balls/Mania*) . . . . . . . . . . . . . . . . .160
cheese (*Planters Cheez Curls*) . . . . . . . . . . . . . . . . . . . . . .150
cheese (*Snyder's* Twist) . . . . . . . . . . . . . . . . . . . . . . . . . . .170
cheese (*Utz* Balls) . . . . . . . . . . . . . . . . . . . . . . . . . . . . . . .170
cheese (*Utz* Curls) . . . . . . . . . . . . . . . . . . . . . . . . . . . . . . .160
cheese, nacho (*Bugles*), 1.1 oz. . . . . . . . . . . . . . . . . . . . . .160

cheese, nacho (*Wahoos* Fiesta) . . . . . . . . . . . . . . . . . . . . .140
cheese twists (*Jax* Crunchy) . . . . . . . . . . . . . . . . . . . . . . . . .160
chili cheese (*Bugles* Chili Con Queso), 1.1 oz. . . . . . . . . . . . .160
chili cheese (*Fritos*) . . . . . . . . . . . . . . . . . . . . . . . . . . . . . .160
hot (*Fritos/Fritos* Sabrositas Flamin') . . . . . . . . . . . . . . . . . .160
lime 'n chili (*Fritos* Sabrositas) . . . . . . . . . . . . . . . . . . . . . .150
pepperoni, toasted (*Corn Nuts*), ⅓ cup . . . . . . . . . . . . . . . .130
tortilla:
(*Bachman* Restaurant) . . . . . . . . . . . . . . . . . . . . . . . . . .130
(*Doritos* Toasted) . . . . . . . . . . . . . . . . . . . . . . . . . . . . . .140
(*Santitas* Restaurant/White) . . . . . . . . . . . . . . . . . . . . . .130
(*Snyder's* White) . . . . . . . . . . . . . . . . . . . . . . . . . . . . . .140
(*Tostitos* Baked/Baked Bite Size) . . . . . . . . . . . . . . . . . .110
(*Tostitos* Crispy Rounds/Restaurant/Santa Fe Gold) . . . .140
(*Tostitos WOW*) . . . . . . . . . . . . . . . . . . . . . . . . . . . . . . . .90
(*Utz* Baked) . . . . . . . . . . . . . . . . . . . . . . . . . . . . . . . . . .120
(*Utz* Restaurant/Round) . . . . . . . . . . . . . . . . . . . . . . . . .140
black bean and salsa (*Bachman*) . . . . . . . . . . . . . . . . . . .140
black bean chili or chili and lime (*Garden of Eatin'*) . . . .140
blue corn (*Garden of Eatin'*) . . . . . . . . . . . . . . . . . . . . . .150
blue corn (*Kettle*) . . . . . . . . . . . . . . . . . . . . . . . . . . . . . .140
brown rice and black bean (*Kettle*) . . . . . . . . . . . . . . . . .120
chili and lime (*Guiltless Gourmet*) . . . . . . . . . . . . . . . . . .110
jalapeño cheddar (*Doritos 3D's*) . . . . . . . . . . . . . . . . . . .130
nacho (*Bachman*) . . . . . . . . . . . . . . . . . . . . . . . . . . . . . .140
nacho (*Doritos Nacho Cheesier/Doritos* Spicier) . . . . . . .140
nacho (*Doritos WOW*) . . . . . . . . . . . . . . . . . . . . . . . . . . . .90
nacho (*Snyder's*) . . . . . . . . . . . . . . . . . . . . . . . . . . . . . . .150
nacho (*Utz* Cheesier) . . . . . . . . . . . . . . . . . . . . . . . . . . .140
picante (*Doritos* Baja) . . . . . . . . . . . . . . . . . . . . . . . . . . .140
quesadilla, spicy (*Tostitos* Bite Size) . . . . . . . . . . . . . . .150
ranch (*Doritos Cooler Ranch/3D's Cooler Ranch*) . . . . . .140
red corn (*Garden of Eatin'* Red Chips/*Salsa Reds*) . . . . .150
salsa and black bean (*Utz*) . . . . . . . . . . . . . . . . . . . . . . .140
salsa and cream cheese (*Tostitos* Baked Bite Size) . . . . .120
salsa verde, sour cream, or taco (*Doritos*) . . . . . . . . . . .140
sesame rye w/caraway (*Kettle*) . . . . . . . . . . . . . . . . . . . .140
yellow corn (*Guiltless Gourmet*) . . . . . . . . . . . . . . . . . . .110
yellow corn (*Kettle/Kettle* 5 Grain) . . . . . . . . . . . . . . . . .140
yellow corn (*Snyder's*) . . . . . . . . . . . . . . . . . . . . . . . . . .140

**Corn dog,** see "Frankfurter, wrapped"
**Corn flake crumbs** (*Kellogg's*), 2 tbsp. . . . . . . . . . . . . . . . . .40
**Corn flour** (*Mascoa*), 1.1 oz. . . . . . . . . . . . . . . . . . . . . . . .110
**Corn fritter,** frozen (*Mrs. Paul's*), 1 pc. . . . . . . . . . . . . . . . .130
**Corn grits,** dry:
(*Quaker* Instant), 1 pkt. . . . . . . . . . . . . . . . . . . . . . . . . . .95
butter flavor or zesty cheddar (*Quaker* Instant), 1 pkt. . . . . .100
w/cheddar flavor, real (*Quaker* Instant), 1 pkt. . . . . . . . . . . .105
w/red-eye gravy, ham bits (*Quaker* Instant), 1 pkt. . . . . . . . .95
white (*Quaker* Quick Hominy), ¼ cup . . . . . . . . . . . . . . . . .130
yellow, hominy (*Quaker* Quick), ¼ cup . . . . . . . . . . . . . . . .125
**Corn relish:**
(*Aunt Nellie's*), 1 tbsp. . . . . . . . . . . . . . . . . . . . . . . . . . .20
(*Mrs. Renfro's*), 1 tbsp. . . . . . . . . . . . . . . . . . . . . . . . . .15
(*Nance's*), 2 tbsp. . . . . . . . . . . . . . . . . . . . . . . . . . . . . .25
**Corn soufflé,** frozen (*Stouffer's* Side Dish), ½ cup . . . . . . .170
**Cornish hen,** fresh or frozen:
raw (*Tyson* Rock Cornish), 4 oz. . . . . . . . . . . . . . . . . . . . .180
whole, cooked, dark (*Perdue*), 3 oz. . . . . . . . . . . . . . . . . . .200
whole, cooked, white (*Perdue*), 3 oz. . . . . . . . . . . . . . . . . .160
**Cornmeal** (see also "Polenta"):
(*Goya* Fine), 3 tbsp. . . . . . . . . . . . . . . . . . . . . . . . . . . . .100
masa harina (*Quaker*), ¼ cup . . . . . . . . . . . . . . . . . . . . . . .110
masa harina (*Quaker* Preparada Para Tortillas), ⅓ cup . . . .160
white (*Quaker* Enriched), 3 tbsp. . . . . . . . . . . . . . . . . . . . .90
yellow (*Quaker* Enriched) . . . . . . . . . . . . . . . . . . . . . . . . .90
**Cornstarch** (*Hodgson Mill*), 2 tsp. . . . . . . . . . . . . . . . . . . .35
**Couscous:**
dry (*Arrowhead Mills*), ¼ cup . . . . . . . . . . . . . . . . . . . . . .170
cooked (*Near East*), 1 cup . . . . . . . . . . . . . . . . . . . . . . . .230
**Couscous dish, mix,** 1 cup*, except as noted:
almond, lentil curry, or Parmesan (*Nile Spice*), 1 pkg. . . . . .200
broccoli and cheese (*Near East*) . . . . . . . . . . . . . . . . . . . .230
chicken herb, curry, or Parmesan (*Near East*) . . . . . . . . . . .220
garlic, roasted (*Marrakesh Express* Grande) . . . . . . . . . . . .250
garlic, roasted, olive oil (*Near East* Meal Cup), 1 pkg. . . . . .280
garlic, roasted, olive oil (*Nile Spice* Cup), 2.8 oz. . . . . . . . . .310
minestrone (*Nile Spice*), 1 pkg. . . . . . . . . . . . . . . . . . . . . .180
mushroom, wild, and herb (*Near East*) . . . . . . . . . . . . . . . .230

sun-dried tomato (*Marrakesh Express* Grande) . . . . . . . . . .250
tomato and lentil (*Near East*) . . . . . . . . . . . . . . . . . . . . . . .220
**Cowpeas, canned or frozen,** see "Black-eyed peas"
**Crab,** meat only:
Alaska king, raw, 4 oz. . . . . . . . . . . . . . . . . . . . . . . . . . . . .95
Alaska king, boiled, poached, or steamed, 4 oz. . . . . . . . . . .110
blue, raw, 4 oz. . . . . . . . . . . . . . . . . . . . . . . . . . . . . . . . .99
blue, boiled, poached, or steamed, 4 oz. . . . . . . . . . . . . . . .116
Dungeness, raw, 4 oz. . . . . . . . . . . . . . . . . . . . . . . . . . . .98
Dungeness, boiled, poached, or steamed, 4 oz. . . . . . . . . . .125
queen, raw, 4 oz. . . . . . . . . . . . . . . . . . . . . . . . . . . . . . .102
queen, boiled, poached, or steamed, 4 oz. . . . . . . . . . . . . .130
**Crab, canned,** 2 oz.:
(*Chicken of the Sea* Fancy) . . . . . . . . . . . . . . . . . . . . . . . .40
lump (*Chicken of the Sea*) . . . . . . . . . . . . . . . . . . . . . . . . .35
white (*Chicken of the Sea*) . . . . . . . . . . . . . . . . . . . . . . . .30
white lump (*Crown Prince Natural*) . . . . . . . . . . . . . . . . . .45
**"Crab," imitation,** frozen or refrigerated, ½ cup:
chunk or flakes (*Louis Kemp Crab Delights*) . . . . . . . . . . . .80
leg style (*Louis Kemp Crab Delights*) . . . . . . . . . . . . . . . . .80
shreds (*Louis Kemp*) . . . . . . . . . . . . . . . . . . . . . . . . . . . .80
**Crab apple,** fresh (*Frieda's*), 5 oz. . . . . . . . . . . . . . . . . .110
**Crab dish, frozen:**
cake (*Chesapeake Bay*), 1 pc. . . . . . . . . . . . . . . . . . . . . . .60
cake (*Fisher Boy*), 1 pc. . . . . . . . . . . . . . . . . . . . . . . . . .110
cake (*Van de Kamp's*), 1 pc. . . . . . . . . . . . . . . . . . . . . . .190
cake, deviled (*Mrs. Paul's*), 1 pc. . . . . . . . . . . . . . . . . . .180
cake, deviled, mini (*Mrs. Paul's*), 6 pcs. . . . . . . . . . . . . . .220
cake, lightly breaded (*Chincoteague* Maryland), 4 oz. . . . . .280
cake, mini (*Van de Kamp's*), 4 pcs. . . . . . . . . . . . . . . . . . .260
cake, unbreaded (*Chincoteague* Maryland), 1 pc. . . . . . . . .170
nuggets, lightly breaded (*Chincoteague* Cocktail), 3 oz. . . . .210
nuggets, unbreaded (*Chincoteague* Cocktail), 6 pcs. . . . . . .180
poppers, cheese (*Mrs. Paul's/Van de Kamp's*), 4 pcs. . . . . .320
**Cracker:**
all varieties (*Toasteds*), 5 pcs., .6 oz. . . . . . . . . . . . . . . .80
bacon (*Nabisco Flavor Crisps*), 15 pcs. . . . . . . . . . . . . . . .160
butter/butter flavor:
(*Harvest Bakery* Country), 2 pcs., .6 oz. . . . . . . . . . . . .70

**Cracker, butter/butter flavor *(cont.)***

(*Hi-Ho/Hi-Ho* Reduced Fat), .5 oz. . . . . . . . . . . . . . . . . . . .70
(*Keebler Club*), 4 pcs., .5 oz. . . . . . . . . . . . . . . . . . . . . . .70
(*Pepperidge Farm*), 4 pcs., .5 oz. . . . . . . . . . . . . . . . . . .70
(*Ritz*), 5 pcs., .6 oz. . . . . . . . . . . . . . . . . . . . . . . . . . . .80
(*Ritz* Mini), 34 pcs., 1.1 oz. . . . . . . . . . . . . . . . . . . . . . .150
(*Ritz* Reduced Fat), 5 pcs., .6 oz. . . . . . . . . . . . . . . . . . .70
(*Ritz Air Crisps*), 24 pcs., 1 oz. . . . . . . . . . . . . . . . . . . .140
(*Town House*), 5 pcs., .6 oz. . . . . . . . . . . . . . . . . . . . . . .80
w/cheese (*Ritz*), 1.4-oz. pkg. . . . . . . . . . . . . . . . . . . . . .200
w/peanut butter (*Ritz*), 1.4-oz. pkg. . . . . . . . . . . . . . . . .190

cheese:

(*BIG Cheeze-It*), 13 pcs., 1 oz. . . . . . . . . . . . . . . . . . . .150
(*Cheez-It*), 27 pcs., 1.1 oz. . . . . . . . . . . . . . . . . . . . . .160
(*Cheez-It* Juniors Mini), 44 pcs., 1 oz. . . . . . . . . . . . . . .140
(*Cheese Nips*), 29 pcs., 1.1 oz. . . . . . . . . . . . . . . . . . . .150
(*Pepperidge Farm* Country), 2 pcs., .6 oz. . . . . . . . . . . . .80
(*SnackWell's* Zesty), 38 pcs., 1.1 oz. . . . . . . . . . . . . . . .130
(*Tid-Bit*), 32 pcs., 1.1 oz. . . . . . . . . . . . . . . . . . . . . . .160
cheddar (*Better Cheddars*), 22 pcs., 1.1 oz. . . . . . . . . . .150
cheddar (*Munch'ems*), 39 pcs., 1.1 oz. . . . . . . . . . . . . . .140
cheddar (*Ritz* Mini), 33 pcs., 1.1 oz. . . . . . . . . . . . . . . .150
cheddar (*Snax Stix*), 20 pcs., 1 oz. . . . . . . . . . . . . . . . .130
cheddar (*Sportz*), 40 pcs., 1.1 oz. . . . . . . . . . . . . . . . . .150
cheddar, extra (*Cheese Nips*), 27 pcs., 1.1 oz. . . . . . . . .140
cheddar, extra (*Goldfish Flavor Blaster*), 1.1 oz. . . . . . . .150
cheddar, mild (*Krispy*), 5 pcs., .5 oz. . . . . . . . . . . . . . . .60
cheddar, white (*Cheez-It*), 26 pcs., 1.1 oz. . . . . . . . . . . .150
cheddar or Parmesan (*Goldfish*), 1.1 oz. . . . . . . . . . . . . .140
hot, spicy (*Cheez-It*), 26 pcs., 1.1 oz. . . . . . . . . . . . . . .150
pizza (*Cheese Nips*), 29 pcs., 1.1 oz. . . . . . . . . . . . . . . .140

cheese sandwich:

(*Keebler Club* Bite Size), 14 pcs., 1.1 oz. . . . . . . . . . . .160
(*Ritz Bits*), 14 pcs., 1.1 oz. . . . . . . . . . . . . . . . . . . . . .170
cheddar, toast (*Nabisco*), 1.4-oz. pkg. . . . . . . . . . . . . . .200
cheddar, wheat (*Keebler*), 1.4-oz. pkg. . . . . . . . . . . . . . .160
nacho (*Doritos* Cheesier), 1 pkg. . . . . . . . . . . . . . . . . . .240
peanut butter (*Planters*), 1.4-oz. pkg. . . . . . . . . . . . . . .190

corn bread (*Harvest Bakery*), 2 pcs., .6 oz. . . . . . . . . . . . . .70
croissant (*Carr's*), 3 pcs., .5 oz. . . . . . . . . . . . . . . . . . . . .70

garlic, roasted (*Health Valley*), 6 pcs., .5 oz. . . . . . . . . . . . . . .60
(*Goldfish* Original), 55 pcs., 1.1 oz. . . . . . . . . . . . . . . . . . . .140
graham cracker, see "Cookie"
herb, garden (*Health Valley*), 6 pcs. .5 oz. . . . . . . . . . . . . . . .60
herb, garden, whole wheat (*Triscuit*), 6 pcs., 1 oz. . . . . . . .130
herb, Italian (*Harvest Crisp*), 13 pcs., 1 oz. . . . . . . . . . . . . .130
lavasch (*Cedar's* Giant), 1 oz. . . . . . . . . . . . . . . . . . . . . . . .40
matzo (*Manischewitz* Everything!/No Salt), 1-oz. pc. . . . . . .110
matzo, garlic, savory (*Manischewitz*), 1-oz. pc. . . . . . . . . . .100
matzo, thins, tea (*Manischewtiz*), .9-oz. pc. . . . . . . . . . . . .100
multigrain (*Harvest Bakery*), 2 pcs., .6 oz. . . . . . . . . . . . . . .70
multigrain (*Harvest Crisp*), 13 pcs., 1.1 oz. . . . . . . . . . . . . .130
multigrain, 7 (*Wheatables*), 12 pcs., 1.1 oz. . . . . . . . . . . . .140
(*Munch'ems* Original), 41 pcs., 1.1 oz. . . . . . . . . . . . . . . . .140
nori-maki (*Eden*), 15 pcs., 1.1 oz. . . . . . . . . . . . . . . . . . . . .110
onion, French (*Health Valley*), 10 pcs., .5 oz. . . . . . . . . . . . .60
onion, French (*Triscuit Thin Crisp*), 14 pcs., 1.1 oz. . . . . . .130
oyster/soup (*Premium*), 23 pcs., .5 oz. . . . . . . . . . . . . . . . . .60
peanut butter sandwich:
(*Keebler Club* Bite Size), 14 pcs., 1.1 oz. . . . . . . . . . . . .150
(*Ritz Bits*), 14 pcs., 1.1 oz. . . . . . . . . . . . . . . . . . . . . . .150
toast (*Keebler*), 1 pkg. . . . . . . . . . . . . . . . . . . . . . . . . . .190
toast (*Peter Pan*), 1 pkg. . . . . . . . . . . . . . . . . . . . . . . . .210
toast (*Planters*), 1.4-oz. pkg. . . . . . . . . . . . . . . . . . . . . .190
pepper, cracked (*SnackWell's*), 5 pcs., .5 oz. . . . . . . . . . . . . .60
pizza flavor (*Goldfish*), 55 pcs., 1.1 oz. . . . . . . . . . . . . . . .140
pizza flavor (*Sportz*) 39 pcs. . . . . . . . . . . . . . . . . . . . . . . .150
poppy, savory (*Barbara's* Rite Lite Rounds),
5 pcs., .5 oz. . . . . . . . . . . . . . . . . . . . . . . . . . . . . . . . . .70
potato, barbecue (*Air Crisps*), 22 pcs., 1 oz. . . . . . . . . . . . .120
potato, sour cream and onion (*Air Crisps*), 1 oz. . . . . . . . . .120
ranch (*Munch'ems*), 40 pcs., 1.1 oz. . . . . . . . . . . . . . . . . . .140
ranch (*Wheat Thins*), 14 pcs., 1.1 oz. . . . . . . . . . . . . . . . . .150
ranch (*Wheat Thins Air Crisps*), 23 pcs., 1.1 oz. . . . . . . . . .130
rice, brown (*Eden*), 5 pcs., 1.1 oz. . . . . . . . . . . . . . . . . . . .120
rice bran (*Health Valley*), 6 pcs., 1 oz. . . . . . . . . . . . . . . . .110
rice wafer, all varieties (*Westbrae Natural*),
7 pcs., .5 oz. . . . . . . . . . . . . . . . . . . . . . . . . . . . . . . . . .50
rye, whole wheat (*Triscuit*), 7 pcs., 1.1 oz. . . . . . . . . . . . . .140
saltine (*Krispy*), 5 pcs., .5 oz. . . . . . . . . . . . . . . . . . . . . . .60

**Cracker** ***(cont.)***
saltine (*Premium*), 5 pcs., .5 oz. . . . . . . . . . . . . . . . . . . . . . . . .60
sesame (*Health Valley*), 5 pcs., .5 oz. . . . . . . . . . . . . . . . . . . . .60
(*Snax Stix* Original), 21 pcs., 1 oz. . . . . . . . . . . . . . . . . . . . .130
(*Sociables*), 7 pcs., .5 oz. . . . . . . . . . . . . . . . . . . . . . . . . . . .80
soda/water:
(*Crown Pilot*), .6-oz. pc. . . . . . . . . . . . . . . . . . . . . . . . . . . .70
cracked pepper (*Carr's*), 5 pcs., .6 oz. . . . . . . . . . . . . . . . . .70
poppy–sesame seeds (*Carr's*), 4 pcs., .6 oz. . . . . . . . . . . .80
roasted garlic and herbs (*Carr's*), 5 pcs., .6 oz. . . . . . . . .70
sour cream and onion (*Ritz* Mini), 33 pcs., 1.1 oz. . . . . . . .150
(*Uneeda* Biscuit), 2 pcs., .5 oz. . . . . . . . . . . . . . . . . . . . . . . .60
vegetable (*Health Valley* Bruschetta), 6 pcs. .5 oz. . . . . . . . .60
vegetable (*Vegetable Thins*), 14 pcs., 1.1 oz. . . . . . . . . . . .160
vegetable, garden (*Harvest Crisps*), 15 pcs., 1.1 oz. . . . . . .130
wheat (*Pepperidge Farm* Hearty), 3 pcs., .6 oz. . . . . . . . . . . .80
wheat (*SnackWell's*), 5 pcs., .5 oz. . . . . . . . . . . . . . . . . . . . .70
wheat (*Toasteds* Reduced Fat), 5 pcs., .5 oz. . . . . . . . . . . . .60
wheat (*Waverly*), 5 pcs., .5 oz. . . . . . . . . . . . . . . . . . . . . . . .70
wheat (*Wheat Thins/Wheat Thins* Big), 1.1 oz. . . . . . . . . . . .140
wheat (*Wheat Thins* Multigrain), 17 pcs., 1.1 oz. . . . . . . . . .130
wheat (*Wheatables*), 12 pcs., 1.1 oz. . . . . . . . . . . . . . . . . . .140
wheat (*Wheatables* Reduced Fat), 13 pcs., 1.1 oz. . . . . . . . .130
wheat (*Wheatsworth*), 5 pcs., .6 oz. . . . . . . . . . . . . . . . . . . . .80
wheat, all varieties (*Barbara's Wheatines*), .5-oz. sq. . . . . . .50
wheat, savory (*Monterey*), 3 pcs., .5 oz. . . . . . . . . . . . . . . . .70
wheat, sesame (*Breton*), 3 pcs., .5 oz. . . . . . . . . . . . . . . . . . .60
wheat, stoned (*Red Oval Farms* Thins), 2 pcs. . . . . . . . . . . .60
wheat, whole (*Health Valley*), 5 pcs., .5 oz. . . . . . . . . . . . . .60
wheat, whole (*Krispy*), 5 pcs., .5 oz. . . . . . . . . . . . . . . . . . . .60
wheat, whole (*Ritz*), 5 pcs., .6 oz. . . . . . . . . . . . . . . . . . . . . .70
wheat, whole (*Triscuit* Original), 7 pcs., 1.1 oz. . . . . . . . . . .140
wheat, whole (*Triscuit Thin Crisps*),
15 pcs., 1.1 oz. . . . . . . . . . . . . . . . . . . . . . . . . . . . . . . . . .130
zwieback (*Nabisco*), 1 pc., .3 oz. . . . . . . . . . . . . . . . . . . . . .35

**Cracker crumbs and meal,** ¼ cup, except as noted:
crumbs (*Ritz*), ⅓ cup . . . . . . . . . . . . . . . . . . . . . . . . . . . . . .140
crumbs, saltine (*Premium* Fat Free) . . . . . . . . . . . . . . . . . . .100
meal (*Nabisco*) . . . . . . . . . . . . . . . . . . . . . . . . . . . . . . . . . . .110
meal, matzo (*Manischewitz*) . . . . . . . . . . . . . . . . . . . . . . . . .130

**Cranberry,** fresh, whole, ½ cup . . . . . . . . . . . . . . . . . . . . . . .23
**Cranberry, dried,** ⅓ cup, 1.4 oz.:
(*Craisins*) . . . . . . . . . . . . . . . . . . . . . . . . . . . . . . .130
(*Frieda's*) . . . . . . . . . . . . . . . . . . . . . . . . . . . . . . .120
(*Sunsweet Fruitlings*) . . . . . . . . . . . . . . . . . . . . . . .140
cherry or orange flavor (*Craisins*) . . . . . . . . . . . . . . . .130
orange flavor (*Sunsweet Fruitlings*) . . . . . . . . . . . . . . .120
**Cranberry bean,** canned, ½ cup . . . . . . . . . . . . . . . . . . .108
**Cranberry drink,** 8 fl. oz.:
(*Snapple* Twist) . . . . . . . . . . . . . . . . . . . . . . . . . . .100
cocktail (*Dole*) . . . . . . . . . . . . . . . . . . . . . . . . . . . .140
cocktail (*Langers*) . . . . . . . . . . . . . . . . . . . . . . . . . .140
cocktail (*Ocean Spray*) . . . . . . . . . . . . . . . . . . . . . . .140
cocktail (*Ocean Spray* Plus) . . . . . . . . . . . . . . . . . . . .160
cocktail (*Ocean Spray Lightstyle*) . . . . . . . . . . . . . . . . .40
cocktail (*Season's Best*) . . . . . . . . . . . . . . . . . . . . . .140
**Cranberry drink blend,** 8 fl. oz.:
apple (*Cranapple*) . . . . . . . . . . . . . . . . . . . . . . . . . .160
apple (*Langers* Fuji) . . . . . . . . . . . . . . . . . . . . . . . .160
berry (*Langers*) . . . . . . . . . . . . . . . . . . . . . . . . . . .135
(*Cran•Cherry*) . . . . . . . . . . . . . . . . . . . . . . . . . . . .160
(*Cran•Currant/Cran•Strawberry*) . . . . . . . . . . . . . . . . .140
(*Cran•Mango/Cran•Tangerine*) . . . . . . . . . . . . . . . . . . .130
(*Cran•Mango Lightstyle*) . . . . . . . . . . . . . . . . . . . . . . .40
grape (*Cran•Grape*) . . . . . . . . . . . . . . . . . . . . . . . . .170
grape (*Cran•Grape Lightstyle*) . . . . . . . . . . . . . . . . . . .40
grape (*Dole*) . . . . . . . . . . . . . . . . . . . . . . . . . . . . .170
grape (*Langers*) . . . . . . . . . . . . . . . . . . . . . . . . . . .165
grape (*Season's Best*) . . . . . . . . . . . . . . . . . . . . . . .170
(*Langers* Caribbean) . . . . . . . . . . . . . . . . . . . . . . . . .135
orange (*Langers*) . . . . . . . . . . . . . . . . . . . . . . . . . . .130
raspberry (*Cran•Raspberry*) . . . . . . . . . . . . . . . . . . . .140
raspberry (*Cran•Raspberry Lightstyle*) . . . . . . . . . . . . . .40
raspberry (*Langers*) . . . . . . . . . . . . . . . . . . . . . . . . .150
raspberry (*Snapple*) . . . . . . . . . . . . . . . . . . . . . . . . .120
**Cranberry fruit blend,** orange or raspberry
(*Cran•Fruit* for Chicken), ¼ cup . . . . . . . . . . . . . . . . . .120
**Cranberry juice** (*Langers*), 8 fl. oz. . . . . . . . . . . . . . . . .140
**Cranberry juice blends,** 8 fl. oz., except as noted:
(*Season's Best* Medley) . . . . . . . . . . . . . . . . . . . . . . .120

**Cranberry juice blends *(cont.)***
apple (*Ocean Spray* Granny Smith) . . . . . . . . . . . . . . . . . . . .130
berry (*Langers*) . . . . . . . . . . . . . . . . . . . . . . . . . . . . .135
grape (*Langers*) . . . . . . . . . . . . . . . . . . . . . . . . . . . . .150
grape (*Ocean Spray* Concord) . . . . . . . . . . . . . . . . . . . . . .150
Key lime, Georgia peach, or raspberry (*Ocean Spray*) . . . . .140
raspberry (*Langers*) . . . . . . . . . . . . . . . . . . . . . . . . . . .145
raspberry grape (*Nantucket Nectars*) . . . . . . . . . . . . . . . . .150
**Cranberry juice cocktail,** see "Cranberry drink"
**Cranberry relish,** ¼ cup:
(*Country Sides*) . . . . . . . . . . . . . . . . . . . . . . . . . . . . .200
orange (*New England*) . . . . . . . . . . . . . . . . . . . . . . . . . .120
**Cranberry sauce, can,** all styles (*Ocean Spray*),
¼ cup . . . . . . . . . . . . . . . . . . . . . . . . . . . . . . . . . . . .110
**Cranberry sauce, refrigerated** (*Marzetti* Homestyle),
¼ cup . . . . . . . . . . . . . . . . . . . . . . . . . . . . . . . . . . . .100
**Crawfish,** frozen, tail meat, cooked (*Ecrevisse Acadienne USA*), 3 oz. . . . . . . . . . . . . . . . . . . . . . . . . . . . . . .90
**Crayfish,** mixed species, meat only:
farmed, raw, 4 oz. . . . . . . . . . . . . . . . . . . . . . . . . . . . . .82
farmed, boiled or steamed, 4 oz. . . . . . . . . . . . . . . . . . . . . .93
wild, raw, 4 oz. . . . . . . . . . . . . . . . . . . . . . . . . . . . . . .87
wild, raw, 8 medium, 1 oz. . . . . . . . . . . . . . . . . . . . . . . . .20
wild, boiled or steamed, 4 oz. . . . . . . . . . . . . . . . . . . . . . .99
**Cream:**
all-purpose (*Hood*), 1 tbsp. . . . . . . . . . . . . . . . . . . . . . . .45
half and half (*Hood*), 2 tbsp. . . . . . . . . . . . . . . . . . . . . . .40
light, coffee or table (*Hood*), 1 tbsp. . . . . . . . . . . . . . . . . .30
medium (25% fat), 1 tbsp. . . . . . . . . . . . . . . . . . . . . . . . . .37
whipping, light, 1 tbsp., 2 tbsp. whipped . . . . . . . . . . . . . . . .44
whipping, heavy, 1 tbsp., 2 tbsp. whipped . . . . . . . . . . . . . . .52
**Cream, sour,** 2 tbsp.:
(*Crowley*) . . . . . . . . . . . . . . . . . . . . . . . . . . . . . . . . . .70
(*Friendship*) . . . . . . . . . . . . . . . . . . . . . . . . . . . . . . . .60
light (*Crowley*) . . . . . . . . . . . . . . . . . . . . . . . . . . . . . . .60
light (*Friendship*) . . . . . . . . . . . . . . . . . . . . . . . . . . . . .40
nonfat (*Crowley*) . . . . . . . . . . . . . . . . . . . . . . . . . . . . . .25
nonfat (*Friendship*) . . . . . . . . . . . . . . . . . . . . . . . . . . . .25
**Cream, sour, flavored,** 2 tbsp.:
roasted garlic (*Friendship*) . . . . . . . . . . . . . . . . . . . . . . .60

onion (*Crowley*) . . . . . . . . . . . . . . . . . . . . . . . . . . . .60
salsa (*Friendship*) . . . . . . . . . . . . . . . . . . . . . . . . . .50
**Cream topping,** 2 tbsp.:
(*Crowley* Real) . . . . . . . . . . . . . . . . . . . . . . . . . . . .25
(*Reddi Wip* Original) . . . . . . . . . . . . . . . . . . . . . . . .20
(*Reddi Wip* Extra Creamy) . . . . . . . . . . . . . . . . . . . .30
(*Reddi Wip* Fat Free) . . . . . . . . . . . . . . . . . . . . . . . .10
(*Reddi Wip* Light) . . . . . . . . . . . . . . . . . . . . . . . . . .15
chocolate (*Reddi Wip*) . . . . . . . . . . . . . . . . . . . . . . .20
**Creamer, nondairy:**
fluid (*Coffee-Mate*), 1 tbsp. . . . . . . . . . . . . . . . . . . . .20
fluid (*Coffee-Mate* Fat Free/Low Fat), 1 tbsp. . . . . . . . . . . . . .10
fluid (*Silk*), 1 tbsp. . . . . . . . . . . . . . . . . . . . . . . . . .15
powder (*Coffee-Mate*), 1 tsp. . . . . . . . . . . . . . . . . . . .10
powder (*Cremora* Fat Free/Lite), 1 tsp. . . . . . . . . . . . . . . .10
powder (*Cremora/Cremora* Royale), 1 tsp. . . . . . . . . . . . . .15
**Creamer, nondairy, flavored:**
fluid, all flavors (*Coffee-Mate*), 1 tbsp. . . . . . . . . . . . . . . .40
fluid, all flavors (*Coffee-Mate* Fat Free), 1 tbsp. . . . . . . . . . .25
fluid, vanilla (*Silk*), 1 tbsp. . . . . . . . . . . . . . . . . . . . . .20
powder, 4 tsp.:
all flavors, except Swiss chocolate (*Coffee-Mate*) . . . . . . .60
chocolate, Swiss (*Coffee-Mate*) . . . . . . . . . . . . . . . . . .50
hazelnut or French vanilla (*Coffee-Mate* Fat Free) . . . . . . .50
**Croaker,** meat only, raw, Atlantic, 4 oz. . . . . . . . . . . . . . .119
**Croissant,** 1 pc.:
butter (*Awrey's*), 3 oz. . . . . . . . . . . . . . . . . . . . . . . .250
butter or margarine (*Awrey's*), 2 oz. . . . . . . . . . . . . . . . .170
margarine (*Awrey's* Sliced), 2.5 oz. . . . . . . . . . . . . . . . . .210
**Croissant, frozen:**
French style (*Sara Lee*), 1 pc. . . . . . . . . . . . . . . . . . . . .170
French style, petite (*Sara Lee*), 2 pcs. . . . . . . . . . . . . . . .230
**Crookneck squash,** fresh:
baby (*Frieda's*), ⅔ cup, 3 oz. . . . . . . . . . . . . . . . . . . . .15
sliced, boiled, drained, ½ cup . . . . . . . . . . . . . . . . . . . .18
**Crookneck squash, canned,** cut, drained, ½ cup . . . . . . . . .14
**Crookneck squash, frozen,** boiled, sliced, ½ cup . . . . . . . . .24
**Croutons,** 2 tbsp. or ¼ cup, except as noted:
Caesar (*Brownberry* Homestyle) . . . . . . . . . . . . . . . . . . .30
Caesar (*Chatham Village*) . . . . . . . . . . . . . . . . . . . . . . .35

**Croutons** ***(cont.)***
Caesar (*Reese* Salad) . . . . . . . . . . . . . . . . . . . . . . . . . .30
cheddar (*Reese*) . . . . . . . . . . . . . . . . . . . . . . . . . . . .30
cheese, sourdough (*Brownberry* Homestyle) . . . . . . . . . . . .30
cheese and garlic (*Chatham Village*) . . . . . . . . . . . . . . . . . .40
garden herb or garlic and butter (*Chatham Village*) . . . . . . . .35
garlic herb or onion garlic (*Brownberry* Homestyle) . . . . . . .30
garlic and onion (*Chatham Village* Fat Free) . . . . . . . . . . . . .25
Italian, zesty (*Arnold/Brownberry* Homestyle) . . . . . . . . . . . .30
onion and garlic (*Reese*) . . . . . . . . . . . . . . . . . . . . . . . .30
seasoned (*Brownberry* Homestyle) . . . . . . . . . . . . . . . . . . .30
sun-dried tomato (*Chatham Village* Fat Free) . . . . . . . . . . . .30
**Cucumber,** fresh, w/peel:
1 medium, 8¼" long . . . . . . . . . . . . . . . . . . . . . . . . . . . .38
sliced, ½ cup . . . . . . . . . . . . . . . . . . . . . . . . . . . . . . . . .7
**Cucumber, Japanese** (*Frieda's* Hothouse), ⅔ cup, 3 oz. . . . .10
**Cucumber–dill dip mix,** dry (*Watkins*), 1 tsp. . . . . . . . . . . . .10
**Cucuzza squash** (*Frieda's*), ¾ cup, 3 oz. . . . . . . . . . . . . . . .10
**Cumin seed,** ground, 1 tsp. . . . . . . . . . . . . . . . . . . . . . . . .8
**Currants,** dried, Zante (*Sun•Maid*), ¼ cup, 1.4 oz. . . . . . . .130
**Curry powder,** 1 tbsp. . . . . . . . . . . . . . . . . . . . . . . . . . .20
**Curry sauce base** (see also "Curry paste"), 1 tsp.:
green (*A Taste of Thai*) . . . . . . . . . . . . . . . . . . . . . . . . . .15
Mussaman or red (*A Taste of Thai*) . . . . . . . . . . . . . . . . . .20
Panang (*A Taste of Thai*) . . . . . . . . . . . . . . . . . . . . . . . . .25
yellow (*A Taste of Thai*) . . . . . . . . . . . . . . . . . . . . . . . . . .30
**Curry seasoning,** dinner (see also "Thai sauce"):
green (*A Taste of Thai* Kit Lite), 3.5 oz. . . . . . . . . . . . . . . . .90
Panang (*A Taste of Thai* Kit Lite), 3.5 oz. . . . . . . . . . . . . . .110
red (*A Taste of Thai* Kit Lite), 3.5 oz. . . . . . . . . . . . . . . . . .90
Mussaman (*A Taste of Thai* Kit Lite), 3.5 oz. . . . . . . . . . . . .100
yellow (*A Taste of Thai* Kit Lite), 3.5 oz. . . . . . . . . . . . . . .110
**Cusk,** meat only:
raw, 4 oz. . . . . . . . . . . . . . . . . . . . . . . . . . . . . . . . . . . .99
baked, broiled, or microwaved, 4 oz. . . . . . . . . . . . . . . . . .127
**Custard apple,** trimmed, 1 oz. . . . . . . . . . . . . . . . . . . . . . .29
**Cuttlefish,** meat only:
raw, 4 oz. . . . . . . . . . . . . . . . . . . . . . . . . . . . . . . . . . . .90
boiled or steamed, 4 oz. . . . . . . . . . . . . . . . . . . . . . . . . .179
**Cuttlefish, canned,** in ink (*Goya*), ¼ cup . . . . . . . . . . . . . .120

# D–E

**FOOD AND MEASURE** | **CALORIES**

**Daikon,** see "Radish, Oriental"
**Dandelion greens,** raw (*Frieda's*), 2 cups, 3 oz. . . . . . . . . . .40
**Danish,** 1 pc., except as noted:
all varieties (*Awrey's* Petite), 1.5 oz. . . . . . . . . . . . . . . . . . .160
apple or cheese (*Awrey's*), 2.75 oz. . . . . . . . . . . . . . . . . . .290
apple, cheese, or strawberry (*Awrey's* Grande),
4.5 oz. . . . . . . . . . . . . . . . . . . . . . . . . . . . . . . . . .470
cheese (*Entenmann's*) . . . . . . . . . . . . . . . . . . . . . . . . .170
cheese (*Sara Lee*), 4.75 oz. . . . . . . . . . . . . . . . . . . . . . .520
cinnamon (*Awrey's* Grande), 4.5 oz. . . . . . . . . . . . . . . . . .480
cinnamon roll (*Awrey's* Homestyle), 3 oz. . . . . . . . . . . . . .270
cinnamon swirl (*Awrey's*), 2.75 oz. . . . . . . . . . . . . . . . . . .300
cinnamon swirl (*Awrey's* Grande), 3.75 oz. . . . . . . . . . . . . .400
raspberry cheese swirl (*Awrey's* Grande), 3.75 oz. . . . . . . .360
strawberry (*Awrey's*), 2.75 oz. . . . . . . . . . . . . . . . . . . . . .290
**Danish, frozen,** crumb (*Sara Lee*), 1 pc. . . . . . . . . . . . . .370
**Danish cake,** see "Cake"
**Date, dried,** pitted:
(*Dole*), 5–6 pcs. . . . . . . . . . . . . . . . . . . . . . . . . . . . . .120
(*Frieda's* Medjool), 2–3 pcs., 1.4 oz. . . . . . . . . . . . . . . . .120
(*Sunsweet*), 1.4 oz., ¼ cup . . . . . . . . . . . . . . . . . . . . . . .120
10 pcs., 2.9 oz. . . . . . . . . . . . . . . . . . . . . . . . . . . . . . .228
chopped (*Sunsweet*), ¼ cup . . . . . . . . . . . . . . . . . . . . . . .120
**Delicata squash** (*Frieda's*), ¾ cup, 3 oz. . . . . . . . . . . . . .30
**Dill dip,** 2 tbsp.:
(*Marzetti* Veggie Dip) . . . . . . . . . . . . . . . . . . . . . . . . . .140
(*Marzetti* Veggie Dip Fat Free) . . . . . . . . . . . . . . . . . . . . .30
**Dill seed,** 1 tsp. . . . . . . . . . . . . . . . . . . . . . . . . . . . . . .6
**Dill weed,** fresh, ½ cup loose-packed . . . . . . . . . . . . . . . . .2
**Dill weed, dried,** 1 tsp. . . . . . . . . . . . . . . . . . . . . . . . . . .3
**Dip** (see also specific listings), 4-layer (*Ortega*), 2 tbsp. . . . .50
**Dolphin fish,** meat only:
raw, 4 oz. . . . . . . . . . . . . . . . . . . . . . . . . . . . . . . . . . . .97
baked, broiled, or microwaved, 4 oz. . . . . . . . . . . . . . . . . .124

***Domino's Pizza,*** 12" medium pie, 2 of 8 slices, except as noted:
deep dish, cheese . . . . . . . . . . . . . . . . . . . . . . . . . .482
w/anchovy . . . . . . . . . . . . . . . . . . . . . . . . . . . . .516
w/extra cheese . . . . . . . . . . . . . . . . . . . . . . . . .531
w/green pepper . . . . . . . . . . . . . . . . . . . . . . . . .486
w/mushrooms . . . . . . . . . . . . . . . . . . . . . . . . . .488
w/olives, ripe . . . . . . . . . . . . . . . . . . . . . . . . . .503
w/onion . . . . . . . . . . . . . . . . . . . . . . . . . . . . . .488
w/pepperoni . . . . . . . . . . . . . . . . . . . . . . . . . . .556
w/sausage . . . . . . . . . . . . . . . . . . . . . . . . . . . .559
hand-tossed, cheese . . . . . . . . . . . . . . . . . . . . . . .375
w/anchovy . . . . . . . . . . . . . . . . . . . . . . . . . . . . .408
w/extra cheese . . . . . . . . . . . . . . . . . . . . . . . . .423
w/green pepper . . . . . . . . . . . . . . . . . . . . . . . . .378
w/mushrooms . . . . . . . . . . . . . . . . . . . . . . . . . .381
w/olives, ripe . . . . . . . . . . . . . . . . . . . . . . . . . .395
w/onion . . . . . . . . . . . . . . . . . . . . . . . . . . . . . .380
w/pepperoni . . . . . . . . . . . . . . . . . . . . . . . . . . .448
w/sausage . . . . . . . . . . . . . . . . . . . . . . . . . . . .451
thin crust, cheese . . . . . . . . . . . . . . . . . . . . . . . .273
w/anchovy . . . . . . . . . . . . . . . . . . . . . . . . . . . . .307
w/extra cheese . . . . . . . . . . . . . . . . . . . . . . . . .321
w/green pepper . . . . . . . . . . . . . . . . . . . . . . . . .277
w/mushrooms . . . . . . . . . . . . . . . . . . . . . . . . . .279
w/olives, ripe . . . . . . . . . . . . . . . . . . . . . . . . . .294
w/onion . . . . . . . . . . . . . . . . . . . . . . . . . . . . . .276
w/pepperoni . . . . . . . . . . . . . . . . . . . . . . . . . . .347
w/sausage . . . . . . . . . . . . . . . . . . . . . . . . . . . .350
6" deep dish, 1 pie
cheese . . . . . . . . . . . . . . . . . . . . . . . . . . . . . . .598
w/anchovy . . . . . . . . . . . . . . . . . . . . . . . . . . . . .643
w/beef . . . . . . . . . . . . . . . . . . . . . . . . . . . . . . .642
w/extra cheese . . . . . . . . . . . . . . . . . . . . . . . . .656
w/green pepper . . . . . . . . . . . . . . . . . . . . . . . . .600
w/mushrooms . . . . . . . . . . . . . . . . . . . . . . . . . .600
w/olives, ripe . . . . . . . . . . . . . . . . . . . . . . . . . .609
w/onion . . . . . . . . . . . . . . . . . . . . . . . . . . . . . .601
w/pepperoni . . . . . . . . . . . . . . . . . . . . . . . . . . .647
w/sausage . . . . . . . . . . . . . . . . . . . . . . . . . . . .642

**Donut,** 1 pc., except as noted:
(*Entenmann's* Donut Dippers) . . . . . . . . . . . . . . . . . . . . .160
plain (*Awrey's*), 1.5 oz. . . . . . . . . . . . . . . . . . . . . . . . .150
plain (*Awrey's*), 2 oz. . . . . . . . . . . . . . . . . . . . . . . . . .210
chocolate iced/frosted:
(*Awrey's*), 1.75 oz. . . . . . . . . . . . . . . . . . . . . . . .200
(*Awrey's* Ring), 2.7 oz. . . . . . . . . . . . . . . . . . . . . .300
(*Entenmann's* Rich) . . . . . . . . . . . . . . . . . . . . . . . .280
(*Entenmann's PopEms*), 4 pcs. . . . . . . . . . . . . . . . . .280
chocolate (*Awrey's*), 1.75 oz. . . . . . . . . . . . . . . . . . .190
custard (*Awrey's* Bismark) . . . . . . . . . . . . . . . . . . . .330
milk chocolate (*Entenmann's*) . . . . . . . . . . . . . . . . . .320
mini (*Entenmann's*) . . . . . . . . . . . . . . . . . . . . . . . . .150
sour cream (*Awrey's*), 3 oz. . . . . . . . . . . . . . . . . . . .310
sour cream (*Awrey's*), 3.75 oz. . . . . . . . . . . . . . . . . .430
cinnamon sugar sour cream (*Awrey's*) . . . . . . . . . . . . . . .260
coconut top (*Awrey's*), 1.75 oz. . . . . . . . . . . . . . . . . . . .210
cruller (*Entenmann's*) . . . . . . . . . . . . . . . . . . . . . . . . . .220
crumb (*Entenmann's*) . . . . . . . . . . . . . . . . . . . . . . . . . .260
crunch (*Awrey's*) . . . . . . . . . . . . . . . . . . . . . . . . . . . .280
crunch-topped (*Awrey's*) . . . . . . . . . . . . . . . . . . . . . . . .160
devil's food, frosted (*Entenmann's*) . . . . . . . . . . . . . . . . .310
devil's food, glazed (*Awrey's*) . . . . . . . . . . . . . . . . . . . .300
glazed (*Entenmann's Little Bites*), 4 pcs. . . . . . . . . . . . . . .220
glazed (*Entenmann's PopEms*), 4 pcs. . . . . . . . . . . . . . . . .210
glazed, sour cream (*Awrey's*), 3 oz. . . . . . . . . . . . . . . . . .240
glazed, sour cream (*Awrey's*), 3.75 oz. . . . . . . . . . . . . . . .420
glazed, stick (*Awrey's* Twin Pack) . . . . . . . . . . . . . . . . . .300
jelly, powdered sugar (*Awrey's* Bismark) . . . . . . . . . . . . . .250
jelly, vanilla-iced (*Awrey's* Bismark) . . . . . . . . . . . . . . . .320
powdered sugar (*Awrey's*), 1.5 oz. . . . . . . . . . . . . . . . . . .160
powdered sugar (*Awrey's*), 2.25 oz. . . . . . . . . . . . . . . . . .240
powdered sugar (*Entenmann's*) . . . . . . . . . . . . . . . . . . . .220
powdered sugar, mini (*Entenmann's Popettes*),
4 pcs. . . . . . . . . . . . . . . . . . . . . . . . . . . . . . . . . . . .280
sour cream (*Awrey's*) . . . . . . . . . . . . . . . . . . . . . . . . . .370
sprinkle-topped (*Awrey's*) . . . . . . . . . . . . . . . . . . . . . . .160
vanilla-iced (*Awrey's* Long John) . . . . . . . . . . . . . . . . . . .370
white-iced (*Awrey's*) . . . . . . . . . . . . . . . . . . . . . . . . . .200

**Drum,** freshwater, meat only:
raw, 4 oz. . . . . . . . . . . . . . . . . . . . . . . . . . . . . . . . . . . . .135
baked, broiled, or microwaved, 4 oz. . . . . . . . . . . . . . . . . .173
**Duck, domesticated,** roasted:
meat w/skin, 4 oz. . . . . . . . . . . . . . . . . . . . . . . . . . . . . . .382
meat only, 4 oz. . . . . . . . . . . . . . . . . . . . . . . . . . . . . . . . .228
**Duck sauce,** see "Sweet and sour sauce"
**Duck sausage,** see "Sausage"
**Dulce de leche topping** (*Smucker's*), 2 tbsp. . . . . . . . . . . .110
**Dumpling,** see "Pasta"
**Dumpling entree,** Oriental style, frozen (*Lean Cuisine Everyday Favorites*), 9 oz. . . . . . . . . . . . . . . . . . . . . . . . .290
**Dumpling squash,** see "Sweet dumpling squash"
**Eclair,** chocolate (*Entennman's*), 1 pc. . . . . . . . . . . . . . . . .260
**Edamame** (see also "Soybean"), fresh (*Yoshinoya*), ½ cup . . . . . . . . . . . . . . . . . . . . . . . . . . . . . . . . . . . . .120
**Edamame,** frozen, in pod (*Cascadian Farm*), ⅔ cup . . . . . .120
**Eel,** meat only:
raw, 4 oz. . . . . . . . . . . . . . . . . . . . . . . . . . . . . . . . . . . . .209
baked, broiled, or microwaved, 4 oz. . . . . . . . . . . . . . . . . .268
**Egg, chicken:**
raw, 1 extra large (*Land O Lakes*) . . . . . . . . . . . . . . . . . . . . . .80
raw, 1 large (*Land O Lakes*) . . . . . . . . . . . . . . . . . . . . . . . . .70
cooked, hard-boiled, chopped, 1 cup . . . . . . . . . . . . . . . . . .210
**Egg, substitute,** ¼ cup:
(*Egg Beaters*) . . . . . . . . . . . . . . . . . . . . . . . . . . . . . . . . . . .30
(*Healthy Choice*) . . . . . . . . . . . . . . . . . . . . . . . . . . . . . . . . .30
(*Morningstar Farms Better'n Eggs*) . . . . . . . . . . . . . . . . . . . .20
(*Morningstar Farms Scramblers*) . . . . . . . . . . . . . . . . . . . . . .35
(*Tofutti Egg Watchers*) . . . . . . . . . . . . . . . . . . . . . . . . . . . . .30
**Egg breakfast,** frozen (see also "Breakfast sandwich" and specific listings), 1 pkg.:
omelette, ham and cheese (*Great Starts*), 5.2 oz. . . . . . . . .250
scrambled, w/sausage (*Great Starts*), 6.25 oz. . . . . . . . . . .360
**Egg roll,** frozen:
chicken (*Chun King/La Choy* Restaurant), 3-oz. roll . . . . . . .210
chicken (*Yu Sing*), 6 rolls, 3 oz. . . . . . . . . . . . . . . . . . . . . .180
chicken, mini (*Chun King/La Choy*), 6 rolls . . . . . . . . . . . . .210
chicken, sweet and sour (*Yu Sing*), 6 rolls, 3 oz. . . . . . . . . .190
pork, sweet and sour (*Yu Sing*), 6 rolls, 3 oz. . . . . . . . . . . .210

pork and shrimp (*Yu Sing*), 6 rolls, 3 oz. . . . . . . . . . . . . . . .200
pork and shrimp, bite-size (*La Choy*), 12 rolls . . . . . . . . . . .210
pork and shrimp, mini (*Chun King/La Choy*), 6 rolls . . . . . .210
shrimp (*Chun King/La Choy* Restaurant), 3-oz. roll . . . . . . .180
shrimp (*Yu Sing*), 6 rolls, 3 oz. . . . . . . . . . . . . . . . . . . . . . .180
shrimp, mini (*Chun King/La Choy*), 6 rolls . . . . . . . . . . . . .190
vegetable w/lobster, mini (*La Choy*), 6 rolls . . . . . . . . . . . .190
**Egg roll, refrigerated,** 1 roll w/sauce pkt.:
shrimp (*Chung's*) . . . . . . . . . . . . . . . . . . . . . . . . . . . . . . . . .140
vegetable (*Chung's*) . . . . . . . . . . . . . . . . . . . . . . . . . . . . . .130
**Egg roll wrapper** (see also "Wrappers"):
(*Frieda's*), 2 pcs. . . . . . . . . . . . . . . . . . . . . . . . . . . . . . . .130
(*Nasoya*), 3 pcs. . . . . . . . . . . . . . . . . . . . . . . . . . . . . . . . .170
**Egg sandwich,** see "Breakfast sandwich"
**Eggnog,** dairy (*Turkey Hill*), ½ cup . . . . . . . . . . . . . . . . . .190
**Eggplant,** fresh:
raw (*Frieda's* Chinese/Japanese), ⅔ cup, 3 oz. . . . . . . . . . . .20
raw, 1" pcs., ½ cup . . . . . . . . . . . . . . . . . . . . . . . . . . . . . . . .11
boiled, drained, 1" cubes, 1 cup . . . . . . . . . . . . . . . . . . . . . .28
**Eggplant appetizer:**
(*Alessi* Caponata), ⅓ cup . . . . . . . . . . . . . . . . . . . . . . . . . .140
(*Cedar's* Baba Ghannouj), 2 tbsp. . . . . . . . . . . . . . . . . . . . . .50
(*Cento* Caponata), 2 tbsp. . . . . . . . . . . . . . . . . . . . . . . . . . . .30
(*Sabra Salads* Babaganoush/Hungarian), 1 oz. . . . . . . . . . . .77
(*Yorgo* Baba Ghannouj), 2 tbsp. . . . . . . . . . . . . . . . . . . . . . .50
marinated (*Casa Visco*), 1 oz. . . . . . . . . . . . . . . . . . . . . . . . .15
**Eggplant dip** (*Victoria*), 2 tbsp. . . . . . . . . . . . . . . . . . . . . .30
**Eggplant dish,** frozen, Parmesan (*Mrs. Paul's*), ½ cup . . . .190
**Eggplant entree,** frozen, 1 pkg., except as noted:
Parmesan (*Wolfgang Puck's*), 9 oz. . . . . . . . . . . . . . . . . . .300
parmigiana (*Celentano*), 10 oz. . . . . . . . . . . . . . . . . . . . . . .350
parmigiana (*DeLuca* Refrigerated), 1 cup . . . . . . . . . . . . . .220
parmigiana, w/linguine (*Michelina's*), 8 oz. . . . . . . . . . . . .270
rollettes (*Celentano*), 10 oz. . . . . . . . . . . . . . . . . . . . . . . . .290
**Empañada,** frozen, beef (*Goya*), 2 pcs. . . . . . . . . . . . . . . . .350
**Enchilada,** frozen, w/sauce, 4.5-oz. pc.:
beef (*El Monterey Family Classics*) . . . . . . . . . . . . . . . . . .180
cheese (*El Monterey Family Classics*) . . . . . . . . . . . . . . . .210
chicken (*El Monterey Family Classics*) . . . . . . . . . . . . . . .190
vegetable, garden (*Cedarlane* Low Fat) . . . . . . . . . . . . . . .140

**Enchilada dinner,** frozen, 1 pkg.:
beef (*Patio*), 11 oz. . . . . . . . . . . . . . . . . . . . . . . . . . . . . .370
beef, and tamales (*Patio*), 12.25 oz. . . . . . . . . . . . . . . . . . .480
cheese (*Patio*), 11 oz. . . . . . . . . . . . . . . . . . . . . . . . . . . . .350
chicken (*Healthy Choice*), 11.3 oz. . . . . . . . . . . . . . . . . . . .270
chicken con queso (*Patio*), 11 oz. . . . . . . . . . . . . . . . . . . . .350
combination (*Patio*), 11 oz. . . . . . . . . . . . . . . . . . . . . . . . .370
**Enchilada entree,** frozen, 1 pkg., except as noted:
beef (*Ortega*), 9⅜ oz. . . . . . . . . . . . . . . . . . . . . . . . . . . . .360
beef (*Patio* Platter), 2 pcs. . . . . . . . . . . . . . . . . . . . . . . . .190
beef and tamale (*Banquet*), 11 oz. . . . . . . . . . . . . . . . . . . . .450
beef and tamale, chili gravy w/ (*Morton*), 10 oz. . . . . . . . . .350
black bean vegetable (*Amy's*), ½ of 9.5-oz. pkg. . . . . . . . . .130
cheese (*Amy's*), ½ of 9.5-oz. pkg. . . . . . . . . . . . . . . . . . . .210
cheese (*Amy's* Family), ⅐ of 35-oz. pkg. . . . . . . . . . . . . . .240
cheese (*Ortega*), 9.75 oz. . . . . . . . . . . . . . . . . . . . . . . . . .410
cheese or chicken (*Banquet*), 11 oz. . . . . . . . . . . . . . . . . . .350
chicken (*Healthy Choice* Solos), 9 oz. . . . . . . . . . . . . . . . . .310
chicken (*Lean Cuisine Everyday Favorites*), 9 oz. . . . . . . . . .280
chicken (*Ortega*), 9.5 oz. . . . . . . . . . . . . . . . . . . . . . . . . .400
chicken and cheese (*Michelina's*), 8 oz. . . . . . . . . . . . . . . .420
combo (*Patio* Platter), 2 pcs. . . . . . . . . . . . . . . . . . . . . . .190
combo, Mexican style (*Banquet*), 11 oz. . . . . . . . . . . . . . . .370
pie, 3-layer (*Cedarlane*), ½ of 10-oz. pkg. . . . . . . . . . . . . .216
vegetarian (*Cascadian Farm*), 10 oz. . . . . . . . . . . . . . . . . . .370
**Enchilada sauce,** ¼ cup:
(*La Victoria*) . . . . . . . . . . . . . . . . . . . . . . . . . . . . . . . . . .25
green chili (*La Victoria*) . . . . . . . . . . . . . . . . . . . . . . . . . .15
green chili (*Las Palmas*) . . . . . . . . . . . . . . . . . . . . . . . . . .25
green chili, mild (*Old El Paso*) . . . . . . . . . . . . . . . . . . . . . .30
hot or mild (*Old El Paso*) . . . . . . . . . . . . . . . . . . . . . . . . . .20
medium (*Hatch*) . . . . . . . . . . . . . . . . . . . . . . . . . . . . . . . . .35
mild or hot (*Hatch*) . . . . . . . . . . . . . . . . . . . . . . . . . . . . . .25
**Enchilada sauce seasoning mix** (*Lawry's*), 2 tsp. . . . . . . . . .20
**Endive, Belgian,** see "Chicory, witloof"
**Escarole,** see "Endive"

# F

**FOOD AND MEASURE** **CALORIES**

**Fajita entree,** frozen:
beef (*Tyson* Meal Kit), ½ pkg. . . . . . . . . . . . . . . . . . . . . . .480
chicken (*Tyson* Meal Kit), ½ pkg. . . . . . . . . . . . . . . . . . . . .460
**Fajita filling,** chicken or steak (*Ortega* Skillet), ½ cup . . . . .35
**Fajita sauce,** 2 tbsp.:
chicken (*Lawry's* Weekday Gourmet) . . . . . . . . . . . . . . . . .20
and marinade, Mexican style (*World Harbors*) . . . . . . . . . . .45
**Fajita seasoning** (*McCormick*), ¼ tsp. . . . . . . . . . . . . . . . . . .0
**Fajita seasoning mix:**
(*Chi-Chi's*), ¼ pkg. . . . . . . . . . . . . . . . . . . . . . . . . . . . . .35
(*El Torito*), ¼ pkg. . . . . . . . . . . . . . . . . . . . . . . . . . . . . .35
(*Lawry's*), 2 tsp. . . . . . . . . . . . . . . . . . . . . . . . . . . . . . .15
(*McCormick*), ⅛ pkg. . . . . . . . . . . . . . . . . . . . . . . . . . . .15
chicken (*Lawry's*), 1 tsp. . . . . . . . . . . . . . . . . . . . . . . . . .10
**Falafel mix** (*Near East*), about 5 fried patties* . . . . . . . . . .230
**Farina, whole-grain** (see also "Cereal"), dry, 1 oz. . . . . . . .105
**Farro,** see "Spelt"
**Fava bean,** see "Broad bean" and "Habas"
**Feijoa,** raw (*Frieda's*), 5 oz. . . . . . . . . . . . . . . . . . . . . . . .70
**Fennel,** bulb, raw:
(*Frieda's*), ¾ cup, 3 oz. . . . . . . . . . . . . . . . . . . . . . . . . . .25
sliced, ½ cup . . . . . . . . . . . . . . . . . . . . . . . . . . . . . . . . . .27
**Fennel seed,** 1 tsp. . . . . . . . . . . . . . . . . . . . . . . . . . . . . . .7
**Fettuccine,** dry, see "Pasta"
**Fettuccine, refrigerated:**
(*Buitoni*), 1¼ cups . . . . . . . . . . . . . . . . . . . . . . . . . . . . .240
spinach (*Buitoni*), 1¼ cups . . . . . . . . . . . . . . . . . . . . . . . .250
**Fettuccine dish, mix:**
Alfredo (*Knorr* Side Dish), ¾ cup . . . . . . . . . . . . . . . . . . . .280
w/creamy basil sauce (*Knorr TasteBreaks* Cup), 1 cont. . . . .220
**Fettuccine entree,** frozen, 1 pkg., except as noted:
Alfredo (*Michelina's*), 9 oz. . . . . . . . . . . . . . . . . . . . . . . . .380
Alfredo (*Stouffer's*), 11.5 oz. . . . . . . . . . . . . . . . . . . . . . . .540
Alfredo, w/broccoli, chicken (*Michelina's*), 8.5 oz. . . . . . . . .310

**Fettuccine entree**, frozen ***(cont.)***
Alfredo, w/4 cheeses (*Budget Gourmet*), 8 oz. . . . . . . . . . .290
Alfredo, w/mushrooms (*Cascadian Farm*), 10 oz. . . . . . . . .360
chicken w/, see "Chicken entree, frozen"
w/chicken (*Michelina's*), 8 oz. . . . . . . . . . . . . . . . . . . . . . .280
primavera (*Lean Cuisine Everyday Favorites*), 10 oz. . . . . . .260
primavera (*Michelina's*), 8 oz. . . . . . . . . . . . . . . . . . . . . . .270
primavera, herb sauce, chicken (*Budget Gourmet*), 8.5 oz. .230
**Fig,** fresh:
1 medium, 1.8 oz. . . . . . . . . . . . . . . . . . . . . . . . . . . . . . .37
California, 2 oz., 4 pcs. . . . . . . . . . . . . . . . . . . . . . . . . .143
**Fig, canned,** Kadota, in heavy syrup (*Oregon*), ½ cup . . . .130
**Fig, dried:**
crown (*Frieda's*), 3 pcs., 1.4 oz. . . . . . . . . . . . . . . . . . . . .100
Kalamata (*Krinos*), 3 pcs., 1.4 oz. . . . . . . . . . . . . . . . . . . .100
Mission (*Frieda's*), ¼ cup, 1.4 oz. . . . . . . . . . . . . . . . . . . .110
Mission (*Sun•Maid Fast Fruit*), 1.5 oz., 3–4 pcs. . . . . . . . . .120
**Filberts:**
raw, diced (*Blue Diamond* Hazelnuts), ¼ cup . . . . . . . . . . .200
dried, 1 oz. . . . . . . . . . . . . . . . . . . . . . . . . . . . . . . . . . . .179
oil-roasted, 1 oz. . . . . . . . . . . . . . . . . . . . . . . . . . . . . . .187
**Filodough,** frozen (*Apollo/Athens*), 2 oz. . . . . . . . . . . . . .180
**Fish,** see specific listings
**"Fish," vegetarian,** frozen (*Worthington* Fillets), 2 pcs. . . .180
**Fish dinner,** frozen, 1 pkg.:
and chips (*Swanson Traditional Favorites*), 10 oz. . . . . . . . .490
herb-baked (*Healthy Choice*), 10.9 oz. . . . . . . . . . . . . . . . .360
**Fish entree,** frozen (see also specific fish listings):
au gratin, baked (*Gorton's*), 1 pc. . . . . . . . . . . . . . . . . . . .130
cakes (*Mrs. Paul's*), 2 pcs. . . . . . . . . . . . . . . . . . . . . . . . .210
w/cheese, salsa (*Oven Poppers*), ½ of 9-oz. pkg. . . . . . . . .130
croquette (*Dr. Praeger's*), 2.2-oz. pc. . . . . . . . . . . . . . . . . .120
fillet, w/macaroni/cheese (*Stouffer's* Homestyle), 9 oz. . . . .410
fillet, battered (*Gorton's*), 2 pcs. . . . . . . . . . . . . . . . . . . . .240
fillet, battered (*Mrs. Paul's*), 1 pc. . . . . . . . . . . . . . . . . . .150
fillet, battered (*Mrs. Paul's* Hearty Size), 1 pc. . . . . . . . . . .200
fillet, battered, lemon pepper (*Gorton's*), 2 pcs. . . . . . . . . .270
fillet, breaded:
(*Dr. Praeger's* Sandwich), 4-oz. pc. . . . . . . . . . . . . . . . .210

(*Gorton's*), 2 pcs. . . . . . . . . . . . . . . . . . . . . . . . . . .250
(*Mrs. Paul's*), 2 pcs. . . . . . . . . . . . . . . . . . . . . . . . .280
(*Mrs. Paul's* Crisp & Healthy), 1 pc. . . . . . . . . . . . . . . . .130
(*Van de Kamp's*), 2 pcs. . . . . . . . . . . . . . . . . . . . . . .260
(*Van de Kamp's* Hearty Size), 1 pc. . . . . . . . . . . . . . . . .150
garlic and herb (*Gorton's*), 2 pcs. . . . . . . . . . . . . . . . . .270
lemon pepper or seasoned (*Gorton's* Skillet), 1 pc. . . . .220
Parmesan (*Gorton's*), 2 pcs. . . . . . . . . . . . . . . . . . . . .250
ranch (*Gorton's*), 2 pcs. . . . . . . . . . . . . . . . . . . . . . .240
fillet, grilled, 1 pc.:
Cajun, garlic butter, or lemon pepper (*Mrs. Paul's*) . . . . .130
char-grilled (*Gorton's Grilled Fillets*) . . . . . . . . . . . . . . .110
garlic butter, lemon butter/pepper (*Van de Kamp's*) . . . .120
Italian herb or lemon pepper (*Gorton's Grilled Fillets*) . . .100
portions, battered (*Van de Kamp's*), 1 pc. . . . . . . . . . . . . .160
portions, breaded (*Fisher Boy*), 2 pcs. . . . . . . . . . . . . . . .200
portions, breaded (*Van de Kamp's*), 3 pcs. . . . . . . . . . . . .360
w/shrimp, crab, vegetables (*Oven Poppers*), 4.5-oz. pc. . . .200
w/spinach, cheese (*Oven Poppers*), 4.5-oz. pc. . . . . . . . . . .160
sticks (*Banquet*), 6.6-oz. pkg. . . . . . . . . . . . . . . . . . . . .270
sticks (*Freezer Queen* Meal), 6.5-oz. pkg. . . . . . . . . . . . . .290
sticks, battered (*Gorton's*), 5 pcs. . . . . . . . . . . . . . . . . . .290
sticks, breaded (*Fisher Boy*), 6 pcs. . . . . . . . . . . . . . . . . .190
sticks, breaded (*Gorton's*), 6 pcs. . . . . . . . . . . . . . . . . . .260
sticks, breaded (*Mrs. Paul's*), 6 pcs. . . . . . . . . . . . . . . . .250
sticks, breaded (*Mrs. Paul's* Crisp & Healthy), 6 pcs. . . . . .190
sticks, breaded (*Van de Kamp's*), 6 pcs. . . . . . . . . . . . . . .290
sticks, breaded, mini (*Gorton's*), 13 pcs. . . . . . . . . . . . . .250
tenders (*Gorton's* Original Batter), 4 oz. . . . . . . . . . . . . . .260
tenders, breaded (*Gorton's* Extra Crunchy), 4 oz. . . . . . . . .270
tenders, lemon herb, breaded (*Gorton's*), 4 oz. . . . . . . . . . .260
**Fish sandwich,** frozen (*Hormel Quick Meal*), 1 pc. . . . . . .420
**Fish seasoning and coating mix:**
(*Old Bay Better Batter*), ¼ cup . . . . . . . . . . . . . . . . . . . .110
fish and chips or seafood (*Don's Chuck Wagon*), ¼ cup . . . .95
fish fry (*Sylvia's*), 3 tbsp. . . . . . . . . . . . . . . . . . . . . . . .100
**Flatfish,** meat only:
raw, 4 oz. . . . . . . . . . . . . . . . . . . . . . . . . . . . . . . . . .104
baked, broiled, or microwaved, 4 oz. . . . . . . . . . . . . . . . . .133

**Flax powder** (*Arrowhead Mills* Nutri), 2 tbsp. . . . . . . . . . . . .70
**Flounder,** fresh, see "Flatfish"
**Flounder entree,** frozen:
au gratin (*Oven Poppers*), 5-oz. pc. . . . . . . . . . . . . . . . . . .220
fillet, breaded (*Mrs. Paul's* Premium), 2.8-oz. pc. . . . . . . . . .170
fillet, breaded (*Van de Kamp's* Premium), 4-oz. pc. . . . . . . .230
stuffed w/broccoli/cheese (*Oven Poppers*), 5-oz. pc. . . . . . .150
stuffed w/crab or garlic/shrimp (*Oven Poppers*),
5-oz. pc. . . . . . . . . . . . . . . . . . . . . . . . . . . . . . . . . . . . .250
**Flour,** see "Wheat flour" and specific listings
**Frankfurter,** 1 link, except as noted:
(*Ball Park* Singles) . . . . . . . . . . . . . . . . . . . . . . . . . . . . .150
(*Boar's Head* Natural Casing/Skinless) . . . . . . . . . . . . . . .150
(*Healthy Choice* 10 Pack), 1.4 oz. . . . . . . . . . . . . . . . . . . .70
(*Healthy Choice* 8 Pack), 1.75 oz. . . . . . . . . . . . . . . . . . . .60
(*Hormel* Fat Free Hot Dogs) . . . . . . . . . . . . . . . . . . . . . . .45
(*Johnsonville* Wieners), 1.7 oz. . . . . . . . . . . . . . . . . . . . .150
(*Light & Lean*) . . . . . . . . . . . . . . . . . . . . . . . . . . . . . . . .45
beef (*Ball Park*), 2 oz. . . . . . . . . . . . . . . . . . . . . . . . . . .180
beef (*Boar's Head* Lite) . . . . . . . . . . . . . . . . . . . . . . . . . .90
beef (*Boar's Head* Natural Casing) . . . . . . . . . . . . . . . . . .160
beef (*Hebrew National*) . . . . . . . . . . . . . . . . . . . . . . . . . .150
beef (*Hebrew National* Family/Party Pack) . . . . . . . . . . . . .180
beef (*Hormel* Natural Casing) . . . . . . . . . . . . . . . . . . . . . .210
beef, cocktail (*Boar's Head*), 5 links . . . . . . . . . . . . . . . .170
beef, cocktail (*Hebrew National*), 5 links, 2 oz. . . . . . . . . . .180
beef, dinner (*Hebrew National* ¼ Pound) . . . . . . . . . . . . . .350
chicken (*Wampler*), 2 oz. . . . . . . . . . . . . . . . . . . . . . . . . .120
smoked (*Oscar Mayer Big & Juicy* Smokie), 2.7 oz. . . . . . .210
smoked (*Wranglers*) . . . . . . . . . . . . . . . . . . . . . . . . . . . .170
turkey (*Jennie-O*) . . . . . . . . . . . . . . . . . . . . . . . . . . . . . .80
turkey (*Jennie-O* Jumbo) . . . . . . . . . . . . . . . . . . . . . . . . .130
(*Wampler*), 1.6 oz. . . . . . . . . . . . . . . . . . . . . . . . . . . . . .90
**Frankfurter, canned** (*Vienna* Big Foot Hot Dog),
2 oz. . . . . . . . . . . . . . . . . . . . . . . . . . . . . . . . . . . . . . . .150
**Frankfurter, wrapped,** 1 pc., except as noted:
beef (*Hebrew National* Franks-in-a-Blanket), 5 pcs. . . . . . . .290
corn dog (*Hormel Quick Meal*) . . . . . . . . . . . . . . . . . . . . .272
corn dog (*State Fair*) . . . . . . . . . . . . . . . . . . . . . . . . . . .170
corn dog, beef or cheese (*State Fair*) . . . . . . . . . . . . . . . .180

corn dog, mini (*Hormel Quick Meal*), 10 pcs. . . . . . . . . . . .490
corn dog, mini (*State Fair*), 4 pcs. . . . . . . . . . . . . . . . . . . .230
corn dog, mini, beef or cheese (*State Fair*), 4 pcs. . . . . . . .250
**French toast breakfast,** frozen, 1 pkg.:
w/sausage (*Great Starts*), 5.5 oz. . . . . . . . . . . . . . . . . . . . .410
w/sausage, cinnamon swirl (*Great Starts*), 5.5 oz. . . . . . . . .440
sticks, w/syrup (*Great Starts*), 4.25 oz. . . . . . . . . . . . . . . . .420
**Frosting,** ready-to-spread, 2 tbsp.:
all varieties, except chocolate and coconut flavors
(*Duncan Hines*) . . . . . . . . . . . . . . . . . . . . . . . . . . . . . . .140
banana creme (*Pillsbury* Creamy Supreme) . . . . . . . . . . . .150
butter cream (*Creamy Deluxe*) . . . . . . . . . . . . . . . . . . . . . .140
butter cream, whipped (*Betty Crocker*) . . . . . . . . . . . . . . . .100
cherry (*Creamy Deluxe*) . . . . . . . . . . . . . . . . . . . . . . . . . . .140
chocolate, all varieties (*Creamy Deluxe*) . . . . . . . . . . . . . . .130
chocolate, all varieties (*Duncan Hines*) . . . . . . . . . . . . . . . .130
chocolate, all varieties (*Pillsbury* Creamy Supreme) . . . . . .140
chocolate, milk, whipped (*Betty Crocker*) . . . . . . . . . . . . . .100
chocolate, whipped (*Betty Crocker*) . . . . . . . . . . . . . . . . . . .90
coconut or coconut pecan (*Duncan Hines*) . . . . . . . . . . . . .150
coconut pecan or cream cheese (*Creamy Deluxe*) . . . . . . . .140
cream cheese (*Pillsbury* Creamy Supreme) . . . . . . . . . . . . .150
cream cheese, whipped (*Betty Crocker*) . . . . . . . . . . . . . . .100
fudge, hot (*Pillsbury* Creamy Supreme) . . . . . . . . . . . . . . .140
lemon (*Creamy Deluxe*) . . . . . . . . . . . . . . . . . . . . . . . . . . .140
lemon, whipped (*Betty Crocker*) . . . . . . . . . . . . . . . . . . . . .100
sour cream, chocolate (*Creamy Deluxe*) . . . . . . . . . . . . . . .130
sour cream, white (*Creamy Deluxe*) . . . . . . . . . . . . . . . . . .140
strawberry, cream cheese (*Creamy Deluxe*) . . . . . . . . . . . .140
strawberry, whipped (*Betty Crocker*) . . . . . . . . . . . . . . . . .100
vanilla, French or regular (*Creamy Deluxe*) . . . . . . . . . . . .140
vanilla, whipped (*Betty Crocker*) . . . . . . . . . . . . . . . . . . . .100
white, fluffy, whipped (*Betty Crocker*) . . . . . . . . . . . . . . . .100
**Frosting mix,** white, fluffy (*Betty Crocker*), 6 tbsp.* . . . . . .100
**Fruit,** see specific listings
**Fruit, mixed, candied** (*Seneca* Glacé Deluxe), 2 tbsp. . . . . .70
**Fruit, mixed, can or chilled** (see also "Fruit cocktail"),
½ cup, except as noted:
in juice (*Del Monte* Fruit Naturals Chunky) . . . . . . . . . . . . . .60
in juice (*Del Monte* Fruit Naturals Snack Cup), 4 oz. . . . . . . .50

**Fruit, mixed, can or chilled *(cont.)***
in juice (*Libby's Lite* Chunky) . . . . . . . . . . . . . . . . . . . . . . . .60
in juice, pineapple/passion, tropical salad (*Del Monte*) . . . . .60
in extra light syrup (*Del Monte* Lite Chunky) . . . . . . . . . . . . .60
in extra light syrup (*Del Monte* Lite Snack Cup), 4 oz. . . . . . .50
in extra light syrup (*Sunfresh* Fruit Salad Chilled) . . . . . . . . .70
in extra light syrup, Ambrosia (*Sunfresh* Chilled) . . . . . . . . .70
in extra light syrup, citrus or tropical (*Sunfresh* Chilled) . . . .80
in light syrup (*Sunfresh* Chilled Mixed Fruit) . . . . . . . . . . . . .90
in light syrup, California (*Del Monte Orchard Select*) . . . . . .80
in light syrup, tropical, w/passion fruit juice (*Del Monte*) . . . .80
in light syrup, tropical (*Dole*) . . . . . . . . . . . . . . . . . . . . . . .80
in heavy syrup (*Del Monte* Chunky) . . . . . . . . . . . . . . . . . .100
in heavy syrup (*Del Monte* Snack Cup), 4 oz. . . . . . . . . . . . . .80
**Fruit, mixed, dried:**
(*Sun•Maid*), ¼ cup . . . . . . . . . . . . . . . . . . . . . . . . . . . . . .110
(*Sunsweet* Fruit Morsels), ¼ cup, 1.4 oz. . . . . . . . . . . . . . . .120
Island mix (*Sunsweet Fruitlings*), ⅓ cup, 1.4 oz. . . . . . . . . .120
tropical (*Sunsweet Fruitlings*), ¼ cup, 1.4 oz. . . . . . . . . . . .140
**Fruit, mixed, frozen:**
(*Big Valley*), ⅔ cup . . . . . . . . . . . . . . . . . . . . . . . . . . . . . .60
(*Birds Eye*), ½ cup . . . . . . . . . . . . . . . . . . . . . . . . . . . . . .90
(*McKenzie's*), ⅓ of 16-oz. pkg. . . . . . . . . . . . . . . . . . . . . . .60
**Fruit bar,** frozen (see also "Sorbet bar"), 1 pc.:
all fruits (*Ocean Spray*) . . . . . . . . . . . . . . . . . . . . . . . . . . .45
all fruits (*Ocean Spray* No Sugar) . . . . . . . . . . . . . . . . . . . .25
all fruits (*Popsicle* Fruit Juicee) . . . . . . . . . . . . . . . . . . . . .60
banana cream (*FrozFruit*) . . . . . . . . . . . . . . . . . . . . . . . . .150
banana cream, chocolate-dipped (*Dreyer's/Edy's*) . . . . . . . .190
banana cream, chocolate-dipped (*FrozFruit*) . . . . . . . . . . . .210
cantaloupe (*FrozFruit*) . . . . . . . . . . . . . . . . . . . . . . . . . . . .60
cherry or watermelon (*FrozFruit*) . . . . . . . . . . . . . . . . . . . . .70
coconut cream (*FrozFruit*) . . . . . . . . . . . . . . . . . . . . . . . . .200
coconut cream, chocolate-dipped (*FrozFruit*) . . . . . . . . . . .240
lemon or pineapple (*FrozFruit*) . . . . . . . . . . . . . . . . . . . . . . .80
lemonade or lime (*Dreyer's/Edy's*) . . . . . . . . . . . . . . . . . . . .80
lime, strawberry, and wildberry (*Dreyer's/Edy's*) . . . . . . . . . .60
lime, tropical, or strawberry (*FrozFruit*) . . . . . . . . . . . . . . . .90
mango (*FrozFruit*) . . . . . . . . . . . . . . . . . . . . . . . . . . . . . . .110
piña colada cream (*FrozFruit*) . . . . . . . . . . . . . . . . . . . . . .180

strawberry (*Dreyer's/Edy's*) . . . . . . . . . . . . . . . . . . . . . . . . .80
strawberry cream (*FrozFruit*) . . . . . . . . . . . . . . . . . . . . . .150
strawberry cream, chocolate-dipped (*Dreyer's/Edy's*) . . . . .190
strawberry cream, chocolate-dipped (*FrozFruit*) . . . . . . . . .200
**Fruit cocktail,** canned, ½ cup:
(*Del Monte Very Cherry*) . . . . . . . . . . . . . . . . . . . . . . . . .90
in juice (*Del Monte* Fruit Naturals) . . . . . . . . . . . . . . . . . .60
in juice (*Libby's Lite*) . . . . . . . . . . . . . . . . . . . . . . . . . . . .60
in extra light syrup (*Del Monte* Lite) . . . . . . . . . . . . . . . . .60
in heavy syrup (*Del Monte*) . . . . . . . . . . . . . . . . . . . . . . .100
**Fruit dip** (see also "Apple dip"), 2 tbsp.:
chocolate (*Marzetti* Fat Free) . . . . . . . . . . . . . . . . . . . . .100
chocolate (*Marzetti* Natural) . . . . . . . . . . . . . . . . . . . . . .120
cream cheese (*Marzetti*) . . . . . . . . . . . . . . . . . . . . . . . . . .70
**Fruit drink blends** (see also specific listings), 8 fl. oz.:
(*Dole* Paradise Blend) . . . . . . . . . . . . . . . . . . . . . . . . . . .120
(*Hawaiian Punch* Juicy Red) . . . . . . . . . . . . . . . . . . . . . .120
(*Snapple* Vitamin Supreme) . . . . . . . . . . . . . . . . . . . . . . .150
punch (*AriZona*) . . . . . . . . . . . . . . . . . . . . . . . . . . . . . . . .110
punch (*Snapple*) . . . . . . . . . . . . . . . . . . . . . . . . . . . . . . . .110
punch (*Tropicana*) . . . . . . . . . . . . . . . . . . . . . . . . . . . . . .130
tropical (*Dole*) . . . . . . . . . . . . . . . . . . . . . . . . . . . . . . . . .160
tropical (*Tropicana Twister*) . . . . . . . . . . . . . . . . . . . . . . .140
**Fruit and nut mix,** see "Trail mix"
**Fruit sauce,** Asian, four (*Heaven and Earth*), 1 tbsp. . . . . . . .20
**Fruit snack,** all varieties:
(*Fruit Roll-Ups*), ½-oz. roll . . . . . . . . . . . . . . . . . . . . . . . . .50
(*Sunkist* Fruit Roll), .75-oz. roll . . . . . . . . . . . . . . . . . . . . .70
**Fruit spread** (see also "Jam and preserves"), all fruits:
(*Cascadian Farm*), 1 tbsp. . . . . . . . . . . . . . . . . . . . . . . . . .40
(*Polaner*), 1 tbsp. . . . . . . . . . . . . . . . . . . . . . . . . . . . . . . .40
**Fudge topping,** see "Chocolate topping"

# G

**FOOD AND MEASURE** | **CALORIES**

**Galanga** (*Frieda's*), ⅔ cup, 3 oz. . . . . . . . . . . . . . . . . . . . .60
**Garbanzo beans,** boiled, ½ cup . . . . . . . . . . . . . . . . . . . .134
**Garbanzo beans,** canned, ½ cup:
(*Bush's Best* Chick Peas) . . . . . . . . . . . . . . . . . . . . . . .130
(*Hain* Organic Chick Peas) . . . . . . . . . . . . . . . . . . . . . .120
**Garbanzo flour** (*Arrowhead Mills*),
¼ cup . . . . . . . . . . . . . . . . . . . . . . . . . . . . . . . . . . . .90
**Garlic,** fresh:
1 clove, .1 oz. . . . . . . . . . . . . . . . . . . . . . . . . . . . . . . .4
granulated or minced, 1 tsp. . . . . . . . . . . . . . . . . . . . . . .13
**Garlic, in jars:**
chopped (*Italian Rose*), 1 tbsp. . . . . . . . . . . . . . . . . . . . .15
marinated (*Frieda's*), 1 oz. . . . . . . . . . . . . . . . . . . . . . . .30
**Garlic, crushed** (*McCormick*), 1 tsp. . . . . . . . . . . . . . . . . .10
**Garlic juice** (*McCormick*), ¼ tsp. . . . . . . . . . . . . . . . . . . . .0
**Garlic oil** (*Watkins* Liquid Spice), 1 tsp. . . . . . . . . . . . . . . .40
**Garlic paste** (*Italia In Tavola*), 1 tbsp. . . . . . . . . . . . . . . . .60
**Garlic salt, pepper, or powder** (*Lawry's*),
¼ tsp. . . . . . . . . . . . . . . . . . . . . . . . . . . . . . . . . . . . .0
**Garlic sauce,** in jars (*Maille* Dipping), 2 tbsp. . . . . . . . . . . .130
**Garlic spread:**
(*Lawry's* Concentrate), 2 tsp. . . . . . . . . . . . . . . . . . . . . . .50
(*McCormick*), ½ tbsp. . . . . . . . . . . . . . . . . . . . . . . . . . . .45
**Gelatin dessert mix*:**
all flavors (*Jell-O*), ½ cup . . . . . . . . . . . . . . . . . . . . . . . .80
all flavors (*Jell-O* Sugar Free), ½ cup . . . . . . . . . . . . . . . . . .10
**Ginger,** trimmed root, sliced, ¼ cup . . . . . . . . . . . . . . . . . . .17
**Ginger, crystallized** (*McCormick*), 1 tsp. . . . . . . . . . . . . . . . .15
**Ginger, ground,** 1 tsp. . . . . . . . . . . . . . . . . . . . . . . . . . . .6
**Ginger, pickled** (*Sushi Chef*), 1 tbsp. . . . . . . . . . . . . . . . . .30
**Ginkgo nut,** canned, drained, 1 oz. . . . . . . . . . . . . . . . . . . .32
**Glaze sauce,** and marinade, Oriental style (*World Harbors*
*Cheriyaki*), 2 tbsp. . . . . . . . . . . . . . . . . . . . . . . . . . . . .50
**Gnocchi,** frozen (*Celentano*), 1 cup . . . . . . . . . . . . . . . . . .210

***Godfather's Pizza,*** 1 slice:
golden:
cheese, medium, ⅛ pie . . . . . . . . . . . . . . . . . . . . . . . . 200
cheese, large, ⅒ pie . . . . . . . . . . . . . . . . . . . . . . . . . . 210
combo, medium, ⅛ pie . . . . . . . . . . . . . . . . . . . . . . . . 250
combo, large, ⅒ pie . . . . . . . . . . . . . . . . . . . . . . . . . . 280
veggie, medium, ⅛ medium or ⅒ large pie . . . . . . . . . 210
original:
cheese, medium, ⅛ pie . . . . . . . . . . . . . . . . . . . . . . . . 230
cheese, large, ⅒ pie . . . . . . . . . . . . . . . . . . . . . . . . . . 260
combo, medium, ⅛ pie . . . . . . . . . . . . . . . . . . . . . . . . 320
combo, large, ⅒ pie . . . . . . . . . . . . . . . . . . . . . . . . . . 350
veggie, medium, ⅛ pie . . . . . . . . . . . . . . . . . . . . . . . . 250
veggie, large, ⅒ pie . . . . . . . . . . . . . . . . . . . . . . . . . . 270
**Goose,** roasted:
meat w/skin, 4 oz. . . . . . . . . . . . . . . . . . . . . . . . . . . . . 346
meat only, 4 oz. . . . . . . . . . . . . . . . . . . . . . . . . . . . . . . 270
**Granola and cereal bar,** 1 bar, except as noted:
all fruits (*Health Valley* Fat Free Fruit/Granola Bar) . . . . . . . . 140
all fruits (*Health Valley* Cobbler/Lowfat Cereal/Tarts) . . . . . . 130
all fruits (*Nutri-Grain* Cereal Bars) . . . . . . . . . . . . . . . . . . . 140
all fruits (*Quaker* Fruit & Oatmeal) . . . . . . . . . . . . . . . . . . 135
all varieties (*Entenmann's* Multi-Grain) . . . . . . . . . . . . . . . 140
apple (*Healthy Valley* Moist & Chewy Granola) . . . . . . . . . . 100
banana (*Nutri-Grain Fruit-full Squares*) . . . . . . . . . . . . . . . 190
banana and strawberry (*Nutri-Grain Twists* Cereal) . . . . . . . 140
berry (*Health Valley* Moist & Chewy Granola) . . . . . . . . . . . 100
berry, mixed (*Nabisco* Fruit 'n Grain) . . . . . . . . . . . . . . . . . 130
w/*Butterfinger* pieces (*Quaker* Chewy Granola) . . . . . . . . . . 120
caramel, chewy (*Hain* Mini Munchie Bar) . . . . . . . . . . . . . . . 90
chocolate chip (*Quaker* Chewy Granola) . . . . . . . . . . . . . . . 120
chocolate peanut butter (*Kashi GoLean*) . . . . . . . . . . . . . . . 290
cinnamon (*Cinnamon Toast Crunch*) . . . . . . . . . . . . . . . . . . 180
cinnamon (*Nature Valley*), 2 bars . . . . . . . . . . . . . . . . . . . 180
cookies and cream (*Kashi GoLean*) . . . . . . . . . . . . . . . . . . . 290
w/*Crunch* pieces (*Quaker* Chewy Granola) . . . . . . . . . . . . . 120
fruit and nut (*Nature Valley* Trail Mix) . . . . . . . . . . . . . . . . 140
honey nut (*Cheerios*) . . . . . . . . . . . . . . . . . . . . . . . . . . . . 160
honey vanilla yogurt (*Kashi GoLean*) . . . . . . . . . . . . . . . . . 290
malted chocolate crisp (*Kashi GoLean*) . . . . . . . . . . . . . . . . 280

**Granola and cereal bar *(cont.)***
marshmallow, all varieties (*Health Valley* Fat Free) . . . . . . . .100
oats 'n honey or peanut butter (*Nature Valley*), 2 bars . . . . . .180
peanut (*Healthy Valley* Moist & Chewy Granola) . . . . . . . . . .110
peanut butter (*Quaker* Chewy Granola) . . . . . . . . . . . . . . . . .110
strawberry vanilla yogurt (*Kashi GoLean*) . . . . . . . . . . . . . . .290
vanilla spice cake (*Kashi GoLean*) . . . . . . . . . . . . . . . . . . . . .280
**Grape,** fresh:
(*Dole*), 1½ cups . . . . . . . . . . . . . . . . . . . . . . . . . . . . . . . . . .90
American type (slipskin), 10 medium . . . . . . . . . . . . . . . . . . .15
American type (slipskin), peeled, seeded, ½ cup . . . . . . . . . .29
champagne (*Frieda's*), ½ cup, 3 oz. . . . . . . . . . . . . . . . . . . . .50
European type (adherent skin), seedless, 10 medium . . . . . . .36
European type (adherent skin), seedless or seeded, ½ cup . . .57
**Grape drink:**
(*Snapple* Grapeade), 8 fl. oz. . . . . . . . . . . . . . . . . . . . . . . . .120
(*Tropicana*), 11.5 fl. oz. . . . . . . . . . . . . . . . . . . . . . . . . . . .200
**Grape juice,** 8 fl. oz.:
(*Season's Best*) . . . . . . . . . . . . . . . . . . . . . . . . . . . . . . . . .160
(*Welch's*) . . . . . . . . . . . . . . . . . . . . . . . . . . . . . . . . . . . . . .170
white (*Welch's*) . . . . . . . . . . . . . . . . . . . . . . . . . . . . . . . . . .160
**Grapefruit,** fresh:
(*Dole*), ½ medium . . . . . . . . . . . . . . . . . . . . . . . . . . . . . . . . .60
pink or red:
  California or Arizona, ½ medium, 3¾" . . . . . . . . . . . . . .46
  California or Arizona, sections w/juice, ½ cup . . . . . . . . .43
  Florida, ½ medium, 3¾" . . . . . . . . . . . . . . . . . . . . . . . . . .37
  Florida, sections w/juice, ½ cup . . . . . . . . . . . . . . . . . . .34
white, California, ½ medium, 3¾" . . . . . . . . . . . . . . . . . . . . .44
white, California, sections w/juice, ½ cup . . . . . . . . . . . . . .42
white, Florida, ½ medium, 3¾" . . . . . . . . . . . . . . . . . . . . . . .38
white, sections w/juice, ½ cup . . . . . . . . . . . . . . . . . . . . . . .38
**Grapefruit, can or chilled,** ½ cup:
in juice, red or white (*Sunfresh* Chilled) . . . . . . . . . . . . . . . .45
in extra light syrup, red (*Sunfresh* Chilled) . . . . . . . . . . . . .70
in light syrup, red or white (*Sunfresh* Can) . . . . . . . . . . . . . .70
**Grapefruit drink,** ruby red, 8 fl. oz., except as noted:
(*Dole*) . . . . . . . . . . . . . . . . . . . . . . . . . . . . . . . . . . . . . . . . .130
(*Ocean Spray*) . . . . . . . . . . . . . . . . . . . . . . . . . . . . . . . . . . .130
(*Season's Best* Cocktail) . . . . . . . . . . . . . . . . . . . . . . . . . . .130

(*Snapple*) . . . . . . . . . . . . . . . . . . . . . . . . . . . . . .120
(*Tropicana Twister*), 10 fl. oz. . . . . . . . . . . . . . . . . . . . .160
**Grapefruit juice,** 8 fl. oz.:
(*Nantucket Nectars*) . . . . . . . . . . . . . . . . . . . . . . . .100
(*Season's Best*) . . . . . . . . . . . . . . . . . . . . . . . . . .90
fresh, pink or white . . . . . . . . . . . . . . . . . . . . . . . . .96
frozen* (*Cascadian Farm*) . . . . . . . . . . . . . . . . . . . . .100
golden or ruby red (*Tropicana Pure Premium*) . . . . . . . . . . .90
ruby red (*Florida's Natural* Calcium) . . . . . . . . . . . . . . . .100
ruby red (*Minute Maid*) . . . . . . . . . . . . . . . . . . . . . . .110
**Gravlax,** see "Salmon, marinated"
**Gravy,** see specific listings
**Great northern bean,** boiled, ½ cup . . . . . . . . . . . . . . . .104
**Great northern bean, canned,** ½ cup:
plain or w/pork (*Bush's Best*) . . . . . . . . . . . . . . . . . . . .110
seasoned (*Glory Foods*) . . . . . . . . . . . . . . . . . . . . . . . .90
**Green bean,** fresh:
raw, ½ cup . . . . . . . . . . . . . . . . . . . . . . . . . . . . . . .17
boiled, drained, ½ cup . . . . . . . . . . . . . . . . . . . . . . . . .22
**Green bean, can or jar,** ½ cup:
all styles (*Libby's*) . . . . . . . . . . . . . . . . . . . . . . . . . .25
all styles, except Italian cut (*Del Monte*) . . . . . . . . . . . . . .20
cut or French style (*Blue Boy*) . . . . . . . . . . . . . . . . . . . .25
cut or French style (*Green Giant*) . . . . . . . . . . . . . . . . . .20
cut or French style (*Veg-All*) . . . . . . . . . . . . . . . . . . . . .20
Italian cut (*Del Monte*) . . . . . . . . . . . . . . . . . . . . . . . .30
seasoned (*Glory Foods*) . . . . . . . . . . . . . . . . . . . . . . . .30
**Green bean, frozen:**
whole (*Green Giant Select*), 1 cup . . . . . . . . . . . . . . . . . .20
whole (*Seabrook Farms*), ¾ cup . . . . . . . . . . . . . . . . . . .25
whole, extra fine (*Bonduelle* Haricot Vert), 3 oz. . . . . . . . . . .30
cut (*Birds Eye*), ½ cup . . . . . . . . . . . . . . . . . . . . . . . .25
cut (*Cascadian Farm*), ⅔ cup . . . . . . . . . . . . . . . . . . . . .40
cut (*John Cope's* 1"), ⅔ cup . . . . . . . . . . . . . . . . . . . . .25
Italian (*Birds Eye* Deluxe), ½ cup . . . . . . . . . . . . . . . . . .35
Szechuan (*Cascadian Farm*), 1 cup . . . . . . . . . . . . . . . . . .60
**Green bean combinations,** canned, ½ cup:
w/potatoes (*Allens/Sunshine*) . . . . . . . . . . . . . . . . . . . . .35
w/potatoes (*Glory Foods*) . . . . . . . . . . . . . . . . . . . . . . .50
and shelly beans (*Bush's Best*) . . . . . . . . . . . . . . . . . . . .45

**Green bean dish,** frozen:
w/almonds (*Cascadian Farm*), ⅔ cup . . . . . . . . . . . . . . . . . . .70
mushroom casserole:
(*Stouffer's Family Style Favorites*), ½ cup . . . . . . . . . . .130
w/mushroom garlic sauce (*Cascadian Farm*), ¾ cup . . . .90
stir-fry (*Birds Eye*), ⅓ of 16-oz. pkg. . . . . . . . . . . . . . . . . .100
**Green peas,** see "Peas, green"
**Greens, mixed,** fresh, see "Salad blend"
**Greens, mixed, canned** (see also specific listings):
(*Bush's Best*), ½ cup . . . . . . . . . . . . . . . . . . . . . . . . . .25
seasoned (*Glory Foods*), ½ cup . . . . . . . . . . . . . . . . . . . . .50
**Grilling sauce** (see also "Barbecue sauce," "Marinade," and specific listings), 2 tbsp.:
(*French's* Grill & Glaze) . . . . . . . . . . . . . . . . . . . . . . . . .60
(*Jack Daniel's* Original No. 7 Barbecue Recipe) . . . . . . . . . . .50
(*Jack Daniel's* Sizzling Smokehouse Recipe) . . . . . . . . . . . . .45
chipotle or roasted pepper (*Texas Best*) . . . . . . . . . . . . . . .50
garlic herb (*McCormick* Flavor Medleys) . . . . . . . . . . . . . . .60
habañero mustard (*Texas Best* Mesa) . . . . . . . . . . . . . . . . .60
hickory mesquite (*Jack Daniel's* Tennessee) . . . . . . . . . . . . .45
Italian, Mediterranean (*World Harbors Amalfi Coast*) . . . . . .25
Italian herb or lemon pepper (*McCormick* Flavor Medleys) . . . . . . . . . . . . . . . . . . . . . . . . . . . . . .50
serrano (*Texas Best* Santa Fe) . . . . . . . . . . . . . . . . . . . . . .35
sun-dried tomato and basil (*McCormick* Flavor Medleys) . . .50
**Grits,** see "Corn grits"
**Grouper,** meat only:
raw, 4 oz. . . . . . . . . . . . . . . . . . . . . . . . . . . . . . . . . . .104
baked, broiled, or microwaved, 4 oz. . . . . . . . . . . . . . . . . .134
**Guacamole,** 2 tbsp.:
(*Dean's*) . . . . . . . . . . . . . . . . . . . . . . . . . . . . . . . . . . .80
(*Marie's*) . . . . . . . . . . . . . . . . . . . . . . . . . . . . . . . . . .90
(*Marzetti*) . . . . . . . . . . . . . . . . . . . . . . . . . . . . . . . . .120
**Guava** (see also "Feijoas") (*Frieda's*), 3-oz. fruit . . . . . . . . . .45
**Guava nectar** (*Goya*), 6 fl. oz. . . . . . . . . . . . . . . . . . . . . .110
**Guinea hen,** raw:
meat w/skin, 4 oz. . . . . . . . . . . . . . . . . . . . . . . . . . . . . .179
meat only, 4 oz. . . . . . . . . . . . . . . . . . . . . . . . . . . . . . .125

# H

| FOOD AND MEASURE | CALORIES |
|---|---|
| **Habas** (*Frieda's*), ½ cup, 3 oz. | 100 |
| **Haddock,** meat only: | |
| raw, 4 oz. | 99 |
| baked, broiled, or microwaved, 4 oz. | 127 |
| smoked, 4 oz. | 132 |
| **Haddock entree,** fillet, frozen: | |
| battered (*Van de Kamp's*), 2 pcs. | 220 |
| breaded (*Mrs. Paul's* Premium), 4.25-oz. pc. | 240 |
| w/shrimp, crab, vegetables (*Oven Poppers*), 4.5-oz. pc. | 210 |
| **Hake,** see "Whiting" | |
| **Halibut,** meat only, 4 oz.: | |
| Atlantic and Pacific, raw | 124 |
| Atlantic and Pacific, baked, broiled, or microwaved | 159 |
| Greenland, raw | 211 |
| Greenland, baked, broiled, or microwaved | 271 |
| **Halibut entree,** frozen, battered, bites or fillet (*Mrs. Friday's*), 4 oz. | 180 |
| **Ham,** fresh, roasted: | |
| whole leg, lean w/fat, 4 oz. | 310 |
| whole leg, lean w/fat, chopped or diced, 1 cup | 369 |
| whole leg, lean only, 4 oz. | 239 |
| whole leg, lean only, chopped or diced, 1 cup | 285 |
| rump half, lean w/fat, 4 oz. | 286 |
| rump half, lean w/fat, chopped or diced, 1 cup | 340 |
| rump half, lean only, 4 oz. | 234 |
| rump half, lean only, chopped or diced, 1 cup | 278 |
| shank half, lean w/fat, 4 oz. | 328 |
| shank half, lean w/fat, chopped or diced, 1 cup | 390 |
| shank half, lean only, 4 oz. | 244 |
| shank half, lean only, chopped or diced, 1 cup | 290 |
| **Ham, cured,** 4 oz., except as noted: | |
| whole leg, lean w/fat, unheated | 279 |
| whole leg, lean w/fat, roasted | 276 |

**Ham, cured** ***(cont.)***
whole leg, lean w/fat, roasted, chopped or diced,
1 cup . . . . . . . . . . . . . . . . . . . . . . . . . . . . . . . . . . . .341
whole leg, lean only, unheated . . . . . . . . . . . . . . . . . . . . . . .167
whole leg, lean only, roasted . . . . . . . . . . . . . . . . . . . . . . .178
whole leg, lean only, roasted, chopped or diced, 1 cup . . . .219
boneless (11% fat), unheated . . . . . . . . . . . . . . . . . . . . . . .206
boneless (11% fat), roasted . . . . . . . . . . . . . . . . . . . . . . . .202
boneless (11% fat), roasted, chopped or diced, 1 cup . . . . .249
boneless, extra lean (5% fat), unheated . . . . . . . . . . . . . . .149
boneless, extra lean (5% fat), roasted . . . . . . . . . . . . . . . . .164
**Ham, deviled,** see "Ham spread"
**Ham, refrigerated or canned,** 3 oz., except as noted:
(*Always Tender*), 4 oz. . . . . . . . . . . . . . . . . . . . . . . . . . . .270
(*Black Label* Refrigerator/Shelf) . . . . . . . . . . . . . . . . . . . .100
(*Krakus* Polish), 2 oz. . . . . . . . . . . . . . . . . . . . . . . . . . . . . .50
(*Light & Lean* 97 Half) . . . . . . . . . . . . . . . . . . . . . . . . . . . . .90
(*Plumrose* Danish), 2 oz. . . . . . . . . . . . . . . . . . . . . . . . . . . .60
(*Spiral Cure 81*) . . . . . . . . . . . . . . . . . . . . . . . . . . . . . . . . .150
chunk (*Hormel*), 2 oz. . . . . . . . . . . . . . . . . . . . . . . . . . . . . .90
maple glazed, baby (*Boar's Head Honey Coat*) . . . . . . . . . . .90
slice (*Boar's Head Sweet Slice*) . . . . . . . . . . . . . . . . . . . . . .100
slice, maple glazed (*Boar's Head Sweet Slice*) . . . . . . . . . . .110
smoked (*Boar's Head* Semi-Boneless) . . . . . . . . . . . . . . . . .130
steak (*Cook's*), 4 oz. . . . . . . . . . . . . . . . . . . . . . . . . . . . . .150
steak (*Oscar Mayer*), 2 oz. . . . . . . . . . . . . . . . . . . . . . . . . . .60
**"Ham," vegetarian,** frozen:
sliced (*Worthington Wham*), 2 slices . . . . . . . . . . . . . . . . . .80
sliced (*Yves* Deli Slices), 2.2 oz. . . . . . . . . . . . . . . . . . . . . .80
steak (*Veggie Master* Vege), ¼ pkg. . . . . . . . . . . . . . . . . . .88
**Ham bologna** (*Boar's Head*), 2 oz. . . . . . . . . . . . . . . . . . . .80
**Ham entree,** frozen:
and cheese (*Healthy Choice* Bread Stuffs), 6.1 oz. . . . . . . . .320
croquette (*Goya*), 3 pcs., 3½ oz. . . . . . . . . . . . . . . . . . . . .280
**Ham glaze** (*Crosse & Blackwell*), 1 tbsp. . . . . . . . . . . . . . .30
**Ham lunch meat,** 2 oz., except as noted:
(*Boar's Head* Deluxe/Tavern) . . . . . . . . . . . . . . . . . . . . . . . .60
(*Citterio Fresca* Rosmarino) . . . . . . . . . . . . . . . . . . . . . . . . .90
(*Healthy Deli* Deluxe/Olde Tyme Tavern/Shattuck) . . . . . . . . .60
baked (*Sara Lee* Homestyle) . . . . . . . . . . . . . . . . . . . . . . . . .60

Black Forest (*Boar's Head*) . . . . . . . . . . . . . . . . . . . . . . . . . .60
boiled (*Oscar Mayer*), 3 slices, 2.2 oz. . . . . . . . . . . . . . . . . .60
brown sugar (*Sara Lee*) . . . . . . . . . . . . . . . . . . . . . . . . . . .70
cappicola (*Boar's Head* Capocollo), 1 oz. . . . . . . . . . . . . . . .80
cappicola (*Daniele* Capocollo), 3 slices, 1 oz. . . . . . . . . . . .80
chopped (*Oscar Mayer*), 1-oz. slice . . . . . . . . . . . . . . . . . . .50
cooked (*Alpine Lace*) . . . . . . . . . . . . . . . . . . . . . . . . . . . .60
cooked (*Hormel* Deli) . . . . . . . . . . . . . . . . . . . . . . . . . . . .60
cooked (*Sara Lee* Old Fashioned) . . . . . . . . . . . . . . . . . . .50
honey (*Alpine Lace*) . . . . . . . . . . . . . . . . . . . . . . . . . . . . .60
honey (*Oscar Mayer*), 3 slices, 2.2 oz. . . . . . . . . . . . . . . . .70
honey (*Sara Lee* Bavarian) . . . . . . . . . . . . . . . . . . . . . . . .70
honey-cured (*Healthy Choice*), 1-oz. slice . . . . . . . . . . . . . .30
honey maple (*Sara Lee*) . . . . . . . . . . . . . . . . . . . . . . . . . .70
honey or hot (*Healthy Deli*) . . . . . . . . . . . . . . . . . . . . . . .60
maple, flame-seared (*Healthy Deli*) . . . . . . . . . . . . . . . . . .70
maple, glazed (*Boar's Head Honey Coat*) . . . . . . . . . . . . . .60
minced, 1 oz. . . . . . . . . . . . . . . . . . . . . . . . . . . . . . . . . . .75
pepper (*Boar's Head*) . . . . . . . . . . . . . . . . . . . . . . . . . . . .70
pepper (*Boar's Head* Gourmet) . . . . . . . . . . . . . . . . . . . . .60
pesto Parmesan, oven-roasted (*Boar's Head*) . . . . . . . . . . . .90
proscuitto, see "Prosciutto"
rosemary (*Black Bear*) . . . . . . . . . . . . . . . . . . . . . . . . . . .70
rosemary and sun-dried tomato (*Boar's Head*) . . . . . . . . . . .70
smoked (*Boar's Head Honey Coat*) . . . . . . . . . . . . . . . . . . .60
smoked (*Sara Lee* Smokehouse) . . . . . . . . . . . . . . . . . . . . .50
smoked, mesquite (*Healthy Choice*) . . . . . . . . . . . . . . . . . .60
spiced (*Boar's Head*) . . . . . . . . . . . . . . . . . . . . . . . . . . .120
Virginia (*Boar's Head*) . . . . . . . . . . . . . . . . . . . . . . . . . . .60
Virginia (*Healthy Choice*) . . . . . . . . . . . . . . . . . . . . . . . . .60
Virginia (*Healthy Deli* Less Sodium) . . . . . . . . . . . . . . . . . .70
Virginia, smoked (*Alpine Lace*) . . . . . . . . . . . . . . . . . . . . .60
**Ham and cheese loaf** (*Oscar Mayer*), 1-oz. slice . . . . . . . . .60
**Ham and cheese pocket/sandwich,** frozen, 1 pc.:
(*Deli Stuffs*), 4.5 oz . . . . . . . . . . . . . . . . . . . . . . . . . . . .320
(*Hot Pockets*), 4.5 oz. . . . . . . . . . . . . . . . . . . . . . . . . . . .310
(*Hot Pockets Toaster Melts*), 2.2 oz. . . . . . . . . . . . . . . . . .160
(*Lean Pockets*). 4.5 oz. . . . . . . . . . . . . . . . . . . . . . . . . . .280
cheddar (*Croissant Pockets*), 4.5 oz. . . . . . . . . . . . . . . . . .330
croissant (*Sara Lee*), 3.7 oz. . . . . . . . . . . . . . . . . . . . . . .300

**Ham spread,** deviled, ¼ cup:
(*Cure 81*) . . . . . . . . . . . . . . . . . . . . . . . . . . . . . . . .150
(*Underwood*) . . . . . . . . . . . . . . . . . . . . . . . . . . . . .140
**Hamburger,** see "Beef sandwich"
**"Hamburger," vegetarian,** see "Burger, vegetarian"
**Hamburger entree mix** (*Hamburger Helper*), 1 cup*:
bacon cheeseburger . . . . . . . . . . . . . . . . . . . . . . . . .380
beef pasta . . . . . . . . . . . . . . . . . . . . . . . . . . . . . . .270
beef Romanoff . . . . . . . . . . . . . . . . . . . . . . . . . . . .300
beef stew . . . . . . . . . . . . . . . . . . . . . . . . . . . . . . .260
beef taco . . . . . . . . . . . . . . . . . . . . . . . . . . . . . . .300
beef teriyaki . . . . . . . . . . . . . . . . . . . . . . . . . . . . .290
cheddar/broccoli . . . . . . . . . . . . . . . . . . . . . . . . . .350
cheddar melt . . . . . . . . . . . . . . . . . . . . . . . . . . . . .300
cheese, 3 . . . . . . . . . . . . . . . . . . . . . . . . . . . . . . .340
cheeseburger macaroni . . . . . . . . . . . . . . . . . . . . . .360
cheesy hash browns . . . . . . . . . . . . . . . . . . . . . . . .400
cheesy shells . . . . . . . . . . . . . . . . . . . . . . . . . . . .340
chili macaroni . . . . . . . . . . . . . . . . . . . . . . . . . . . .300
fettuccine Alfredo . . . . . . . . . . . . . . . . . . . . . . . . .300
Italian, zesty . . . . . . . . . . . . . . . . . . . . . . . . . . . . .300
Italian Parmesan . . . . . . . . . . . . . . . . . . . . . . . . . .300
lasagna . . . . . . . . . . . . . . . . . . . . . . . . . . . . . . . . .270
lasagna, 4-cheese . . . . . . . . . . . . . . . . . . . . . . . . .350
pizza, double cheese . . . . . . . . . . . . . . . . . . . . . . .320
pizza, pepperoni . . . . . . . . . . . . . . . . . . . . . . . . . . .310
pizza pasta, w/cheese topping . . . . . . . . . . . . . . . . .280
Philly cheese steak . . . . . . . . . . . . . . . . . . . . . . . . .330
potatoes Stroganoff . . . . . . . . . . . . . . . . . . . . . . . .260
ravioli w/cheese topping . . . . . . . . . . . . . . . . . . . . .310
rice Oriental . . . . . . . . . . . . . . . . . . . . . . . . . . . . .280
Salisbury . . . . . . . . . . . . . . . . . . . . . . . . . . . . . . . .270
spaghetti . . . . . . . . . . . . . . . . . . . . . . . . . . . . . . . .270
Stroganoff . . . . . . . . . . . . . . . . . . . . . . . . . . . . . . .320
**Hard sauce,** brandied (*Crosse & Blackwell*), 2 tbsp. . . . . . .180
***Hardee's,*** 1 serving:
breakfast:
biscuit, apple cinnamon 'N' raisin . . . . . . . . . . . . . . . . .250
biscuit, bacon, egg, cheese . . . . . . . . . . . . . . . . . . . . .520

biscuit, chicken .590
biscuit, ham .410
biscuit, ham, country .440
biscuit, jelly .440
biscuit, *Made From Scratch* .390
biscuit, sausage .550
biscuit, sausage and egg .620
biscuit, steak .580
*Biscuit 'N' Gravy* .530
*Frisco* sandwich, ham .450
*Hash Rounds,* regular .230
*Omelet* Biscuit .550

sandwiches:
All-Star burger .660
bacon Swiss crispy chicken .670
*Big Roast Beef* .410
chicken, grilled .350
chicken fillet .480
Famous Star burger .570
*Fisherman's Fillet* .530
*Frisco* burger .720
hamburger .270
hot dog, w/condiments .450
Hot Ham 'N Cheese .300
*Monster Burger* 1,060
roast beef, monster .610
roast beef, regular .310
Super Star burger .790

chicken breast .370
chicken leg .170
chicken thigh .330
chicken wing .200

sides:
coleslaw, 4 oz. .240
*Crispy Curls,* large .520
*Crispy Curls,* medium .340
*Crispy Curls,* monster .590
fries, large .440
fries, monster .510

***Hardee's*, sides *(cont.)***
fries, regular ............................340
gravy, 1.5 oz. ............................20
mashed potatoes, small ....................70
desserts/shakes:
apple turnover ............................270
peach cobbler .............................310
shake, chocolate ..........................370
shake, vanilla ............................350
twist cone ................................180
**Hazelnut,** see "Filberts"
**Hazelnut spread** (*Nutella*), 2 tbsp. ..................160
**Head cheese** (*Oscar Mayer*), 1 oz. ....................50
**Herbs,** see specific listings
**Herring,** fresh, meat only, 4 oz.:
Atlantic, raw, 4 oz. ..............................180
Atlantic, baked, broiled, or microwaved, 4 oz. ...........230
lake, see "Cisco"
Pacific, raw, 4 oz. ...............................224
Pacific, baked, broiled, or microwaved, 4 oz. ............284
**Herring, canned,** see "Sardine"
**Herring, kippered, canned,** ¼ cup:
in mustard (*Crown Prince* Natural) ..................100
in salsa picante (*Crown Prince*) .....................90
smoked (*Crown Prince* Natural) ......................110
**Herring, pickled, in jars:**
in dill sauce (*Vita*), ¼ cup .........................100
slices (*Vita* Lunch), 2 oz. ..........................130
in sour cream (*Elf*), ¼ cup ..........................110
in wine sauce (*Fish Market*), ¼ cup .................100
in wine sauce (*Vita* Party Snacks Tastee Bits), 2 oz. ......120
**Hoisin sauce** (*House of Tsang*), 1 tsp. ...............15
**Hollandaise sauce mix:**
(*Knorr* Classic), 1 tsp. ............................10
(*McCormick Produce Partners*), ⅒ pkt. ................20
**Homestyle gravy mix** (*McCormick*), ¼ cup* .............25
**Hominy,** dry, white (*Goya*), ¼ cup ....................180
**Hominy, canned,** ½ cup:
golden (*Bush's Best*) ...............................60
golden, w/red and green pepper (*Bush's Best*) ...........70

Mexican (*Allens/Uncle William* Pepi) . . . . . . . . . . . . . . . . . . 120
white (*Bush's Best* Pozole Blanco) . . . . . . . . . . . . . . . . . . 70
white (*Juanita's* Mexican) . . . . . . . . . . . . . . . . . . . . . . . . . 60
white, w/red and green pepper (*Bush's Best*) . . . . . . . . . . . . 80
**Hominy grits,** dry, see "Corn grits"
**Honey,** 1 tbsp. . . . . . . . . . . . . . . . . . . . . . . . . . . . . . . . . 60
**Honey mustard sauce,** Dijon (*World Harbors* Mont
St. Michel), 2 tbsp. . . . . . . . . . . . . . . . . . . . . . . . . . . . . 30
**Honey roll sausage,** beef, 1 oz. . . . . . . . . . . . . . . . . . . . . . 52
**Honeycomb** (*Frieda's*), ½ cup, 3 oz. . . . . . . . . . . . . . . . . . 260
**Honeydew,** 1/10 melon, 7" × 2" . . . . . . . . . . . . . . . . . . . . . . . 46
**Horned melon** (*Frieda's*), 3.5-oz. melon . . . . . . . . . . . . . . . 25
**Horseradish,** fresh:
leafy tips, boiled, drained, chopped, ½ cup . . . . . . . . . . . . . . 13
pods, boiled, drained, sliced, ½ cup . . . . . . . . . . . . . . . . . . . 21
**Horseradish, prepared,** 1 tsp. . . . . . . . . . . . . . . . . . . . . . . . 0
**Horseradish root** (*Frieda's*), 1 tbsp. . . . . . . . . . . . . . . . . . . 0
**Horseradish sauce:**
(*Bennetts*), 1 tbsp. . . . . . . . . . . . . . . . . . . . . . . . . . . . . . 50
(*Boar's Head* Pub Style), 1 tsp. . . . . . . . . . . . . . . . . . . . . . 15
(*Heinz*), 1 tsp. . . . . . . . . . . . . . . . . . . . . . . . . . . . . . . . . 20
**Hot dog,** see "Frankfurter"
**Hot dog sauce,** see "Chili sauce"
**Hot fudge sauce,** see "Chocolate topping"
**Hot sauce,** 1 tsp., except as noted:
(*Louisiana*) . . . . . . . . . . . . . . . . . . . . . . . . . . . . . . . . . . . . 0
(*Tabasco*) . . . . . . . . . . . . . . . . . . . . . . . . . . . . . . . . . . . . . 0
jalapeño or picante (*Búfalo*) . . . . . . . . . . . . . . . . . . . . . . . . 0
**Hummus,** 2 tbsp., except as noted:
(*Athenos* Original) . . . . . . . . . . . . . . . . . . . . . . . . . . . . . . 60
(*Sabra Salads* Chumus), 1 oz. . . . . . . . . . . . . . . . . . . . . . . 69
(*Tribe of Two Sheiks*) . . . . . . . . . . . . . . . . . . . . . . . . . . . . 50
all varieties (*Cedar's*) . . . . . . . . . . . . . . . . . . . . . . . . . . . 50
all varieties (*Yorgo*) . . . . . . . . . . . . . . . . . . . . . . . . . . . . . 50
cucumber dill (*Athenos*) . . . . . . . . . . . . . . . . . . . . . . . . . . . 60
eggplant, roasted (*Athenos*) . . . . . . . . . . . . . . . . . . . . . . . . 45
garlic, black olive, pesto, or scallion (*Athenos*) . . . . . . . . . . . 50
red pepper, roasted, or spicy 3 pepper (*Athenos*) . . . . . . . . . 60
**Hummus and pita,** 2 tbsp. hummus and 2 pcs. pita:
(*Athenos* Travelers Original) . . . . . . . . . . . . . . . . . . . . . . . 130

eggplant, roasted (*Athenos* Travelers) . . . . . . . . . . . . . . . . . .120
garlic, roasted or spicy 3 pepper (*Athenos* Travelers) . . . . .130
red pepper, roasted (*Athenos* Travelers) . . . . . . . . . . . . . . . .140
**Hunter gravy mix,** see "Mushroom gravy mix"
**Hush puppies,** frozen (*McKenzie's*),•2 oz. . . . . . . . . . . . . . . .190
**Hush puppies, mix** (*Sylvia's*), ⅓ cup . . . . . . . . . . . . . . . . . .130

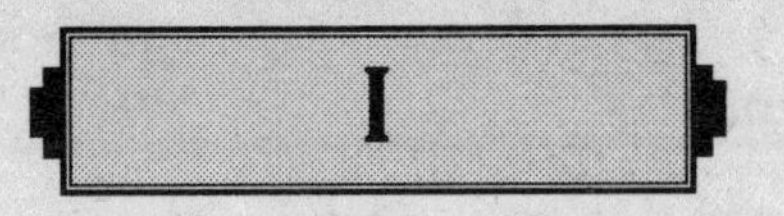

| FOOD AND MEASURE | CALORIES |
|---|---|
| **Ice bar,** see "Fruit bar" and "Iced confection bar" | |
| **Ice cream,** ½ cup: | |
| almond (*Darigold* Avalanche) | 170 |
| apple pie, deep dish (*Dreamery*) | 280 |
| banana (*Dreamery Banana Boogie*) | 290 |
| banana fudge chunk (*Breyers* Special Edition) | 170 |
| banana nut (*Blue Bell*) | 170 |
| banana split (*Breyers Ice Cream Parlor*) | 180 |
| banana split (*Healthy Choice*) | 130 |
| (*Ben & Jerry's* Peanut Turtles) | 320 |
| (*Ben & Jerry's Aloha Macadamia*) | 330 |
| (*Ben & Jerry's Apple Crumble*) | 280 |
| (*Ben & Jerry's Bovinity Divinity*) | 290 |
| (*Ben & Jerry's Chubby Hubby*) | 350 |
| (*Ben & Jerry's Chunky Monkey/Nutty Waffle Cone*) | 310 |
| (*Ben & Jerry's Concession Obsession/Festivus*) | 300 |
| (*Ben & Jerry's Phish Food/2-Twisted This is Nuts*) | 300 |
| (*Ben & Jerry's 2-Twisted S.N.A.F.U.*) | 250 |
| Black Forest (*Breyers Ice Cream Parlor*) | 150 |
| blackberry swirl (*Edy's* Grand) | 140 |
| butter almond (*Turkey Hill*) | 180 |
| butter pecan (*Breyers/Breyers Homemade*) | 170 |
| butter pecan (*Turkey Hill*) | 170 |
| butter pecan crunch (*Healthy Choice*) | 120 |
| candy bar sundae (*Breyers Ice Cream Parlor*) | 170 |
| cappuccino (*Cascadian Farm*) | 175 |
| cappuccino chocolate crunch (*Healthy Choice*) | 120 |
| cappuccino mocha crunch (*Healthy Choice*) | 140 |
| caramel (*Ben & Jerry's Triple Caramel Chunk*) | 290 |
| caramel creme (*Stonyfield Farm*) | 250 |
| caramel creme, pecan (*Häagen-Dazs*) | 320 |
| caramel fudge pecan (*Blue Bell*) | 200 |
| caramel praline sundae (*Blue Bell*) | 190 |
| cashew praline (*Dreamery Parfait*) | 260 |

**Ice cream *(cont.)***

cherry, black, chunk (*Darigold*) .140
cherry chocolate chip (*Breyers* Special Edition) .160
cherry chocolate chunk (*Healthy Choice*) .120
cherry fudge chip (*Ben & Jerry's Cherry Garcia*) .260
cherry vanilla (*Häagen-Dazs*) .240
cherry vanilla (*Stonyfield Farm*) .250
cherry vanilla, black (*Edy's* Grand) .140
chocolate (*Ben & Jerry's World's Best*) .280
chocolate (*Blue Bell* Decadence) .190
chocolate (*Häagen-Dazs*) .270
chocolate, double (*Cascadian Farm*) .195
chocolate, Dutch (*Turkey Hill*) .150
chocolate, French (*Breyers* Light) .140
chocolate, triple (*Blue Bell*) .180
chocolate, triple (*Edy's Triple Chocolate Thunder*) .160
chocolate almond (*Breyers Hershey's Ice Cream Parlor*) .170
chocolate almond bar (*Dreamery*) .300
chocolate almond marshmallow (*Blue Bell*) .200
chocolate brownie walnut (*Häagen-Dazs*) .290
chocolate cake, German (*Häagen-Dazs*) .290
chocolate caramel nut (*Breyers* Special Edition) .190
chocolate caramel swirl (*Dreyer's/Edy's* Grand) .170
chocolate cheesecake (*Häagen-Dazs*) .300
chocolate chip (*Blue Bell*) .170
chocolate chip (*Green's*) .180
chocolate chip, chocolate (*Häagen-Dazs*) .300
chocolate cookie dough (*Blue Bell*) .190
chocolate cookie dough (*Turkey Hill*) .190
chocolate cookie dough, double (*Blue Bell*) .210
chocolate fudge brownie (*Healthy Choice*) .110
chocolate malt, double (*Breyers Ice Cream Parlor*) .160
chocolate marshmallow (*Turkey Hill*) .160
chocolate raspberry (*Stonyfield Farm*) .250
coconut (*Häagen-Dazs* Gelato) .240
coconut cream pie (*Green's*) .160
coffee (*Blue Bell*) .160
coffee (*Häagen-Dazs*) .270
coffee (*Starbucks* Classic) .230
coffee (*Stonyfield Farm* Decaf) .250

coffee (*Turkey Hill* Colombian) .......................... 140
coffee almond fudge (*Healthy Choice*) ................ 110
coffee mocha chip (*Häagen-Dazs*) ..................... 290
cookies and cream (*Breyers*) ........................... 170
cookies and cream (*Breyers Oreo Ice Cream Parlor*) ...... 160
(*Dreamery Coney Island Waffle Cone*) ................ 300
(*Dreamery Nuts About Malt*) .......................... 280
(*Dreamery White Out*) ................................ 320
dulce de leche (*Blue Bell*) ............................ 170
dulce de leche (*Dreamery*) ............................ 270
dulce de leche (*Healthy Choice*) ..................... 110
eggnog (*Green's*) ...................................... 150
fudge brownie (*Breyers Ice Cream Parlor Sundae*) ....... 200
fudge ripple (*Turkey Hill*) ............................ 140
fudge sundae, hot (*Blue Bell*) ........................ 180
honey almond (*Häagen-Dazs* Gelato) .................... 250
ice cream sandwich (*Breyers Ice Cream Parlor*) ......... 160
Irish cream (*Häagen-Dazs Baileys*) .................... 270
latte (*Starbucks* Low Fat) ............................. 170
mango (*Häagen-Dazs*) ................................... 250
mint (*Dreamery* Cool Mint) ............................. 280
mint chip (*Häagen-Dazs*) ............................... 300
mint chocolate chip (*Ben & Jerry's*) ................... 280
mint chocolate chip (*Blue Bell*) ...................... 170
mint chocolate chip (*Turkey Hill*) .................... 180
mint chocolate cookie (*Breyers Oreo Ice Cream Parlor*) ... 160
Mississippi mud (*Breyers Ice Cream Parlor*) ............ 180
mocha almond fudge (*Blue Bell*) ....................... 180
mocha almond fudge (*Breyers* Special Edition) .......... 180
mocha biscotti (*Stonyfield Farm*) ..................... 260
mud pie (*Starbucks*) ................................... 240
Neapolitan (*Blue Bell*) ................................ 160
Neapolitan (*Turkey Hill*) .............................. 150
peach (*Dreamery* Harvest) .............................. 220
peach (*Green's* Just Peachy) ........................... 140
peanut butter chunk, chocolate (*Dreamery*) ............ 310
peanut butter cup (*Breyers Reese's Ice Cream Parlor*) .... 180
peanut butter fudge chunk (*Häagen-Dazs*) ............. 340
pecan caramel (*Ben & Jerry's Southern Pecan Pie*) ....... 290
peppermint (*Blue Bell*) ................................ 160

**Ice cream *(cont.)***

pineapple passion fruit (*Ben & Jerry's Island Paradise*) . . . .240
pistachio (*Ben & Jerry's Pistachio Pistachio*) . . . . . . . . . . .240
raspberry (*Häagen-Dazs* Gelato) . . . . . . . . . . . . . . . . . . . . .240
raspberry, black (*Dreamery* Avalanche) . . . . . . . . . . . . . . . .250
raspberry, black (*Turkey Hill*) . . . . . . . . . . . . . . . . . . . . . . .140
raspberry brownie (*Dreamery* à la Mode) . . . . . . . . . . . . . .270
raspberry cheesecake (*Dreyer's/Edy's* Grand) . . . . . . . . . . .150
rocky road (*Blue Bell*) . . . . . . . . . . . . . . . . . . . . . . . . . . . .180
rocky road (*Turkey Hill*) . . . . . . . . . . . . . . . . . . . . . . . . . .170
rum raisin (*Häagen-Dazs*) . . . . . . . . . . . . . . . . . . . . . . . . .270
spumoni (*Edy's* Grand) . . . . . . . . . . . . . . . . . . . . . . . . . . .150
strawberry (*Breyers*) . . . . . . . . . . . . . . . . . . . . . . . . . . . . .130
strawberry (*Breyers Ice Cream Parlor Sundae*) . . . . . . . . . .140
strawberry (*Dreamery Strawberry Fields*) . . . . . . . . . . . . . .220
strawberry cheesecake (*Blue Bell*) . . . . . . . . . . . . . . . . . . .170
strawberry shortcake (*Breyers Ice Cream Parlor*) . . . . . . . .160
strawberry shortcake (*Dreyer's/Edy's Grand Light*) . . . . . . .110
tin Lizzie sundae (*Turkey Hill* Light) . . . . . . . . . . . . . . . . .140
tin roof sundae (*Healthy Choice*) . . . . . . . . . . . . . . . . . . . .120
tiramisu (*Dreamery*) . . . . . . . . . . . . . . . . . . . . . . . . . . . . .270
tiramisu (*Häagen-Dazs* Gelato) . . . . . . . . . . . . . . . . . . . . .250
toffee, English (*Breyers Heath Ice Cream Parlor*) . . . . . . . .180
turtle sundae (*Breyers Ice Cream Parlor*) . . . . . . . . . . . . . .170
vanilla (*Ben & Jerry's World's Best*) . . . . . . . . . . . . . . . . .250
vanilla (*Breyers*) . . . . . . . . . . . . . . . . . . . . . . . . . . . . . . .150
vanilla (*Breyers* Light Natural) . . . . . . . . . . . . . . . . . . . . .110
vanilla (*Cascadian Farm*) . . . . . . . . . . . . . . . . . . . . . . . . .180
vanilla (*Dreamery*) . . . . . . . . . . . . . . . . . . . . . . . . . . . . . .260
vanilla (*Häagen-Dazs*) . . . . . . . . . . . . . . . . . . . . . . . . . . .270
vanilla (*Stonyfield Farm*) . . . . . . . . . . . . . . . . . . . . . . . . .250
vanilla (*Turkey Hill*) . . . . . . . . . . . . . . . . . . . . . . . . . . . . .170
vanilla, French (*Breyers*) . . . . . . . . . . . . . . . . . . . . . . . . .160
vanilla, French or bean (*Turkey Hill*) . . . . . . . . . . . . . . . . .140
vanilla caramel almond (*Cascadian Farm*) . . . . . . . . . . . . . .210
vanilla caramel almond fudge (*Ben & Jerry's*) . . . . . . . . . . .300
vanilla–chocolate (*Turkey Hill*) . . . . . . . . . . . . . . . . . . . . .150
vanilla–chocolate–strawberry (*Breyers*) . . . . . . . . . . . . . . .140
vanilla fudge (*Breyers Ice Cream Parlor Sundae*) . . . . . . . . .160

vanilla fudge brownie (*Stonyfield Farm*) . . . . . . . . . . . . . . .260
vanilla fudge swirl (*Green's*) . . . . . . . . . . . . . . . . . . . . . . . . .150
vanilla Swiss almond (*Häagen-Dazs*) . . . . . . . . . . . . . . . . . . .300
**"Ice cream," nondairy,** ½ cup:
cappuccino, carob, or chocolate (*Rice Dream*) . . . . . . . . . . .150
cappuccino almond fudge (*Rice Dream* Supreme) . . . . . . . . .170
carob almond (*Rice Dream*) . . . . . . . . . . . . . . . . . . . . . . . . .170
cherry chocolate chunk (*Rice Dream* Supreme) . . . . . . . . . .170
cherry vanilla (*Rice Dream*) . . . . . . . . . . . . . . . . . . . . . . . .150
chocolate (*Soy Dream*) . . . . . . . . . . . . . . . . . . . . . . . . . . . .140
chocolate almond chunk (*Rice Dream* Supreme) . . . . . . . . . .170
chocolate chip or cookies (*Rice Dream*) . . . . . . . . . . . . . . .170
cocoa marble fudge or Neapolitan (*Rice Dream*) . . . . . . . . . .150
espresso bean, double (*Rice Dream* Supreme) . . . . . . . . . . .160
mint carob or chocolate chip (*Rice Dream*) . . . . . . . . . . . . .170
mint chocolate cookie (*Rice Dream* Supreme) . . . . . . . . . . . .170
peanut butter cup (*Rice Dream* Supreme) . . . . . . . . . . . . . . .180
praline (*Rice Dream* Supreme Pralines N' Dream) . . . . . . . .180
strawberry (*Rice Dream*) . . . . . . . . . . . . . . . . . . . . . . . . . .140
vanilla or orange vanilla swirl (*Rice Dream*) . . . . . . . . . . . .150
vanilla almond, Swiss (*Rice Dream*) . . . . . . . . . . . . . . . . . .180
**Ice cream bar** (see also "Iced confection bar"), 1 pc.:
all flavors (*Blue Bell* Créme Pops Reduced Fat) . . . . . . . . . . .60
almond (*Klondike Big Bear*) . . . . . . . . . . . . . . . . . . . . . . . .310
almond, toasted (*Good Humor* Single) . . . . . . . . . . . . . . . . .230
(*Ben & Jerry's Phish Stick*) . . . . . . . . . . . . . . . . . . . . . . . .260
(*Ben & Jerry's Phish Stick* Single) . . . . . . . . . . . . . . . . . . .290
candy center (*Good Humor* Crunch) . . . . . . . . . . . . . . . . . .300
cappuccino (*Klondike*) . . . . . . . . . . . . . . . . . . . . . . . . . . . .290
cherry, dark chocolate (*Cascadian Farm*) . . . . . . . . . . . . . .220
cherry fudge (*Ben & Jerry's Cherry Garcia*) . . . . . . . . . . . . .250
chocolate (*Klondike* Variety Pack) . . . . . . . . . . . . . . . . . . .240
chocolate and almonds (*Häagen-Dazs* Single) . . . . . . . . . . .380
chocolate chocolate (*Klondike*) . . . . . . . . . . . . . . . . . . . . . .280
chocolate w/dark chocolate (*Cascadian Farm*) . . . . . . . . . . .230
chocolate w/dark chocolate (*Häagen-Dazs* Single) . . . . . . . .350
chocolate éclair (*Col. Crunch*) . . . . . . . . . . . . . . . . . . . . . .150
chocolate éclair (*Good Humor* Single) . . . . . . . . . . . . . . . .220
coffee (*Frappuccino*) . . . . . . . . . . . . . . . . . . . . . . . . . . . . .110

**Ice cream bar** ***(cont.)***
coffee almond, milk chocolate (*Cascadian Farm*) . . . . . . . . .230
coffee almond crunch (*Häagen-Dazs* Single) . . . . . . . . . . . .370
cookies and cream (*Good Humor*) . . . . . . . . . . . . . . . . . . .190
cookies and cream crunch (*Häagen-Dazs* Single) . . . . . . . .370
dulce de leche (*Häagen-Dazs* Single) . . . . . . . . . . . . . . . . .370
(*Good Humor* Number 1) . . . . . . . . . . . . . . . . . . . . . . . . .190
(*Klondike Krunch*) . . . . . . . . . . . . . . . . . . . . . . . . . . . . .270
raspberry, dark chocolate (*Cascadian Farm*) . . . . . . . . . . . .220
strawberry shortcake (*Good Humor* Single) . . . . . . . . . . . .220
vanilla w/chocolate (*Dove Bar* Single) . . . . . . . . . . . . . . . . .320
vanilla w/chocolate (*Good Humor* Premium) . . . . . . . . . . . .240
vanilla w/chocolate (*Klondike* Original) . . . . . . . . . . . . . . .290
vanilla w/chocolate (*Popsicle*) . . . . . . . . . . . . . . . . . . . . .160
vanilla w/dark chocolate (*Cascadian Farm*) . . . . . . . . . . . .220
vanilla w/dark chocolate (*Good Humor*) . . . . . . . . . . . . . . .180
vanilla w/milk chocolate (*Ben & Jerry's*) . . . . . . . . . . . . . .330
vanilla w/milk chocolate (*Good Humor*) . . . . . . . . . . . . . . .180
vanilla w/milk chocolate (*Häagen-Dazs* Single) . . . . . . . . . .340
vanilla w/milk chocolate, almond (*Cascadian Farm*) . . . . . . .230
(*York* Peppermint Pattie Bar) . . . . . . . . . . . . . . . . . . . . . .290
**"Ice cream" bar or pie, nondairy,** 1 pc.:
bar, chocolate or vanilla (*Rice Dream*) . . . . . . . . . . . . . . .270
bar, strawberry (*Rice Dream*) . . . . . . . . . . . . . . . . . . . . . .250
pie, all flavors (*Rice Dream*) . . . . . . . . . . . . . . . . . . . . . .320
**Ice cream cake,** 2.4-oz. slice:
cappuccino or vanilla (*Viennetta*) . . . . . . . . . . . . . . . . . . .190
chocolate, triple (*Viennetta*) . . . . . . . . . . . . . . . . . . . . . .180
**Ice cream cone,** filled, 1 pc.:
(*Good Humor Giant King Cone*) . . . . . . . . . . . . . . . . . . . . .390
(*Klondike Kone*) . . . . . . . . . . . . . . . . . . . . . . . . . . . . . . .330
rocky road sundae (*Turkey Hill*) . . . . . . . . . . . . . . . . . . . .310
sundae (*Good Humor*) . . . . . . . . . . . . . . . . . . . . . . . . . . .140
sundae, caramel or fudge center (*Klondike Big Bear*) . . . . .340
sundae, vanilla (*Klondike Big Bear*) . . . . . . . . . . . . . . . . . .330
tin roof sundae (*Turkey Hill*) . . . . . . . . . . . . . . . . . . . . . .290
vanilla (*Good Humor King Cone*) . . . . . . . . . . . . . . . . . . . .270
**Ice cream cone/cup,** unfilled, 1 pc.:
bowl, waffle (*Keebler*) . . . . . . . . . . . . . . . . . . . . . . . . . . .50
cone, chocolate (*Oreo*) . . . . . . . . . . . . . . . . . . . . . . . . . . .50

cone, sugar or waffle (*Keebler*) . . . . . . . . . . . . . . . . . . . . . .50
cone, fudge-dipped (*Keebler*) . . . . . . . . . . . . . . . . . . . . . . .35
cup (*Keebler*) . . . . . . . . . . . . . . . . . . . . . . . . . . . . . . .15
**Ice cream cup,** filled, 1 pc.:
chocolate, Dutch (*Blue Bell*), 3 fl. oz. . . . . . . . . . . . . . . . . . .180
cookies and cream (*Popsicle* Zone) . . . . . . . . . . . . . . . . . . .360
fudge (*Fudgsicle Frostee*) . . . . . . . . . . . . . . . . . . . . . . . . .280
(*Good Humor Sundae Twist*) . . . . . . . . . . . . . . . . . . . . . . .160
sundae (*Klondike*) . . . . . . . . . . . . . . . . . . . . . . . . . . . . .280
vanilla (*Blue Bell* Homemade) . . . . . . . . . . . . . . . . . . . . . .170
**Ice cream sandwich,** 1 pc:
cookie (*Good Humor* Premium) . . . . . . . . . . . . . . . . . . . . . .290
cookie (*Klondike Oreo*) . . . . . . . . . . . . . . . . . . . . . . . . . .240
(*Klondike Choco Taco*) . . . . . . . . . . . . . . . . . . . . . . . . . .300
mint chocolate chip (*Turkey Hill*) . . . . . . . . . . . . . . . . . . . .200
Mississippi mud (*Good Humor* Giant) . . . . . . . . . . . . . . . . . .310
Neapolitan (*Good Humor* Giant) . . . . . . . . . . . . . . . . . . . . .250
vanilla (*Good Humor* Single) . . . . . . . . . . . . . . . . . . . . . . .180
vanilla (*Good Humor* Giant) . . . . . . . . . . . . . . . . . . . . . . . .250
vanilla (*Turkey Hill*) . . . . . . . . . . . . . . . . . . . . . . . . . . . .190
vanilla–chocolate (*Turkey Hill* Double Decker) . . . . . . . . . . .200
**Iced confection bar** (see also “Sherbet bar”), 1 pc.:
banana fudge (*Blue Bell* Single) . . . . . . . . . . . . . . . . . . . . .120
chocolate fudge (*Fudgsicle* 8 Pack/Single) . . . . . . . . . . . . . . .90
chocolate fudge (*Fudgsicle* Fat Free) . . . . . . . . . . . . . . . . . . .60
chocolate fudge (*Fudgsicle* Fudge/Original Pop) . . . . . . . . . . .60
chocolate–vanilla (*Popsicle* Pop) . . . . . . . . . . . . . . . . . . . . .100
chocolate–vanilla swirl (*Fudgsicle* Variety Pack) . . . . . . . . . .120
**Icing,** cake, see “Frosting”
**Italian sausage,** see “Sausage”

# J-K

**FOOD AND MEASURE** | **CALORIES**

**Jackfruit**, trimmed, 1 oz. . . . . . . . . . . . . . . . . . . . . . . . . . . .27
**Jackfruit, dried** (*Frieda's*), ½ cup, 3 oz. . . . . . . . . . . . . . . . . .80
**Jalapeño**, see "Pepper, jalapeño"
**Jam and preserves** (see also "Fruit spreads"), 1 tbsp.:
all fruits (*Smucker's*) . . . . . . . . . . . . . . . . . . . . . . . . . . .50
all fruits (*Smucker's* Low Sugar) . . . . . . . . . . . . . . . . . . . . . .25
all fruits (*Smucker's* Sugar Free) . . . . . . . . . . . . . . . . . . . . . .10
berry, twin (*Watkins Preserves*) . . . . . . . . . . . . . . . . . . . . . . .50
ginger (*Chivers*) . . . . . . . . . . . . . . . . . . . . . . . . . . . . . .50
kiwi (*Frieda's*) . . . . . . . . . . . . . . . . . . . . . . . . . . . . . . .35
mango (*Goya*) . . . . . . . . . . . . . . . . . . . . . . . . . . . . . . . .40
marmalade, orange (*Crosse & Blackwell*) . . . . . . . . . . . . . . . . . .60
papaya (*Goya*) . . . . . . . . . . . . . . . . . . . . . . . . . . . . . . . .45
raspberry or strawberry (*Cascadian Farm* Conserve) . . . . . . .40
**Java plum**, seeded, ½ cup . . . . . . . . . . . . . . . . . . . . . . . . . .41
**Jelly**, all fruits (*Smucker's*), 1 tbsp. . . . . . . . . . . . . . . . . . . . .50
**Jerk sauce** (see also "Marinade"), 2 tbsp.:
dipping (*Helen's Tropical Exotics* Jamaican) . . . . . . . . . . . . .45
Jamaican style (*World Harbors*) . . . . . . . . . . . . . . . . . . . . . . .70
**Jerusalem artichoke** (*Frieda's Sunchoke*), ½ cup,
3 oz. . . . . . . . . . . . . . . . . . . . . . . . . . . . . . . . . . . . . .70
**Jicama**, see "Yam bean tuber"
**Jujube**, dried, 1 oz. . . . . . . . . . . . . . . . . . . . . . . . . . . . . .81
**Kale**, fresh, 1 cup:
raw, chopped . . . . . . . . . . . . . . . . . . . . . . . . . . . . . . . . .34
boiled, drained, chopped . . . . . . . . . . . . . . . . . . . . . . . . . . .36
**Kale, canned**, ½ cup:
chopped (*Bush's Best*) . . . . . . . . . . . . . . . . . . . . . . . . . . . .30
seasoned (*Glory Foods*) . . . . . . . . . . . . . . . . . . . . . . . . . . .50
**Kale, Scotch**, ½ cup:
raw, chopped . . . . . . . . . . . . . . . . . . . . . . . . . . . . . . . . .14
boiled, drained, chopped . . . . . . . . . . . . . . . . . . . . . . . . . . .18
**Kamut flakes**, see "Cereal"
**Kasha**, see "Buckwheat groats"

**Ketchup,** 1 tbsp.:
(*Heinz*) .......... 15
(*Heinz* Hot) .......... 20
(*Hunt's*) .......... 15
(*Smucker's*) .......... 25
***KFC,*** 1 serving:
chicken, 1 pc.:
*Original Recipe,* breast .......... 400
*Original Recipe,* drumstick .......... 140
*Original Recipe,* thigh .......... 250
*Original Recipe,* whole wing .......... 140
*Extra Crispy,* breast .......... 470
*Extra Crispy,* drumstick .......... 195
*Extra Crispy,* thigh .......... 380
*Extra Crispy,* whole wing .......... 250
Hot & Spicy, breast .......... 505
Hot & Spicy, drumstick .......... 175
Hot & Spicy, thigh .......... 355
Hot & Spicy, whole wing .......... 210
chicken pot pie .......... 770
chicken *Twister* .......... 600
*Crispy Strips, Colonel's,* 3 pcs. .......... 300
*Crispy Strips,* spicy, 3 pcs. .......... 335
honey barbecue, 6 pcs. .......... 607
*Hot Wings,* 6 pcs. .......... 471
popcorn chicken, large .......... 620
popcorn chicken, small .......... 362
sandwiches:
*Original Recipe* .......... 450
*Original Recipe,* w/out sauce .......... 360
honey barbecue .......... 310
honey barbecue crunch melt .......... 556
*Tender Roast* .......... 350
*Tender Roast,* w/out sauce .......... 270
*Triple Crunch* .......... 490
*Triple Crunch,* w/out sauce .......... 390
*Triple Crunch Zinger* .......... 550
*Triple Crunch Zinger,* w/out sauce .......... 390
sides and vegetables:
baked beans, BBQ .......... 190

***KFC*, sides and vegetables *(cont.)***
biscuit, 1 pc. . . . . . . . . . . . . . . . . . . . . . . . . . . . . . .180
coleslaw, 5 oz. . . . . . . . . . . . . . . . . . . . . . . . . . . . .232
corn on the cob . . . . . . . . . . . . . . . . . . . . . . . . . . .150
macaroni & cheese . . . . . . . . . . . . . . . . . . . . . . . .180
potato salad . . . . . . . . . . . . . . . . . . . . . . . . . . . . .230
potato wedges . . . . . . . . . . . . . . . . . . . . . . . . . . .280
potatoes, mashed, w/gravy . . . . . . . . . . . . . . . . . .120
desserts:
*Colonel's* pie, apple . . . . . . . . . . . . . . . . . . . . . . .310
*Colonel's* pie, pecan . . . . . . . . . . . . . . . . . . . . . .490
*Colonel's* pie, strawberry creme . . . . . . . . . . . . . . . .280
double chocolate chip cake . . . . . . . . . . . . . . . . . .320
*Little Bucket* parfait, chocolate cream . . . . . . . . . . . .290
*Little Bucket* parfait, fudge brownie . . . . . . . . . . . . . .280
*Little Bucket* parfait, lemon creme . . . . . . . . . . . . . . .410
strawberry shortcake . . . . . . . . . . . . . . . . . . . . . . .200
**Kidney,** beef, braised, 4 oz. . . . . . . . . . . . . . . . . . . . .163
**Kidney beans,** mature, boiled, ½ cup . . . . . . . . . . . . . . .112
**Kidney beans, can or jar,** ½ cup:
red (*Blue Boy*) . . . . . . . . . . . . . . . . . . . . . . . . . . . . .120
red (*Trappey's* Creole Style) . . . . . . . . . . . . . . . . . . .100
red (*Westbrae Natural* Fat Free) . . . . . . . . . . . . . . . . . .80
red, dark (*Bush's Best*) . . . . . . . . . . . . . . . . . . . . . . .130
red, dark (*Hain* Organic) . . . . . . . . . . . . . . . . . . . . . .120
red, light (*Bush's Best*) . . . . . . . . . . . . . . . . . . . . . . .110
red, light (*Joan of Arc*) . . . . . . . . . . . . . . . . . . . . . . . .110
red, w/bacon (*Trappey's* New Orleans Style) . . . . . . . . . . .110
red, w/chili gravy or jalapeño (*Trappey's*) . . . . . . . . . . . .110
white (*Progresso* Cannellini) . . . . . . . . . . . . . . . . . . . .100
**Kielbasa** (see also "Polish sausage"):
(*Healthy Choice* Polska), 2 oz. . . . . . . . . . . . . . . . . . . .80
(*Thorn Apple Valley*), 3.2-oz. link . . . . . . . . . . . . . . . . .280
grilled (*Johnsonville*), 3-oz. link . . . . . . . . . . . . . . . . .290
turkey (*Jennie-O*), 2 oz. . . . . . . . . . . . . . . . . . . . . . . . .70
turkey (*Louis Rich* Polska), 2 oz. . . . . . . . . . . . . . . . . . .90
**Kimchee,** in jars (*Frieda's*), ¼ cup, 2 oz. . . . . . . . . . . . . .15
**Kiwi:**
(*Dole*), 2 medium, 5.2 oz. . . . . . . . . . . . . . . . . . . . . . .100
(*Frieda's*), 5 oz. . . . . . . . . . . . . . . . . . . . . . . . . . . . . .90

1 large, 3.7 oz. . . . . . . . . . . . . . . . . . . . . . . . . . .56
1 medium, 3.1 oz. . . . . . . . . . . . . . . . . . . . . . . . . .46
**Kiwi, dried** (*Sonoma*), 7–8 pcs., 1 oz. . . . . . . . . . . . . . . . . .90
**Kiwi drink blend,** strawberry (*Snapple*), 8 fl. oz. . . . . . . . . . .110
**Kiwi–lime topping** (*Smucker's Plate Scrapers*), 2 tbsp. . . .100
**Knockwurst,** beef, 1 link:
(*Boar's Head*), 4 oz. . . . . . . . . . . . . . . . . . . . . . . .310
(*Hebrew National*), 3 oz. . . . . . . . . . . . . . . . . . . . .260
(*Shofar*), 3 oz. . . . . . . . . . . . . . . . . . . . . . . . . . .210
jalapeño (*Hebrew National*), 3 oz. . . . . . . . . . . . . . . .260
**Kohlrabi,** fresh:
raw (*Frieda's*), ⅔ cup, 3 oz. . . . . . . . . . . . . . . . . . . .25
boiled, drained, sliced, ½ cup . . . . . . . . . . . . . . . . . . .24
***Krispy Kreme*** Doughnuts, 1 pc.:
blueberry, glazed . . . . . . . . . . . . . . . . . . . . . . . . . .300
blueberry-filled, powdered . . . . . . . . . . . . . . . . . . . .270
cake, traditional . . . . . . . . . . . . . . . . . . . . . . . . . .200
cinnamon apple-filled . . . . . . . . . . . . . . . . . . . . . . .280
cinnamon bun . . . . . . . . . . . . . . . . . . . . . . . . . . . .220
cinnamon twist . . . . . . . . . . . . . . . . . . . . . . . . . . .220
creme-filled, glazed . . . . . . . . . . . . . . . . . . . . . . . .350
cruller, glazed . . . . . . . . . . . . . . . . . . . . . . . . . . . .250
devil's food, glazed . . . . . . . . . . . . . . . . . . . . . . . .390
fudge-iced, cake . . . . . . . . . . . . . . . . . . . . . . . . . .230
fudge-iced, creme-filled . . . . . . . . . . . . . . . . . . . . .340
fudge-iced, custard-filled . . . . . . . . . . . . . . . . . . . .310
fudge-iced, sprinkles . . . . . . . . . . . . . . . . . . . . . . .220
fudge, glazed . . . . . . . . . . . . . . . . . . . . . . . . . . . .280
fudge, glazed cruller . . . . . . . . . . . . . . . . . . . . . . .240
lemon-filled, glazed . . . . . . . . . . . . . . . . . . . . . . . .280
maple-iced, glazed . . . . . . . . . . . . . . . . . . . . . . . . .200
original glazed . . . . . . . . . . . . . . . . . . . . . . . . . . .210
raspberry-filled, glazed . . . . . . . . . . . . . . . . . . . . . .270
**Kumquat:**
(*Frieda's*), 5 oz. . . . . . . . . . . . . . . . . . . . . . . . . . .90
1 medium, .7 oz. . . . . . . . . . . . . . . . . . . . . . . . . . .12
seeded, 1 oz. . . . . . . . . . . . . . . . . . . . . . . . . . . . .18

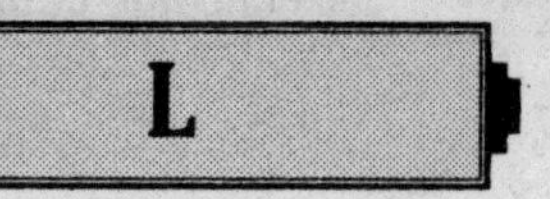

| FOOD AND MEASURE | CALORIES |
|---|---|
| **Lamb,** choice, meat only, trimmed to ¼" fat, 4 oz., except as noted: | |
| cubed, leg and shoulder, braised, lean only | 253 |
| cubed, leg and shoulder, broiled, lean only | 211 |
| ground, raw | 320 |
| ground, broiled | 321 |
| ground, broiled, 1 cup | 328 |
| foreshank, braised, lean w/fat | 276 |
| foreshank, braised, lean only | 212 |
| leg, whole, roasted, lean w/fat | 293 |
| leg, whole, roasted, w/fat, 1 slice, 3" diam. × ¼" | 73 |
| leg, whole, roasted, lean only | 217 |
| leg, whole, roasted, lean only, 1 slice, 3" diam. × ¼" | 54 |
| leg, shank half, roasted, lean w/fat | 255 |
| leg, shank half, roasted, lean only | 204 |
| leg, sirloin half, roasted, lean w/fat | 331 |
| leg, sirloin half, roasted, lean only | 231 |
| loin, roasted, lean w/fat | 350 |
| loin, roasted, lean only | 229 |
| loin chop, broiled, lean w/fat | 358 |
| loin chop, broiled, lean w/fat, 2.25 oz. (4.2 oz. raw w/bone) | 201 |
| loin chop, broiled, lean only, 1.6 oz. (4.2 oz. raw w/bone and fat) | 100 |
| rib, broiled, lean w/fat | 409 |
| rib, broiled, lean only | 266 |
| rib, roasted, lean w/fat | 407 |
| rid, roasted, lean only | 263 |
| shoulder, whole, braised, lean w/fat | 390 |
| shoulder, whole, braised, lean only | 321 |
| shoulder, whole, broiled, lean w/fat | 315 |
| shoulder, whole, broiled, lean only | 238 |
| shoulder, whole, roasted, lean w/fat | 313 |
| shoulder, whole, roasted, lean only | 231 |

shoulder arm chop:
braised, lean w/fat ....................................393
braised, lean only .....................................316
broiled, lean w/fat ....................................319
broiled, lean w/fat, 3.2 oz. (5.6 oz. raw w/bone) .......261
broiled, lean only .....................................227
broiled, lean only, 2.6 oz. (5.6 oz. raw w/bone and fat) . .148
roasted, lean w/fat ....................................316
roasted, lean only .....................................218
shoulder, blade, braised, lean w/fat ....................391
shoulder, blade, braised, lean only .....................327
shoulder, blade, broiled, lean w/fat ....................315
shoulder, blade, broiled, lean only .....................239
shoulder, blade, roasted, lean w/fat ....................319
shoulder, blade, roasted, lean only .....................237
**Lamb's-quarter,** boiled, drained, chopped, ½ cup .........29
**Lard,** pork, 1 tbsp. ..................................115
**Lasagna,** see "Pasta" and "Pasta, frozen"
**Lasagna entree, can or pkg.:**
(*Dinty Moore American Classics*), 1 bowl ..............340
w/meat sauce (*Chef Boyardee*), 1 cup ...................270
w/meat sauce (*Hormel* Microcup), 1 cup .................210
**Lasagna entree, frozen,** 1 pkg., except as noted:
bake (*Healthy Choice* Solos), 13.5 oz. ..................280
bake (*Stouffer's*), 11.5 oz. ...........................450
cheese (*Celentano* Low Fat), 10 oz. ....................290
cheese (*Lean Cuisine Everyday Favorites*), 10 oz. ........240
cheese, extra (*Marie Callender's*), 15 oz. ...............590
cheese, 5 (*Stouffer's*), 10¾ oz. ........................340
cheese, 4 (*Marie Callender's*), 10.75 oz. ...............330
cheese, 4 (*Wolfgang Puck's*), 12 oz. ....................480
chicken (*Lean Cuisine Cafe Classics*), 10 oz. ............270
chicken (*Lean Cuisine Everyday Favorites*), 10 oz. ........280
chicken (*Michelina's* Pollo), 8 oz. ......................280
chicken (*Stouffer's Family Style Favorites*), 1 cup ........310
chicken, spicy (*Wolfgang Puck's*), 12 oz. ...............470
meat (*Healthy Choice* Medley), 10.6 oz. .................360
meat (*Marie Callender's*), 10.5 oz. .....................350
meat (*Marie Callender's* 21 oz.), 1 cup ..................280
meat (*Marie Callender's* Family 40/96 oz.), 1 cup ........310

**Lasagna entree, frozen *(cont.)***
meat (*Wolfgang Puck's*), 12 oz. . . . . . . . . . . . . . . . . . . . . . . .490
meat sauce (*Banquet*), 11 oz. . . . . . . . . . . . . . . . . . . . . . . . .320
meat sauce (*Banquet* Family), 1 cup . . . . . . . . . . . . . . . . . . .270
meat sauce (*Budget Gourmet*), 8.5 oz. . . . . . . . . . . . . . . . . .250
meat sauce (*Freezer Queen* Deluxe Family), 1 cup . . . . . . . .270
meat sauce (*Marie Callender's*), 15 oz. . . . . . . . . . . . . . . . .630
meat sauce (*Michelina's*), 8 oz. . . . . . . . . . . . . . . . . . . . . . .240
meat sauce (*Michelina's*), 10 oz. . . . . . . . . . . . . . . . . . . . . .410
meat sauce (*Stouffer's*), 10.5 oz. . . . . . . . . . . . . . . . . . . . .370
meat sauce (*Stouffer's* 21 oz.), 1 cup or ⅓ pkg. . . . . . . . . .270
mozzarella (*Budget Gourmet*), 8 oz. . . . . . . . . . . . . . . . . . . .300
mushroom (*Wolfgang Puck's*), 12 oz. . . . . . . . . . . . . . . . . . .410
pomodoro (*Michelina's*), 8 oz. . . . . . . . . . . . . . . . . . . . . . . .270
primavera (*Celentano*), 10 oz. . . . . . . . . . . . . . . . . . . . . . . .260
primavera (*Michelina's*), 8 oz. . . . . . . . . . . . . . . . . . . . . . .270
spinach (*Cascadian Farm*), 11 oz. . . . . . . . . . . . . . . . . . . . .330
tomato sauce and sausage (*Stouffer's*), 10⅞ oz. . . . . . . . . .420
vegetable (*Amy's*), 9.5 oz. . . . . . . . . . . . . . . . . . . . . . . . . .300
vegetable (*Lean Cuisine Everyday Favorites*), 10.5 oz. . . . . .260
vegetable (*Michelina's*), 8 oz. . . . . . . . . . . . . . . . . . . . . . . .210
vegetable (*Stouffer's*), 10.5 oz. . . . . . . . . . . . . . . . . . . . . .410
vegetable, garden (*Cedarlane*), 10 oz. . . . . . . . . . . . . . . . . .280
vegetable, Italian (*Wolfgang Puck's*), 12 oz. . . . . . . . . . . . .440
**Leek,** fresh:
raw (*Frieda's*), 1 cup, 3 oz. . . . . . . . . . . . . . . . . . . . . . . . . .50
raw, 9.9-oz. leek . . . . . . . . . . . . . . . . . . . . . . . . . . . . . . . . .76
boiled, drained, chopped, ½ cup . . . . . . . . . . . . . . . . . . . . . .16
**Leek, freeze-dried,** 1 tbsp. . . . . . . . . . . . . . . . . . . . . . . . . .1
**Lemon:**
(*Dole*), 1 medium . . . . . . . . . . . . . . . . . . . . . . . . . . . . . . . . .15
2⅛" lemon, 3.8 oz. . . . . . . . . . . . . . . . . . . . . . . . . . . . . . . . .22
**Lemon butter dill sauce,** 2 tbsp.:
(*Golden Dipt*) . . . . . . . . . . . . . . . . . . . . . . . . . . . . . . . . . . .120
(*Golden Dipt* Fat Free) . . . . . . . . . . . . . . . . . . . . . . . . . . . . .35
**Lemon curd** (*Dickinson's*), 2 tbsp. . . . . . . . . . . . . . . . . . . . .65
**Lemongrass,** fresh, ½ cup . . . . . . . . . . . . . . . . . . . . . . . . . . .33
**Lemongrass hearts,** in jars (*A Taste of Thai*), .3-oz. pc. . . . . .0
**Lemon herb sauce mix** (*Knorr* Classic), 1 tbsp. . . . . . . . . . .30

**Lemon juice,** fresh, 1 tbsp. . . . . . . . . . . . . . . . . . . . . . . . . .4
**Lemon peel, candied,** diced (*Seneca* Glacé), 2 tbsp. . . . . . .70
**Lemon pepper/pepper salt** (*McCormick*), ¼ tsp. . . . . . . . . . .0
**Lemon sauce,** Oriental (*Ka•Me*), 1 tbsp. . . . . . . . . . . . . . . . .45
**Lemonade,** 8 fl. oz.:
(*Horizon* Organic) . . . . . . . . . . . . . . . . . . . . . . . . . .110
(*Newman's Own*) . . . . . . . . . . . . . . . . . . . . . . . . . . .110
(*Snapple*) . . . . . . . . . . . . . . . . . . . . . . . . . . . . . . .120
(*Tropicana*) . . . . . . . . . . . . . . . . . . . . . . . . . . . . . .110
(*Turkey Hill*) . . . . . . . . . . . . . . . . . . . . . . . . . . . . .120
pink (*AriZona*) . . . . . . . . . . . . . . . . . . . . . . . . . . . .110
pink (*Snapple*) . . . . . . . . . . . . . . . . . . . . . . . . . . . .110
frozen* (*Cascadian Farm*) . . . . . . . . . . . . . . . . . . . . .110
**Lemonade fruit blends,** raspberry or strawberry kiwi
(*Turkey Hill*), 8 fl. oz. . . . . . . . . . . . . . . . . . . . . . . .120
**Lentil:**
dry, green or red (*Arrowhead Mills*), ¼ cup . . . . . . . . . . . .150
cooked, ½ cup . . . . . . . . . . . . . . . . . . . . . . . . . . . . . .115
**Lentil, canned,** ½ cup:
(*Eden* Organic) . . . . . . . . . . . . . . . . . . . . . . . . . . . . .90
(*Westbrae Natural*) . . . . . . . . . . . . . . . . . . . . . . . . . .80
**Lentil dish, mix,** dahl:
(*Neera's* Chaunk), 1 cup* . . . . . . . . . . . . . . . . . . . . . .140
(*Neera's* Urad and Channa), 1 cup* . . . . . . . . . . . . . . . .105
**Lentil entree,** packaged, w/rice, 1 pkg.:
chili (*Tamarind Tree* Dal Makhani) . . . . . . . . . . . . . . . . .330
w/vegetables (*Tamarind Tree* Channa Dal Masala) . . . . . . . .340
**Lentil rice loaf,** frozen (*Natural Touch*), 1" slice, 3.2 oz. . . .170
**Lettuce** (see also "Salad blend" and "Salad kit"):
(*Dole* Greener Selection/Just Lettuce), 3 oz. . . . . . . . . . . . .15
bibb or Boston, 1 head, 5" diam. . . . . . . . . . . . . . . . . . . .21
bibb or Boston, 2 inner leaves . . . . . . . . . . . . . . . . . . . . .2
butterhead (*Frieda's* Limestone), ⅔ cup, 3 oz. . . . . . . . . . . .10
iceberg (*Dole* Classic Salad/Shredded), 3 oz. . . . . . . . . . . .15
iceberg, 1 head, 6" diam. . . . . . . . . . . . . . . . . . . . . . . . .70
leaf, shredded (*Dole*), 1½ cups . . . . . . . . . . . . . . . . . . . .15
looseleaf, shredded, ½ cup . . . . . . . . . . . . . . . . . . . . . . . .5
romaine (*Dole*), 6 leaves, 3 oz. . . . . . . . . . . . . . . . . . . . .20
romaine (*Dole* Classic Salad), 3 oz. . . . . . . . . . . . . . . . . . .15

**Lettuce** ***(cont.)***
romaine or cos, 1 inner leaf . . . . . . . . . . . . . . . . . . . . . . . . . .2
romaine hearts (*Dole/Dole* Organic Blend Mix), 3 oz. . . . . . . .15
romaine hearts, jumbo (*Andy Boy*), 6 leaves, 3 oz. . . . . . . . . .20
**Lima beans,** ½ cup, except as noted:
fresh, raw, trimmed . . . . . . . . . . . . . . . . . . . . . . . . . . . . . .88
boiled, drained . . . . . . . . . . . . . . . . . . . . . . . . . . . . . . . . .104
mature, dry, baby or large (*Jack Rabbit*), ¼ cup . . . . . . . . . . .70
mature, boiled, baby, ½ cup . . . . . . . . . . . . . . . . . . . . . . . .115
mature, boiled, large, ½ cup . . . . . . . . . . . . . . . . . . . . . . . .108
**Lima beans, can or jar,** ½ cup:
(*Aunt Nellie's* Reber Butter Beans) . . . . . . . . . . . . . . . . . .140
(*Libby's* Lima) . . . . . . . . . . . . . . . . . . . . . . . . . . . . . . . . . .80
(*Stubb's* Butterbeans) . . . . . . . . . . . . . . . . . . . . . . . . . . . .120
baby (*Bush's Best* Butterbeans) . . . . . . . . . . . . . . . . . . . . .120
green (*Del Monte*) . . . . . . . . . . . . . . . . . . . . . . . . . . . . . . . .80
green, baby (*Veg-All* Limas) . . . . . . . . . . . . . . . . . . . . . . . . .90
green or speckled (*Bush's Best* Butterbeans) . . . . . . . . . . .110
large (*Bush's Best* Butterbeans) . . . . . . . . . . . . . . . . . . . . .100
w/bacon, baby, green (*Trappey's* Limas) . . . . . . . . . . . . . . .120
w/bacon, baby, white (*Trappey's* Limas) . . . . . . . . . . . . . . .130
seasoned (*Glory Foods* Butter Beans) . . . . . . . . . . . . . . . . .120
seasoned (*Glory Foods* Limas) . . . . . . . . . . . . . . . . . . . . . .140
**Lima beans, frozen,** ½ cup, except as noted:
(*Birds Eye* Southern/Speckled Butter Beans) . . . . . . . . . . . .100
(*McKenzie's* Butter Beans/Speckled Butter Beans) . . . . . . . .100
baby (*Birds Eye*) . . . . . . . . . . . . . . . . . . . . . . . . . . . . . . . .130
baby (*John Cope's*) . . . . . . . . . . . . . . . . . . . . . . . . . . . . . .110
baby (*McKenzie's*) . . . . . . . . . . . . . . . . . . . . . . . . . . . . . . .110
baby (*Seabrook Farms* Petite) . . . . . . . . . . . . . . . . . . . . . . .110
Fordhook (*Birds Eye*) . . . . . . . . . . . . . . . . . . . . . . . . . . . . .100
**Lime,** fresh, 2"-diam. lime . . . . . . . . . . . . . . . . . . . . . . . . . .20
**Lime juice:**
fresh, 1 tbsp. . . . . . . . . . . . . . . . . . . . . . . . . . . . . . . . . . . . .4
from concentrate (*Key Largo*), 1 tsp. . . . . . . . . . . . . . . . . . . .0
sweetened (*Rose's*), 1 tbsp. . . . . . . . . . . . . . . . . . . . . . . . . .90
unsweetened (*Rose's*), 2 tbsp. . . . . . . . . . . . . . . . . . . . . . . .10
**Limeade,** frozen (*Minute Maid*), 8 fl. oz.* . . . . . . . . . . . . .100
**Ling,** meat only:
raw, 4 oz. . . . . . . . . . . . . . . . . . . . . . . . . . . . . . . . . . . . . . .99

baked, broiled, or microwaved, 4 oz. . . . . . . . . . . . . . . . . . .126
**Ling cod,** meat only:
raw, 4 oz. . . . . . . . . . . . . . . . . . . . . . . . . . . . . . . . . .96
baked, broiled, or microwaved, 4 oz. . . . . . . . . . . . . . . . . . .124
**Linguica sausage** (*Caspers*), 2 oz. . . . . . . . . . . . . . . . . . . . .120
**Linguine:**
dry, see "Pasta"
refrigerated (*Buitoni*), 1¼ cups . . . . . . . . . . . . . . . . . . . . . .240
**Linguine pasta dish, mix,** 1 cup*:
chicken and broccoli (*Pasta Roni*) . . . . . . . . . . . . . . . . . . . . .380
chicken Parmesan, creamy (*Pasta Roni*) . . . . . . . . . . . . . . .410
**Linguine entree,** frozen, 1 pkg.:
w/clams and sauce (*Michelina's*), 8.5 oz. . . . . . . . . . . . . . .290
w/clams and shrimp (*Budget Gourmet*), 8 oz. . . . . . . . . . .300
**Liquor**[1], 1 fl. oz.:
80 proof . . . . . . . . . . . . . . . . . . . . . . . . . . . . . . . . . . . . .65
90 proof . . . . . . . . . . . . . . . . . . . . . . . . . . . . . . . . . . . . .74
100 proof . . . . . . . . . . . . . . . . . . . . . . . . . . . . . . . . . . . .83
**Litchi,** see "Lychee"
**Liver:**
beef, pan-fried, 4 oz. . . . . . . . . . . . . . . . . . . . . . . . . . . . .246
chicken, simmered, 4 oz. . . . . . . . . . . . . . . . . . . . . . . . . . .178
chicken, simmered, chopped, 1 cup . . . . . . . . . . . . . . . . . . . .219
duck, raw, 1 oz. . . . . . . . . . . . . . . . . . . . . . . . . . . . . . . . . .39
goose, raw, 1 oz. . . . . . . . . . . . . . . . . . . . . . . . . . . . . . . . .38
lamb, pan-fried, 4 oz. . . . . . . . . . . . . . . . . . . . . . . . . . . . . .270
pork, braised, 4 oz. . . . . . . . . . . . . . . . . . . . . . . . . . . . . . .187
turkey, simmered, chopped, 1 cup . . . . . . . . . . . . . . . . . . . . .237
veal (calves'), braised, 4 oz. . . . . . . . . . . . . . . . . . . . . . . . .187
veal (calves'), pan-fried, 4 oz. . . . . . . . . . . . . . . . . . . . . . . .278
**Liver pâté,** see "Pâté"
**"Liver" spread,** vegetarian (*Sabra Salads*), 1 oz. . . . . . . . . .70
**Liverwurst** (see also "Braunschweiger" and "Pâté"), 2 oz.:
(*Boar's Head* Strassburger/Smoked) . . . . . . . . . . . . . . . . . .170
(*Hansel 'n Gretel*) . . . . . . . . . . . . . . . . . . . . . . . . . . . . . . .170
**Lo bok,** see "Radish, Chinese"
**Lobster** (see also "Spiny lobster"), northern, meat only:
raw, 1 lobster, 5.3 oz. . . . . . . . . . . . . . . . . . . . . . . . . . . . .135

[1]Includes all pure distilled liquors: bourbon, brandy, gin, rum, scotch, tequila, vodka, etc.

raw, 4 oz. . . . . . . . . . . . . . . . . . . . . . . . . . . . . . . . . .102
boiled or steamed, 4 oz. . . . . . . . . . . . . . . . . . . . . . . . .111
boiled or steamed, 1 cup, 5.1 oz. . . . . . . . . . . . . . . . . . . .142
**"Lobster," imitation,** chunk or salad (*Louis Kemp Lobster Delights*), ½ cup, 3 oz. . . . . . . . . . . . . . . . . . . .80
**Lobster sauce** (*Progresso*), ½ cup . . . . . . . . . . . . . . . . . .100
**Loganberry,** fresh, 1 cup . . . . . . . . . . . . . . . . . . . . . . . .89
**Loganberry, frozen,** ½ cup . . . . . . . . . . . . . . . . . . . . . . .40
**Long bean,** see "Yard-long bean"
**Longan,** shelled, dried, 1 oz. . . . . . . . . . . . . . . . . . . . . .81
**Loquat** (*Frieda's*), 5 oz. . . . . . . . . . . . . . . . . . . . . . . . . .70
**Lotus root,** raw (*Frieda's*), 1 cup, 3 oz. . . . . . . . . . . . . . . .50
**Lotus seed,** dried, 1 oz. . . . . . . . . . . . . . . . . . . . . . . . . .94
**Lox,** see "Salmon, smoked"
**Lunch meat,** loaf (see also specific listings):
Dutch brand (*Oscar Mayer*), 2 oz. . . . . . . . . . . . . . . . . . . .150
honey (*Oscar Mayer*), 1-oz. slice . . . . . . . . . . . . . . . . . . . .35
jalapeño (*Hansel 'n Gretel*) . . . . . . . . . . . . . . . . . . . . . . .150
macaroni and cheese (*Hansel 'n Gretel*) . . . . . . . . . . . . . .160
mother's loaf, pork, 1 oz. . . . . . . . . . . . . . . . . . . . . . . . . .80
old-fashioned (*Oscar Mayer*), 1-oz. slice . . . . . . . . . . . . . .70
olive (*Boar's Head*), 2 oz. . . . . . . . . . . . . . . . . . . . . . . . .130
olive (*Oscar Mayer*), 1-oz. slice . . . . . . . . . . . . . . . . . . . .70
pickle and pepper (*Boar's Head*) . . . . . . . . . . . . . . . . . . .150
pickle and pimiento (*Oscar Mayer*), 1-oz. slice . . . . . . . . . .70
pickle and pimiento (*Russer* Light P&P) . . . . . . . . . . . . . . .100
spiced (*Hansel 'n Gretel*) . . . . . . . . . . . . . . . . . . . . . . . .180
spiced (*Oscar Mayer*), 1-oz. slice . . . . . . . . . . . . . . . . . . .60
**Lunch meat, canned,** 2 oz.:
(*Spam* Lite) . . . . . . . . . . . . . . . . . . . . . . . . . . . . . . . . .110
(*Spam/Spam* Smoked/Less Salt) . . . . . . . . . . . . . . . . . . . .170
(*Treet*) . . . . . . . . . . . . . . . . . . . . . . . . . . . . . . . . . . . .130
turkey (*Spam*) . . . . . . . . . . . . . . . . . . . . . . . . . . . . . . . .70
**Lupin,** boiled, ½ cup . . . . . . . . . . . . . . . . . . . . . . . . . . .98
**Lychee,** fresh:
whole (*Frieda's*), 1 fruit . . . . . . . . . . . . . . . . . . . . . . . . .60
raw, shelled and seeded, ½ cup . . . . . . . . . . . . . . . . . . . . .66
**Lychee, dried,** 1 oz. . . . . . . . . . . . . . . . . . . . . . . . . . . . .78
**Lychee juice blend** (*Ceres*), 5.25 fl. oz. . . . . . . . . . . . . . . .87
**Lyonnaise gravy mix** (*Knorr* Classic), 2 tsp. . . . . . . . . . . . .20

# M

**FOOD AND MEASURE** | **CALORIES**

**Macadamia nut,** shelled:
(*Mauna Loa*), 1 oz. .210
(*Mauna Loa* Unsalted), 1 oz. .220
dry-roasted, diced (*Blue Diamond*), ¼ cup .240
oil-roasted, 1 oz. .204
**Macaroni** (see also "Pasta"), uncooked, dry:
elbow, 2 oz. .210
elbow, 1 cup .389
**Macaroni, cooked** (see also "Pasta, cooked"), 1 cup:
elbow .197
small shells, protein fortified, or spirals .189
vegetable (tricolor) .172
whole wheat .174
**Macaroni entree, can or pkg.,** 1 cup, except as noted:
and beef (*Chef Boyardee Beefaroni*) .260
and beef (*Chef Boyardee Beefaroni*), 7-oz. can .190
and beef (*Kid's Kitchen* Beefy) .190
and cheese (*Chef Boyardee*), ½ of 15-oz. can .180
and cheese (*Hormel*), 7.5-oz. can .270
and cheese (*Hormel* Microcup) .270
and cheese w/ham (*Dinty Moore American Classics/Cure 81*), 1 bowl .330
**Macaroni entree, frozen,** 1 pkg., except as noted:
and beef (*Lean Cuisine Everyday Favorites*), 10 oz. .250
and beef (*Michelina's*), 8 oz. .250
and beef (*Michelina's* Family), 1 cup .200
and beef (*Stouffer's*), 11.5 oz. .380
and cheese (*Banquet* Family), 1 cup .230
and cheese (*Boston Market* Home Style), 10 oz. .430
and cheese (*Budget Gourmet* Homestyle), 8 oz. .340
and cheese (*Freezer Queen* Homestyle), 8 oz. .350
and cheese (*Healthy Choice* Solos), 9 oz. .250
and cheese (*Lean Cuisine Everyday Favorites*), 10 oz. .290
and cheese (*Marie Callender's*), 12 oz. .540

**Macaroni entree, frozen *(cont.)***
and cheese (*Michelina's*), 8 oz. . . . . . . . . . . . . . . . . . . . . . . .270
and cheese (*Stouffer's*), ½ of 12-oz. pkg. . . . . . . . . . . . . . .320
and cheese (*Stouffer's* 20 oz.), 1 cup . . . . . . . . . . . . . . . . .340
and cheese (*Swanson*), 6 oz. . . . . . . . . . . . . . . . . . . . . . . . .200
and cheese, w/broccoli (*Stouffer's*), 10.5 oz. . . . . . . . . . . . .350
and cheese, cheddar/Romano (*Budget Gourmet*), 8 oz. . . .270
and cheese, 4 (*Wolfgang Puck's*), 12 oz. . . . . . . . . . . . . . . . .650
and cheese, w/ham (*Michelina's*), 8 oz. . . . . . . . . . . . . . . . . .340
and "cheese," nondairy (*Tofutti*), 6 oz. . . . . . . . . . . . . . . . . .194
and cheese pie (*Morton*), 6.5 oz. . . . . . . . . . . . . . . . . . . . . .210
vegetarian (*Yves* Veggie Macaroni), 10.5 oz. . . . . . . . . . . . .230
**Macaroni entree mix,** and cheese, dry, except as noted:
(*Annie's* Microwaveable Single Serve), ¾ cup* . . . . . . . . . .230
(*Annie's* Original Shells), 1 cup* . . . . . . . . . . . . . . . . . . . . .270
(*Bowl Appétit!*), 1 bowl . . . . . . . . . . . . . . . . . . . . . . . . . . .370
(*Land O Lakes*), 2.5 oz. . . . . . . . . . . . . . . . . . . . . . . . . . . .260
(*Land O Lakes* Deluxe Plus), 3.5 oz. . . . . . . . . . . . . . . . . . .360
Alfredo (*Annie's*), ⅔ cup . . . . . . . . . . . . . . . . . . . . . . . . . .270
Alfredo (*Annie's* Organic), 1 cup* . . . . . . . . . . . . . . . . . . . .280
cheddar (*Annie's/Annie's* Cheddar Mac), 1 cup* . . . . . . . . . .270
cheddar, white (*Annie's* Organic Shells), 1 cup* . . . . . . . . . .280
cheddar, whole-wheat shells (*Annie's* Organic), 1 cup* . . . .270
Mexican, mild (*Annie's*), ⅔ cup . . . . . . . . . . . . . . . . . . . . . .270
whole wheat (*Hodgson Mill*), ⅓ pkg. . . . . . . . . . . . . . . . . . .250
**Macaroni and cheese,** see "Macaroni entree"
**Macaroni salad,** refrigerated (*Blue Ridge Farms*), ½ cup . . .230
**Mace,** ground, 1 tsp. . . . . . . . . . . . . . . . . . . . . . . . . . . . . . .8
**Mackerel,** meat only, 4 oz.:
Atlantic, raw . . . . . . . . . . . . . . . . . . . . . . . . . . . . . . . . . . . .230
Atlantic, baked, broiled, or microwaved . . . . . . . . . . . . . . . .297
king, raw . . . . . . . . . . . . . . . . . . . . . . . . . . . . . . . . . . . . . . .119
king, baked, broiled, or microwaved . . . . . . . . . . . . . . . . . . .152
Pacific/jack, raw . . . . . . . . . . . . . . . . . . . . . . . . . . . . . . . . .179
Pacific/jack, baked, broiled, or microwaved . . . . . . . . . . . . .228
Spanish, raw . . . . . . . . . . . . . . . . . . . . . . . . . . . . . . . . . . . .158
Spanish, baked, broiled, or microwaved . . . . . . . . . . . . . . . .179
**Mackerel, canned:**
jack (*Chicken of the Sea*), 2 oz. . . . . . . . . . . . . . . . . . . . . . . .90
jack, boneless, drained, 4 oz. . . . . . . . . . . . . . . . . . . . . . . . .177

fillets (*Crown Prince*), 1 can, 3.1 oz. . . . . . . . . . . . . . . . . . .130
in oil (*Royal Crown*), ¼ cup . . . . . . . . . . . . . . . . . . . . . . . . .80
in oil, smoked (*3 Diamonds*), 2 oz. . . . . . . . . . . . . . . . . . . . .160
**Mackerel, smoked,** fillets, 2 oz.:
(*Belweder*) . . . . . . . . . . . . . . . . . . . . . . . . . . . . . . . . . .150
(*Spence & Co.*) . . . . . . . . . . . . . . . . . . . . . . . . . . . . . .180
**Mahi mahi,** see "Dolphin fish"
**Mai Tai drink mixer,** bottled (*Trader Vic's*), 4 fl. oz. . . . . . .130
**Malanga** (*Frieda's*), ⅔ cup, 3 oz. . . . . . . . . . . . . . . . . . . . . .90
**Mandarin orange,** see "Tangerine"
**Mandioca,** see "Yuca"
**Mango,** fresh:
(*Dole*), ½ medium, 3.7 oz. . . . . . . . . . . . . . . . . . . . . . . . . . .70
10.6-oz. fruit, 7.3 oz. trimmed . . . . . . . . . . . . . . . . . . . . . . .135
peeled, sliced, ½ cup . . . . . . . . . . . . . . . . . . . . . . . . . . . . . .54
**Mango, can or jar:**
in extra light syrup (*Sunfresh* Chilled), ½ cup . . . . . . . . . . .100
in light syrup (*Sunfresh* Can), ½ cup . . . . . . . . . . . . . . . . . . .90
in syrup (*Herdez*), 2 pcs. . . . . . . . . . . . . . . . . . . . . . . . . . .170
**Mango, dried** (*Setton Farms*), 6 pcs., 1.4 oz. . . . . . . . . . . .160
**Mango–orange topping** (*Smucker's Plate Scrapers*),
2 tbsp. . . . . . . . . . . . . . . . . . . . . . . . . . . . . . . . . . . . . . . .100
**Mango drink:**
(*AriZona* Mucho), 8 fl. oz. . . . . . . . . . . . . . . . . . . . . . . . . . .100
(*Libby's*), 8 fl. oz. . . . . . . . . . . . . . . . . . . . . . . . . . . . . . . .140
(*Libby's*), 11.5-fl.-oz. can . . . . . . . . . . . . . . . . . . . . . . . . . .210
(*Snapple Mango Madness*), 8 fl. oz. . . . . . . . . . . . . . . . . . . .110
**Mango juice blend:**
(*Ceres*), 5.25 fl. oz. . . . . . . . . . . . . . . . . . . . . . . . . . . . . . . .87
orange guanabana (*Nantucket Nectars*), 8 fl. oz. . . . . . . . . . .130
**Manicotti entree,** frozen, 1 pkg.:
cheese (*Celentano*), 10 oz. . . . . . . . . . . . . . . . . . . . . . . . . . .340
cheese (*Stouffer's*), 9 oz. . . . . . . . . . . . . . . . . . . . . . . . . . . .360
cheese, 3 (*Healthy Choice* Solos), 11 oz. . . . . . . . . . . . . . . .300
cheese, 3, marinara (*Budget Gourmet*), 8.5 oz. . . . . . . . . . . . .290
cheese/spinach (*Lean Cuisine Hearty Portions*), 15.5 oz. . . .350
**Maple syrup** (*Maple Grove Farms*), ¼ cup . . . . . . . . . . . . . .200
**Margarine,** 1 tbsp., except as noted:
(*I Can't Believe It's Not Butter*) . . . . . . . . . . . . . . . . . . . . . . .90
(*I Can't Believe It's Not Butter* Squeeze) . . . . . . . . . . . . . . . .80

**Margarine *(cont.)***
(*Land O Lakes/Land O Lakes* Country Morning Blend) . . . .100
(*Mazola* Premium) . . . . . . . . . . . . . . . . . . . . . . . . . .100
(*Parkay* Tub, Soft) . . . . . . . . . . . . . . . . . . . . . . . . .100
light (*I Can't Believe It's Not Butter* Light/Sweet
Cream/Calcium) . . . . . . . . . . . . . . . . . . . . . . . . . . .50
light (*Land O Lakes* Country Morning Blend) . . . . . . . . . . . .50
light (*Mazola* 40% Corn Oil Diet Reduced Calorie) . . . . . . . . .50
light (*Smart Balance*) . . . . . . . . . . . . . . . . . . . . . . . . . .45
light (*Smart Beat* Trans-Fat Free) . . . . . . . . . . . . . . . . . .20
spread (*Country Morning* Soft/Stick) . . . . . . . . . . . . . . . .100
spread (*Country Morning* Soft/Stick Light) . . . . . . . . . . . . .50
spread (*Land O Lakes* w/Sweet Cream, Soft) . . . . . . . . . . . .80
spread (*Land O Lakes* w/Sweet Cream, Stick) . . . . . . . . . . . .90
spread (*Mazola* 40% Corn Oil Light) . . . . . . . . . . . . . . . . . .50
**Margarita drink mixer:**
bottled (*Mr & Mrs T*), 4 fl. oz. . . . . . . . . . . . . . . . . . . . . .130
bottled, strawberry (*Trader Vic's*), 4 fl. oz. . . . . . . . . . . . . . .160
frozen (*Bacardi*), 2 fl. oz. . . . . . . . . . . . . . . . . . . . . . . . . .90
**Marinade** (see also "Grilling sauce," and specific listings):
Cajun or chipotle pepper (*Cardini's*), 1 tbsp. . . . . . . . . . . . . .10
citrus grill w/orange juice (*Lawry's*), 1 tbsp. . . . . . . . . . . . . .15
Dijon, white wine (*Golden Dipt*), 1 tbsp. . . . . . . . . . . . . . . . .10
Dijon/honey, Hawaiian, or hickory (*Lawry's*), 1 tbsp. . . . . . . .20
garlic, roasted, and herb (*Cardini's*), 1 tbsp. . . . . . . . . . . . . .10
garlic herb or ginger teriyaki (*Golden Dipt*), 1 tbsp. . . . . . . .60
herb and garlic or lemon pepper (*Lawry's*), 1 tbsp. . . . . . . . . .10
honey Dijon (*Cardini's*), 1 tbsp. . . . . . . . . . . . . . . . . . . . . . .20
honey hickory (*World Harbors* Ember Wisp), 2 tbsp. . . . . . .45
honey soy (*Golden Dipt*), 1 tbsp. . . . . . . . . . . . . . . . . . . . . .30
Indian style, mango (*World Harbors Bengali*), 2 tbsp. . . . . . .45
jerk, Caribbean, w/papaya juice (*Lawry's*), 1 tbsp. . . . . . . . . .25
lemon herb (*Golden Dipt*), 2 tbsp. . . . . . . . . . . . . . . . . . . . .80
lemon pepper garlic (*World Harbors* Maine's Own),
2 tbsp. . . . . . . . . . . . . . . . . . . . . . . . . . . . . . . . . . . . . . .35
lemon pepper, zesty (*Cardini's*), 1 tbsp. . . . . . . . . . . . . . . .15
London broil (*Lawry's Weekday Gourmet*), 1 tbsp. . . . . . . . .10
mesquite (*Golden Dipt*), 1 tbsp. . . . . . . . . . . . . . . . . . . . . . .10
mesquite, fajita (*Cardini's*), 1 tbsp. . . . . . . . . . . . . . . . . . . .10
tequila lime w/lime juice (*Lawry's*), 1 tbsp. . . . . . . . . . . . . . .15

teriyaki, and sauce (*Kikkoman*) . . . . . . . . . . . . . . . . . . . . . . . .15
teriyaki, and sauce, roasted garlic (*Kikkoman*) . . . . . . . . . . .25
teriyaki, steak (*Lawry's Weekday Gourmet*) . . . . . . . . . . . .25
Thai ginger w/lime juice (*Lawry's*) . . . . . . . . . . . . . . . . . . .10
**Marinade seasoning mix** (see also specific listings):
Cajun, garlic, or mesquite (*Adolph's For the Grill*), 1 tsp. . . . .5
meat (*McCormick*), ½ cup* . . . . . . . . . . . . . . . . . . . . . . . . . .15
steak or meat (*Adolph's Marinade in Minutes*), ¾ tsp. . . . . . .5
**Marjoram,** dried, 1 tsp. . . . . . . . . . . . . . . . . . . . . . . . . . . . .2
**Marmalade,** see "Jam and preserves"
**Marshmallow topping** (*Marshmallow Fluff*), 2 tbsp. . . . . . . .60
**Matzo,** see "Crackers"
**Matzo balls,** in jars (*Manischewitz*), 1 cup . . . . . . . . . . . . .220
**Mayonnaise,** in jars, 1 tbsp.:
(*Hellmann's/Best Foods* Real/Extra Heavy) . . . . . . . . . . . . .100
(*Hellmann's/Best Foods* Light) . . . . . . . . . . . . . . . . . . . . . . . .50
(*Hollywood* Canola) . . . . . . . . . . . . . . . . . . . . . . . . . . . . . . .100
(*Kraft*) . . . . . . . . . . . . . . . . . . . . . . . . . . . . . . . . . . . . . . . .100
(*Smart Balance* Light) . . . . . . . . . . . . . . . . . . . . . . . . . . . . .50
**Mayonnaise dressing,** in jars, 1 tbsp.:
(*Hain* Eggless) . . . . . . . . . . . . . . . . . . . . . . . . . . . . . . . . . .100
(*Hellmann's/Best Foods* Deli Blend Whipped Dressing) . . . . .60
(*Hellmann's/Best Foods* Low Fat) . . . . . . . . . . . . . . . . . . . . .15
(*Hellmann's/BestFoods/Just 2 Good!* Reduced Fat) . . . . . . . .25
(*Kraft Light*) . . . . . . . . . . . . . . . . . . . . . . . . . . . . . . . . . . . .50
(*Miracle Whip*) . . . . . . . . . . . . . . . . . . . . . . . . . . . . . . . . . . .70
tofu (*Nayonaise*) . . . . . . . . . . . . . . . . . . . . . . . . . . . . . . . . .35
***McDonald's,*** 1 serving:
breakfast:
bagel, ham and egg, cheese . . . . . . . . . . . . . . . . . . . . . . .550
bagel, Spanish omelet . . . . . . . . . . . . . . . . . . . . . . . . . . . .690
bagel, steak and egg, cheese . . . . . . . . . . . . . . . . . . . . . .700
biscuit, plain . . . . . . . . . . . . . . . . . . . . . . . . . . . . . . . . . . .290
biscuit, bacon, egg, cheese . . . . . . . . . . . . . . . . . . . . . . . .540
biscuit, sausage . . . . . . . . . . . . . . . . . . . . . . . . . . . . . . . .470
biscuit, sausage and egg . . . . . . . . . . . . . . . . . . . . . . . . . .550
breakfast burrito . . . . . . . . . . . . . . . . . . . . . . . . . . . . . . . .290
*Egg McMuffin* . . . . . . . . . . . . . . . . . . . . . . . . . . . . . . . . . .290
eggs, scrambled, 2 . . . . . . . . . . . . . . . . . . . . . . . . . . . . . .160
English muffin, plain . . . . . . . . . . . . . . . . . . . . . . . . . . . . .140

***McDonald's*, breakfast *(cont.)***

hash browns . . . . . 130
hot cakes, plain . . . . . 340
hot cakes, w/syrup, margarine . . . . . 600
sausage . . . . . 170
*Sausage McMuffin* . . . . . 360
*Sausage McMuffin*, w/egg . . . . . 440

danish and muffin:

apple bran muffin, low-fat . . . . . 300
apple danish . . . . . 340
cheese danish . . . . . 400
cinnamon roll . . . . . 390

sandwiches:

*Big Mac* . . . . . 590
*Big N' Tasty* . . . . . 540
*Big N' Tasty* w/cheese . . . . . 590
cheeseburger . . . . . 330
*Chicken McGrill* . . . . . 450
*Chicken McGrill* w/out mayo . . . . . 340
crispy chicken . . . . . 550
*Filet-O-Fish* . . . . . 470
hamburger . . . . . 280
*Quarter Pounder* . . . . . 430
*Quarter Pounder* w/cheese . . . . . 530

*Chicken McNuggets*, 4 pcs. . . . . . 190
*Chicken McNuggets*, 6 pcs. . . . . . 290
*Chicken McNuggets*, 9 pcs. . . . . . 430

*McNuggets* sauce pkt.:

barbeque or honey . . . . . 45
honey mustard or sweet and sour . . . . . 50
hot mustard . . . . . 60
mayonnaise, light . . . . . 40

french fries, large . . . . . 540
french fries, medium . . . . . 450
french fries, small . . . . . 210
french fries, *Super Size* . . . . . 610

salads, w/out dressing:

chef salad . . . . . 150
garden salad . . . . . 100
grilled chicken Caesar salad . . . . . 100

croutons, 1 pkt. . . . . . . . . . . . . . . . . . . . . . . . . . . . .50
dressing, 1 pkt.:
Caesar . . . . . . . . . . . . . . . . . . . . . . . . . . . . . . . . .150
herb vinaigrette, fat-free . . . . . . . . . . . . . . . . . . . . .35
honey mustard . . . . . . . . . . . . . . . . . . . . . . . . . . .160
ranch . . . . . . . . . . . . . . . . . . . . . . . . . . . . . . . . . .170
red French, reduced calorie, or Thousand Island . . . . . .130
desserts/shakes:
baked apple pie . . . . . . . . . . . . . . . . . . . . . . . . . . .260
chocolate chip cookie, 1 pkg. . . . . . . . . . . . . . . . . . .280
*Fruit 'n Yogurt Parfait* . . . . . . . . . . . . . . . . . . . . . .380
*Fruit 'n Yogurt Parfait* w/out granola . . . . . . . . . . . . .280
*McDonaldland Cookies,* 1 pkg. . . . . . . . . . . . . . . . . .230
*McFlurry, Butterfinger* . . . . . . . . . . . . . . . . . . . . . .620
*McFlurry, M&M* . . . . . . . . . . . . . . . . . . . . . . . . . . .630
*McFlurry, Nestlé Crunch* . . . . . . . . . . . . . . . . . . . . .630
*McFlurry, Oreo* . . . . . . . . . . . . . . . . . . . . . . . . . . .570
shake, chocolate, strawberry, or vanilla, small . . . . . . . .360
sundae, hot caramel . . . . . . . . . . . . . . . . . . . . . . . . .360
sundae, hot fudge . . . . . . . . . . . . . . . . . . . . . . . . . .340
sundae, strawberry . . . . . . . . . . . . . . . . . . . . . . . . .290
sundae nuts . . . . . . . . . . . . . . . . . . . . . . . . . . . . . . .40
vanilla cone, reduced fat . . . . . . . . . . . . . . . . . . . . .150
**Meat,** see specific listings
**Meat, potted,** see "Meat spread"
**Meat loaf,** refrigerated (*Always Tender*), 5 oz. . . . . . . . . . .240
**Meat loaf dinner,** frozen, 1 pkg.:
(*Healthy Choice*), 12 oz. . . . . . . . . . . . . . . . . . . . . . . . .330
(*Stouffer's* HomeStyle), 17 oz. . . . . . . . . . . . . . . . . . . .560
(*Swanson Traditional Favorites*), 10.75 oz. . . . . . . . . . . . .380
**Meat loaf entree,** frozen, 1 pkg.:
(*Banquet*), 9.5 oz. . . . . . . . . . . . . . . . . . . . . . . . . . . .240
(*Freezer Queen* Meal), 9.5 oz. . . . . . . . . . . . . . . . . . . .310
(*Stouffer's* HomeStyle), 9⅞ oz. . . . . . . . . . . . . . . . . . .390
and gravy (*Marie Callender's*), 14 oz. . . . . . . . . . . . . . . .540
and gravy, w/mashed potato (*Michelina's*), 8 oz. . . . . . . . . .340
and gravy, w/mashed potato (*Michelina's*), 10.5 oz. . . . . . .390
and gravy, savory (*Banquet* Family), 1 patty w/gravy . . . . . .190
w/mashed potato, gravy (*Marie Callender's* Family), 1 patty,
gravy, ½ cup potato . . . . . . . . . . . . . . . . . . . . . . . . .280

**Meat loaf entree, frozen *(cont.)***
in port wine sauce (*Wolfgang Puck's*), 12 oz. . . . . . . . . . . . .540
tomato sauce and (*Freezer Queen* Family), ⅙ pkg. . . . . . . . .200
w/whipped potato (*Lean Cuisine Cafe Classics*), 9⅜ oz. . . .260
**Meat loaf seasoning mix,** 1 tbsp.:
(*Adolph's Meal Makers*), 1 tbsp. . . . . . . . . . . . . . . . . . . . . .25
(*Lawry's*), 1 tbsp. . . . . . . . . . . . . . . . . . . . . . . . . . . . . . .35
(*McCormick*), ⅒ pkg. . . . . . . . . . . . . . . . . . . . . . . . . . . .15
**Meat spread** (see also specific listings):
(*Spam* Spread), 4 tbsp. . . . . . . . . . . . . . . . . . . . . . . . . .140
potted meat (*Armour*), ¼ cup . . . . . . . . . . . . . . . . . . . . . .80
potted meat (*Hormel*), 4 tbsp., 2 oz. . . . . . . . . . . . . . . . . .100
**Meat tenderizer** (*Adolph's* Original No MSG), ¼ tsp. . . . . . . .0
**Meatball,** frozen or refrigerated:
baked (*DeLuca*), 2 pcs., ¼ cup sauce . . . . . . . . . . . . . . . . .180
chicken, Italian style (*Tyson* Family Pack), 6 pcs., 3 oz. . . . .150
Italian (*Home Market*), 3 pcs., 3 oz. . . . . . . . . . . . . . . . . . .230
Italian (*Master Choice*), about 4 pcs., 3 oz. . . . . . . . . . . . . .230
Italian (*Rosina*), 6 small or 1 large, 3 oz. . . . . . . . . . . . . . .250
Swedish (*Rosina*), 6 pcs., 3 oz. . . . . . . . . . . . . . . . . . . . . .260
turkey (*Rosina*), 3 pcs., 3 oz. . . . . . . . . . . . . . . . . . . . . . .170
turkey, Italian (*Shady Brook Farms*), 3 pcs., 3 oz. . . . . . . . .130
**Meatball entree, canned,** stew (*Dinty Moore*), 1 cup . . . . .250
**Meatball entree, frozen,** 1 pkg.:
Italian style (*Healthy Choice* Bread Stuffs), 6.1 oz. . . . . . . .330
mashed potatoes and (*Michelina's*), 8.5 oz. . . . . . . . . . . . . .280
Stroganoff (*Country Skillet*),¼ of 32-oz. pkg. . . . . . . . . . . .340
Swedish (*Banquet*), 10.25 oz. . . . . . . . . . . . . . . . . . . . . . .400
Swedish (*Budget Gourmet*), 10 oz. . . . . . . . . . . . . . . . . . . .530
Swedish (*Marie Callender's*), 10.25 oz. . . . . . . . . . . . . . . . .450
Swedish (*Stouffer's*), 10.5 oz. . . . . . . . . . . . . . . . . . . . . . .520
Swedish, w/gravy (*Michelina's* Family), 1 cup . . . . . . . . . . .290
**Meatball pocket,** frozen, 4.5-oz. pc.:
(*Lean Pockets*) . . . . . . . . . . . . . . . . . . . . . . . . . . . . . . . .300
and mozzarella (*Hot Pockets*) . . . . . . . . . . . . . . . . . . . . . .320
**Melon,** see specific listings
**Melon, mixed, dried** (*Sunsweet Fruitlings*), ⅓ cup . . . . . . .130
**Melon balls,** frozen, cantaloupe/honeydew, ½ cup . . . . . . . .28
**Melon salad,** chilled, in light syrup (*Sunfresh*), ½ cup . . . . .45
**Melogold,** fresh (*Frieda's*), ½ fruit, 5.9 oz. . . . . . . . . . . . . . .50

**Menudo,** see "Soup, canned, ready-to-serve"
**Mexican beans** (see also "Chili beans"), canned:
(*Allens/Brown Beauty* Chili), ½ cup . . . . . . . . . . . . . . . . .120
(*Old El Paso* Mexe), ½ cup . . . . . . . . . . . . . . . . . . . . . . .110
**Mexican dinner** (see also specific listings), frozen, 1 pkg.:
(*Swanson Hungry-Man*), 20 oz. . . . . . . . . . . . . . . . . . . . . .710
combo (*Swanson Traditional Favorites*), 13.25 oz. . . . . . . .470
**Mexican squash** (*Frieda's*), ½ cup, 3 oz. . . . . . . . . . . . . . .35
**Milk,** dairy, 8 fl. oz.:
buttermilk, cultured . . . . . . . . . . . . . . . . . . . . . . . . . . . .99
whole, 3.3% fat . . . . . . . . . . . . . . . . . . . . . . . . . . . . . .150
reduced/low fat, 2% fat . . . . . . . . . . . . . . . . . . . . . . . . .121
reduced/low fat, 2%, protein-fortified . . . . . . . . . . . . . . .137
reduced/low fat, 1% fat . . . . . . . . . . . . . . . . . . . . . . . . .102
1%, protein-fortified . . . . . . . . . . . . . . . . . . . . . . . . . . .119
skim/fat-free . . . . . . . . . . . . . . . . . . . . . . . . . . . . . . . .86
**Milk, canned,** 2 tbsp.:
condensed, sweetened (*Carnation*) . . . . . . . . . . . . . . . . .130
evaporated (*Pet*) . . . . . . . . . . . . . . . . . . . . . . . . . . . . .40
evaporated skim (*Pet*) . . . . . . . . . . . . . . . . . . . . . . . . . .25
**Milk, chocolate,** see "Milk, flavored"
**Milk, dry:**
buttermilk, sweet cream, 1 tbsp. . . . . . . . . . . . . . . . . . . .25
whole, 1 tbsp. . . . . . . . . . . . . . . . . . . . . . . . . . . . . . . .40
nonfat, regular, 1 tbsp. . . . . . . . . . . . . . . . . . . . . . . . . .27
nonfat, instant, 1 tbsp. . . . . . . . . . . . . . . . . . . . . . . . . .15
**Milk, flavored,** 8 fl. oz.:
banana (*Nesquik* Reduced Fat) . . . . . . . . . . . . . . . . . . . .200
berry (*DariGo* Blast Reduced Fat) . . . . . . . . . . . . . . . . . .220
chocolate:
  (*Hershey's*) . . . . . . . . . . . . . . . . . . . . . . . . . . . . . . .230
  (*Hershey's* Fat Free) . . . . . . . . . . . . . . . . . . . . . . . . .150
  (*Nesquik*) . . . . . . . . . . . . . . . . . . . . . . . . . . . . . . . .230
  (*Nesquik* Fat Free) . . . . . . . . . . . . . . . . . . . . . . . . . .160
  (*Parmalat* 2%) . . . . . . . . . . . . . . . . . . . . . . . . . . . . .180
  (*Turkey Hill* 1%) . . . . . . . . . . . . . . . . . . . . . . . . . . .180
orange cream (*Turkey Hill Cool Moos*) . . . . . . . . . . . . . . .190
strawberry (*Nesquik*) . . . . . . . . . . . . . . . . . . . . . . . . . .230
strawberry or vanilla (*Turkey Hill Cool Moos*) . . . . . . . . . .160
**Milk, goat's** (*Meyenberg*), 8 fl. oz. . . . . . . . . . . . . . . . . .140

**"Milk," nondairy,** see "Rice beverage" and "Soy beverage"
**Milk, sheep's,** 1 cup . . . . . . . . . . . . . . . . . . . . . . . . . . . .264
**Milkfish,** meat only:
raw, 4 oz. . . . . . . . . . . . . . . . . . . . . . . . . . . . . . . . . . . . .168
baked, broiled, or microwaved, 4 oz. . . . . . . . . . . . . . . . . .215
**Millet,** hulled (*Arrowhead Mills*), ¼ cup . . . . . . . . . . . . . . .150
**Mincemeat,** see "Pie filling"
**Mirin** (*Sushi Chef*), 1 tbsp. . . . . . . . . . . . . . . . . . . . . . . . .50
**Miso,** soy (*Eden/Eden* Organic Hacho), 1 tbsp. . . . . . . . . . . .35
**Molasses,** 1 tbsp.:
blackstrap (*New Morning*) . . . . . . . . . . . . . . . . . . . . . . . . . .60
regular, mild or robust (*Grandma's*) . . . . . . . . . . . . . . . . . . .50
**Mole sauce** (*Doña Maria*), 2 tbsp. . . . . . . . . . . . . . . . . . . .230
**Monkfish,** meat only:
raw, 4 oz. . . . . . . . . . . . . . . . . . . . . . . . . . . . . . . . . . . . .86
baked, broiled, or microwaved, 4 oz. . . . . . . . . . . . . . . . . .110
**Mortadella,** 2 oz.:
(*Boar's Head*) . . . . . . . . . . . . . . . . . . . . . . . . . . . . . . . . .160
(*Daniele*) . . . . . . . . . . . . . . . . . . . . . . . . . . . . . . . . . . . .150
w/pistachios (*Boar's Head*) . . . . . . . . . . . . . . . . . . . . . . . . .170
**Mothbean,** boiled, 4 oz. . . . . . . . . . . . . . . . . . . . . . . . . . .133
**Muffin,** 1 pc., except as noted:
apple (*Awrey's* 2.5 oz.) . . . . . . . . . . . . . . . . . . . . . . . . . . .230
apple, banana nut, or blueberry (*Awrey's* 1.5 oz.) . . . . . . . .130
banana nut (*Awrey's* Grande 4 oz.) . . . . . . . . . . . . . . . . . . .410
banana walnut, mini (*Hostess*), 3 pcs. . . . . . . . . . . . . . . . .160
blueberry (*Awrey's* 2.5 oz.) . . . . . . . . . . . . . . . . . . . . . . . .210
blueberry (*Awrey's* Grande 4 oz.) . . . . . . . . . . . . . . . . . . . .380
blueberry (*Entenmann's* Light) . . . . . . . . . . . . . . . . . . . . . .130
blueberry, mini (*Entenmann's Little Bites*), 4 pcs. . . . . . . . .190
blueberry, mini (*Hostess*), 3 pcs. . . . . . . . . . . . . . . . . . . . .150
cheese streusel (*Awrey's* Grande) . . . . . . . . . . . . . . . . . . . .380
chocolate chip chocolate (*Awrey's* Grande) . . . . . . . . . . . . .480
chocolate chip or cinnamon apple, mini (*Hostess*),
3 pcs. . . . . . . . . . . . . . . . . . . . . . . . . . . . . . . . . . . . . . .160
corn (*Awrey's* 1.25 oz.) . . . . . . . . . . . . . . . . . . . . . . . . . . .130
corn (*Awrey's* 4 oz.) . . . . . . . . . . . . . . . . . . . . . . . . . . . . .410
corn (*Entenmann's*) . . . . . . . . . . . . . . . . . . . . . . . . . . . . . .210
cranberry nut (*Awrey's*) . . . . . . . . . . . . . . . . . . . . . . . . . . .150
English (*Bays*) . . . . . . . . . . . . . . . . . . . . . . . . . . . . . . . . . .140

English (*Thomas'*) .......................... 120
English (*Thomas'* Super Size) .......................... 190
English (*Vermont Bread*) .......................... 120
English, blueberry (*Thomas'*) .......................... 140
English, blueberry (*Vermont Bread*) .......................... 120
English, cinnamon (*Thomas'*) .......................... 150
English, cinnamon raisin or maple (*Vermont Bread*) ...... 130
English, honey wheat or oat bran (*Thomas'*) ............ 130
English, maple French toast (*Thomas'*) ................ 150
English, sourdough (*Bays*) .......................... 130
English, sourdough (*Thomas'*) .......................... 120
lemon poppy seed (*Awrey's* 4 oz.) .......................... 420
lemon poppy seed (*Awrey's* Petite), 2 pcs. ............. 160
oat bran (*Hostess*) .......................... 160
raisin bran (*Awrey's* 1.5 oz.) .......................... 110
raisin bran (*Awrey's* 2.5 oz.) .......................... 200
raisin bran (*Awrey's* 4 oz.) .......................... 350
**Muffin, frozen,** 1 pc.:
blueberry (*Sara Lee*) .......................... 220
corn (*Sara Lee*) .......................... 260
**Muffin mix** (see also "Bread mix, sweet"), 1 pc.*, except as noted:
apple cinnamon (*Betty Crocker*) .......................... 170
apple cinnamon (*Duncan Hines* All Bran) ............. 140
apple cinnamon (*Sweet Rewards*) .......................... 140
apple cinnamon (*Sweet Rewards* Fat Free) ........... 120
apple streusel (*Betty Crocker*) .......................... 210
banana nut (*Betty Crocker* Box/Pouch) ............. 170
blueberry (*Betty Crocker* Pouch) .......................... 160
blueberry (*Duncan Hines* All Bran) .......................... 140
blueberry (*Duncan Hines* Streusel) .......................... 190
blueberry, twice (*Betty Crocker* Box) .......................... 140
blueberry, wild (*Betty Crocker* Box) .......................... 170
blueberry, wild (*Sweet Rewards*) .......................... 130
bran (*Hodgson Mill*), ¼ cup mix .......................... 130
bran w/dates (*"Jiffy"*), ¼ cup mix .......................... 150
chocolate, double (*Betty Crocker*) .......................... 200
chocolate chip (*Betty Crocker*) .......................... 170
chocolate chip (*Duncan Hines*) .......................... 190
cinnamon swirl (*Duncan Hines*) .......................... 200

**Muffin mix** ***(cont.)***
corn (*Glory Foods*), ¼ cup mix .......................150
corn, golden (*Betty Crocker*) ........................160
cranberry orange (*Betty Crocker*) ....................150
cranberry orange (*Duncan Hines*) .....................150
lemon poppy seed (*Betty Crocker* Box) ................190
lemon poppy seed (*Betty Crocker* Pouch) ..............180
strawberry or wildberry (*Pillsbury*), ⅓ cup mix .........170
whole grain (*Arrowhead Mills*), ⅓ cup mix .............150
whole wheat (*Hodgson Mill*), ¼ cup mix ...............130
**Muffin sandwich,** see "Breakfast sandwich"
**Mulberry,** ½ cup .................................31
**Mullet,** striped, meat only:
raw, 4 oz. .........................................133
baked, broiled, or microwaved, 4 oz. ...................170
**Mung bean,** dry (*Arrowhead Mills*), ¼ cup .............160
**Mung bean sprouts,** raw (*Jonathan's*), 1 cup ...........30
**Mushroom,** white or common, fresh:
raw, pcs., ½ cup .....................................9
boiled, drained, pcs., ½ cup ..........................21
**Mushroom, can or jar:**
whole or sliced (*Giorgio*), ½ cup w/liquid ...............20
whole, sliced, or pcs. (*Green Giant*), ½ cup .............30
whole, marinated (*Giorgio*), 1 oz., about 6 whole .........10
sliced (*BinB*), 1 can ................................30
stems and pieces (*Libby's*), ½ cup .....................25
**Mushroom, chanterelle,** dried (*Frieda's*), 2 pcs. ..........15
**Mushroom, enoki,** fresh (*Frieda's*), ¼ pkg., .9 oz. ........10
**Mushroom, morel,** dried (*Frieda's*), 3 pcs. ..............15
**Mushroom, oyster:**
fresh (*Frieda's*), 3 oz. ..............................20
dried (*Epicurean Specialty*), ⅓ oz. .....................12
dried (*Frieda's*), 3 pcs. .............................15
**Mushroom, padi straw,** dried (*Frieda's*), 6 pcs. ..........15
**Mushroom, porcini,** dried:
(*Epicurean Specialty*), ⅓ oz. .........................12
(*Frieda's*), 5 pcs. ..................................15
**Mushroom, portobello,** dried (*Frieda's*), 7 pcs. ...........5
**Mushroom, shiitake:**
fresh, cooked, 4 medium or ½ cup pcs. ..................40

dried (*Frieda's*), ¼ cup . . . . . . . . . . . . . . . . . . . . . . . . . . .10
dried, 4 medium, ½ oz. . . . . . . . . . . . . . . . . . . . . . . . . . . . .44
**Mushroom, wood ear,** dried (*Frieda's*), 3 pcs. . . . . . . . . . . .15
**Mushroom batter mix** (*Don's Chuck Wagon*), ¼ cup . . . . . .95
**Mushroom gravy,** rich (*Heinz* Homestyle), ¼ cup . . . . . . . . .25
**Mushroom gravy mix:**
(*Loma Linda Gravy Quik*), ¼ cup* . . . . . . . . . . . . . . . . . . .15
• (*Knorr* Classic Hunter), 1 tbsp. . . . . . . . . . . . . . . . . . . . .25
(*McCormick*), ¼ cup* . . . . . . . . . . . . . . . . . . . . . . . . . . .20
**Mushroom sauce:**
carciofi or porcini (*Italia In Tavola*), 2 tbsp. . . . . . . . . . . . .110
shiitake (*Annie Chun's*), 1 tbsp. . . . . . . . . . . . . . . . . . . . . .15
**Mussels,** blue, meat only:
raw, 4 oz. . . . . . . . . . . . . . . . . . . . . . . . . . . . . . . . . . . .90
raw, 1 cup . . . . . . . . . . . . . . . . . . . . . . . . . . . . . . . . . . .119
boiled, poached, or steamed, 4 oz. . . . . . . . . . . . . . . . . . . .195
**Mussels, smoked** (*Ducktrap River*), ¼ cup . . . . . . . . . . . .140
**Mussels dish,** frozen, 3 oz.:
half shell (*Southern Seafoods* New Zealand Greenshell) . . .100
in tomato sauce (*Plumpy*), 3 oz. . . . . . . . . . . . . . . . . . . . .100
**Mustard,** prepared, 1 tsp.:
(*Boar's Head* Deli) . . . . . . . . . . . . . . . . . . . . . . . . . . . . . .0
(*Grey Poupon* Spicy Brown/Hickory Smoke) . . . . . . . . . . . . .5
(*Gulden's* Spicy Brown) . . . . . . . . . . . . . . . . . . . . . . . . . . .5
(*Hebrew National* Deli) . . . . . . . . . . . . . . . . . . . . . . . . . . .4
(*Hellmann's/Best Foods* Deli) . . . . . . . . . . . . . . . . . . . . . . .5
(*Jack Daniel's* Old No. 7/Hickory Smoke) . . . . . . . . . . . . . .5
(*Plochman's Premium* Stoneground/Dijon/Bavarian) . . . . . . . .5
Dijon, w/white wine (*Grey Poupon*) . . . . . . . . . . . . . . . . . . .5
hot (*Nance's*) . . . . . . . . . . . . . . . . . . . . . . . . . . . . . . . . .15
hot (*Plochman's Premium Spicy Peppa*) . . . . . . . . . . . . . . . .0
sharp and creamy (*Nance's*) . . . . . . . . . . . . . . . . . . . . . . .15
yellow, mild (*Plochman's*) . . . . . . . . . . . . . . . . . . . . . . . . .0
**Mustard blend,** 1 tsp., except as noted:
chili (*Plochman's Premium Chili Dog*) . . . . . . . . . . . . . . . . .0
honey (*Hellmann's/Best Foods*) . . . . . . . . . . . . . . . . . . . . .10
honey (*Nance's*) . . . . . . . . . . . . . . . . . . . . . . . . . . . . . . .15
honey Dijon (*Jack Daniel's*) . . . . . . . . . . . . . . . . . . . . . . . .10
honey Dijon or spicy (*Plochman's Premium*) . . . . . . . . . . . .10
horseradish (*Grey Poupon*) . . . . . . . . . . . . . . . . . . . . . . . . .5

**Mustard blend** ***(cont.)***
horseradish (*Jack Daniel's*) . . . . . . . . . . . . . . . . . . . . . . . . . . . .5
mayonnaise (*Dijonnaise*), 1 tbsp. . . . . . . . . . . . . . . . . . . . . . .20
**Mustard greens,** fresh:
chopped, raw, 1 oz. or ½ cup . . . . . . . . . . . . . . . . . . . . . . . . . .7
boiled, drained, ½ cup . . . . . . . . . . . . . . . . . . . . . . . . . . . . . .11
**Mustard greens, canned,** ½ cup:
(*Stubb's*) . . . . . . . . . . . . . . . . . . . . . . . . . . . . . . . . . . . . . . .30
chopped (*Bush's Best*) . . . . . . . . . . . . . . . . . . . . . . . . . . . . . .25
seasoned (*Glory Foods*) . . . . . . . . . . . . . . . . . . . . . . . . . . . . .50
**Mustard greens, frozen,** chopped (*Birds Eye*), 1 cup . . . . . .30
**Mustard powder,** 1 tsp. . . . . . . . . . . . . . . . . . . . . . . . . . . . . .9
**Mustard seeds,** 1 tsp. . . . . . . . . . . . . . . . . . . . . . . . . . . . . .15
**Mustard spinach:**
raw, chopped, ½ cup . . . . . . . . . . . . . . . . . . . . . . . . . . . . . . .17
boiled, drained, chopped, ½ cup . . . . . . . . . . . . . . . . . . . . . .14

# N–O

**FOOD AND MEASURE** | **CALORIES**

**Nacho dip,** see "Cheese dip"
**Nacho entree,** see specific listings
**Nacho snack,** stuffed, beef, frozen, 6 pcs.:
(*Totino's* Grande) . . . . . . . . . . . . . . . . . . . . . . . . . . . . .210
and cheese (*Totino's*) . . . . . . . . . . . . . . . . . . . . . . . . . . .210
nacho cheese or taco flavor (*Totino's*) . . . . . . . . . . . . . . . .220
**Nacho topping,** ¼ cup:
beef fiesta flavor (*Tostitos*) . . . . . . . . . . . . . . . . . . . . . . .120
chicken quesadilla flavor (*Tostitos*) . . . . . . . . . . . . . . . . . .90
**Name yam,** fresh (*Frieda's*), ¾ cup, 3 oz. . . . . . . . . . . . . . .100
**Natto,** ½ cup . . . . . . . . . . . . . . . . . . . . . . . . . . . . . . . . .187
**Navy beans,** boiled, ½ cup . . . . . . . . . . . . . . . . . . . . . . . .129
**Navy beans, canned,** ½ cup:
(*Bush's Best*) . . . . . . . . . . . . . . . . . . . . . . . . . . . . . . . . .110
Creole, bacon or bacon and jalapeño (*Trappey's*) . . . . . . . . .110
**Nectarine:**
(*Dole*), 1 medium, 4.9 oz. . . . . . . . . . . . . . . . . . . . . . . . . . .70
1 medium, 2½" diam. . . . . . . . . . . . . . . . . . . . . . . . . . . . . . .67
sliced, ½ cup . . . . . . . . . . . . . . . . . . . . . . . . . . . . . . . . . . .34
**Noodle, Asian,** 2 oz. dry, except as noted:
cellophane or long rice . . . . . . . . . . . . . . . . . . . . . . . . . . .200
Chinese style (*Nasoya*), 1 cup . . . . . . . . . . . . . . . . . . . . . .210
chow mein (*Annie Chun's* Original) . . . . . . . . . . . . . . . . . . .200
chow mein (*La Choy*), ½ cup . . . . . . . . . . . . . . . . . . . . . . .140
crispy (*Frieda's*), ½ cup, 1 oz. . . . . . . . . . . . . . . . . . . . . . .160
Japanese style (*Nasoya*), 1 cup . . . . . . . . . . . . . . . . . . . . .210
pad Thai, rice, basil or original (*Annie Chun's*) . . . . . . . . . .210
rice (*Annie Chun's* Original/Hunan) . . . . . . . . . . . . . . . . . .210
rice (*A Taste of Thai*) . . . . . . . . . . . . . . . . . . . . . . . . . . . .200
soba (*Eden* Organic Traditional) . . . . . . . . . . . . . . . . . . . .200
soba, buckwheat (*Eden*) . . . . . . . . . . . . . . . . . . . . . . . . . .200
soba, lotus root, mugwort, or wild yam (*Eden*) . . . . . . . . . . .190
soba, cooked, 1 cup . . . . . . . . . . . . . . . . . . . . . . . . . . . . . .113
somen (*Eden* Organic Traditional) . . . . . . . . . . . . . . . . . . . .200

**Noodle, Asian *(cont.)***
somen, cooked, 1 cup .230
spinach (*Azumaya/Nasoya*), 1 cup .210
thin cut (*Azumaya*), 1 cup .210
udon (*Eden* Organic Traditional) .200
udon, brown rice (*Eden*) .190
wide cut (*Azumaya*), 1 cup .210
**Noodle, egg:**
dry, all styles (*Mueller's*), 2 oz. .220
cooked, 1 cup .212
cooked, spinach, 1 cup .211
**Noodle, egg, frozen:**
(*Aunt Vi's*), 2 oz. .150
(*Reames* Homestyle), ½ cup .170
(*Reames* Quick Cook), 1 cup .230
flat dumplings (*Reames* Homestyle), ½ cup .190
precooked (*Aunt Vi's* Heat-N-Serve), 4 oz. .150
yolk-free (*Aunt Vi's*), 4 oz. .80
**Noodle, Japanese or Thai,** see "Noodle, Asian"
**Noodle dish, mix,** ⅓ box:
chow mein, w/garlic scallion sauce (*Annie Chun's*) .250
w/garlic black bean sauce (*Annie Chun's*) .260
soba, w/soy ginger sauce (*Annie Chun's*) .210
**Noodle entree, can or pkg.:**
and beef, Stroganoff (*Dinty Moore* Microwave Cup) .240
and chicken (*Hormel* Microcup) .200
**Noodle entree, frozen,** 1 pkg., except as noted:
Alfredo (*Michelina's*), 8 oz. .330
w/beef (*Freezer Queen* Family), 1 cup .200
w/beef and gravy (*Banquet* Family), 1 cup .150
w/chicken (*Michelina's*), 8 oz. .300
w/chicken (*Michelina's* Noodles 'n Chicken), 8 oz. .290
w/chicken, creamy (*Kid Cuisine* Bowl), 8 oz. .220
w/chicken, escalloped (*Marie Callender's*), 13 oz. .740
w/chicken, escalloped (*Marie Callender's* Family), 1 cup .280
w/chicken, homestyle (*Banquet*), 12 oz. .390
Japanese, and vegetables (*Cascadian Farm Veggie Bowl*), 9 oz. .180
Romanoff (*Stouffer's*), 12 oz. .490

Romanoff, w/meatballs (*Michelina's*), 10 oz. . . . . . . . . . . . . 310
stir-fry, Asian (*Amy's*), 10 oz. . . . . . . . . . . . . . . . . . . . . . . 240
**Nopale,** fresh, cooked, 1 cup . . . . . . . . . . . . . . . . . . . . . . 22
**Nopale, canned** (*La Costeña* Nopalitos), 1 cup . . . . . . . . . . 20
**Nutmeg,** ground, 1 tsp. . . . . . . . . . . . . . . . . . . . . . . . . . . 12
**Nuts,** see specific listings
**Nuts, mixed,** 1 oz., except as noted:
(*Fisher*) . . . . . . . . . . . . . . . . . . . . . . . . . . . . . . . . . . . . 180
(*Planters* Deluxe) . . . . . . . . . . . . . . . . . . . . . . . . . . . . . . 170
w/peanuts (*Blue Diamond* Deluxe), ¼ cup . . . . . . . . . . . . . 210
w/peanuts (*Planters*) . . . . . . . . . . . . . . . . . . . . . . . . . . . 170
w/out peanuts (*Blue Diamond* Extra Fancy), ¼ cup . . . . . . . 210
cinnamon, honey, or vanilla (*Planters* Sweet Roasts) . . . . . 160
dry-roasted, w/peanuts . . . . . . . . . . . . . . . . . . . . . . . . . . 169
honey-roasted (*Planters*) . . . . . . . . . . . . . . . . . . . . . . . . . 160
oil-roasted, w/peanuts . . . . . . . . . . . . . . . . . . . . . . . . . . . 175
**Oat** (see also "Cereal"):
flakes, rolled (*Arrowhead Mills*), ⅓ cup . . . . . . . . . . . . . . 130
rolled or oatmeal, dry, 1 oz. . . . . . . . . . . . . . . . . . . . . . . . 109
**Oat bran,** dry (*Arrowhead Mills*), ⅓ cup . . . . . . . . . . . . . 150
**Oat flour** (*Arrowhead Mills*), ⅓ cup . . . . . . . . . . . . . . . . 120
**Oca,** fresh (*Frieda's*), ½ cup, 3 oz. . . . . . . . . . . . . . . . . . . 70
**Ocean perch,** Atlantic, meat only:
raw, 4 oz. . . . . . . . . . . . . . . . . . . . . . . . . . . . . . . . . . . . . 107
baked, broiled, or microwaved, 4 oz. . . . . . . . . . . . . . . . . 137
**Ocean perch entree,** frozen, battered fillet
(*Van de Kamp's*), 2 pcs., 3.7 oz. . . . . . . . . . . . . . . . . . . . . 220
**Octopus,** meat only:
raw, 4 oz. . . . . . . . . . . . . . . . . . . . . . . . . . . . . . . . . . . . . . 93
boiled or steamed, 4 oz. . . . . . . . . . . . . . . . . . . . . . . . . . . 186
**Octopus, canned:**
(*Goya*), ¼ cup . . . . . . . . . . . . . . . . . . . . . . . . . . . . . . . . . 140
spiced, in red sauce (*Reese*), 2 oz. . . . . . . . . . . . . . . . . . . 120
**Oheloberry,** ½ cup . . . . . . . . . . . . . . . . . . . . . . . . . . . . . . 20
**Oil,** vegetable, nut, or grain, 1 tbsp. . . . . . . . . . . . . . . . . 120
**Okra,** fresh:
raw, sliced, ½ cup . . . . . . . . . . . . . . . . . . . . . . . . . . . . . . . 19
boiled, drained, 8 pods, 3" × ⅝" . . . . . . . . . . . . . . . . . . . . 27
boiled, drained, sliced, ½ cup . . . . . . . . . . . . . . . . . . . . . . 25

**Okra, canned,** ½ cup:
cut (*Glory Foods*) . . . . . . . . . . . . . . . . . . . . . . . . . . . . .25
gumbo (*Trappey's* Creole) . . . . . . . . . . . . . . . . . . . . . . . .35
w/tomatoes or tomatoes and corn (*Allens/Trappey's*) . . . . . .30
**Okra, cocktail,** hot (*Trappey's*), 1.1 oz. . . . . . . . . . . . . . . . .10
**Okra, frozen:**
whole (*Birds Eye*), 9 pods . . . . . . . . . . . . . . . . . . . . . . . .25
whole (*McKenzie's*), 3 oz. . . . . . . . . . . . . . . . . . . . . . . . .25
cut (*McKenzie's*), ¾ cup . . . . . . . . . . . . . . . . . . . . . . . . .25
and tomatoes (*Birds Eye*), ¾ cup . . . . . . . . . . . . . . . . . . .25
and tomatoes (*McKenzie's*), ¾ cup . . . . . . . . . . . . . . . . . .20
**Old**-fashioned loaf, see "Lunch meat"
**Olive,** pickled, can or jar:
black, see "ripe," below
Calamata (*Krinos*), 3 pcs., .5 oz. . . . . . . . . . . . . . . . . . . . .45
Greek, black (*Krinos/Krinos* Alfonso), 2 pcs., .5 oz. . . . . . . . .35
Greek, black, 10 medium . . . . . . . . . . . . . . . . . . . . . . . . .65
green, w/pits, 10 small . . . . . . . . . . . . . . . . . . . . . . . . . .33
green, w/pits, 10 large . . . . . . . . . . . . . . . . . . . . . . . . . .45
green, pitted, 1 oz. . . . . . . . . . . . . . . . . . . . . . . . . . . . . .33
green, pitted, Spanish (*Early California*), 5 pcs., .5 oz. . . . . .25
ripe, pitted (*Lindsay*), 6 small, 5 medium, or 4 large . . . . . . .25
ripe, pitted, chopped (*Black Pearls*), 1⅓ tbsp. . . . . . . . . . . . .25
ripe, pitted, sliced (*Lindsay*), 2 tbsp. . . . . . . . . . . . . . . . . .25
ripe, w/pits (*Lindsay*), 5 medium or 4 large . . . . . . . . . . . . .25
stuffed w/almonds (*Reese*), 4 pcs., .5 oz. . . . . . . . . . . . . . . .35
stuffed w/anchovies (*Reese*), 4 pcs., .5 oz. . . . . . . . . . . . . . .20
stuffed w/pimento (*Pompeian*), 6 pcs., .5 oz. . . . . . . . . . . . .25
**Olive–jalapeño spread,** in jars (*D. L. Jardine's* Texas
Caviar), .5 oz. . . . . . . . . . . . . . . . . . . . . . . . . . . . . . . . .15
**Olive loaf,** see "Lunch meat"
**Olive oil,** see "Oil"
**Olive salad** (*Progresso*), 2 tbsp. . . . . . . . . . . . . . . . . . . . .25
**Olive sauce,** green (*Italia in Tavola*), 2 tbsp. . . . . . . . . . . . .90
**Onion,** fresh/stored:
raw (*Frieda's* Boiler/Cipolline), 3 pcs., 3 oz. . . . . . . . . . . . . .30
raw (*Frieda's* Hawaiian Maui), ⅓ cup, 3 oz. . . . . . . . . . . . . . .10
raw (*Lucinda's* Pearl Red/White), 1 oz., about 1 pc. . . . . . . . .20
raw, chopped, 1 tbsp. . . . . . . . . . . . . . . . . . . . . . . . . . . . .4
boiled, drained, chopped, ½ cup . . . . . . . . . . . . . . . . . . . . .47

**Onion, can or jar:**
whole (*Aunt Nellie's/Lohmann*), ½ cup . . . . . . . . . . . . . . . . .35
whole (*Hanover*), ½ cup . . . . . . . . . . . . . . . . . . . . . . . . . .25
pickled, sour (*London Pub*), ¼ cup, 1.1 oz. . . . . . . . . . . . . .10
**Onion, dried,** minced, 1 tsp. . . . . . . . . . . . . . . . . . . . . . . .30
**Onion, frozen** (see also "Onion rings"):
whole, small (*Birds Eye*), 17 pcs. . . . . . . . . . . . . . . . . . . . . .30
diced (*Birds Eye*), ⅔ cup . . . . . . . . . . . . . . . . . . . . . . . . .30
chopped (*Seabrook Farms*), ⅔ cup . . . . . . . . . . . . . . . . . . . .30
boiled, drained, 1 tbsp. . . . . . . . . . . . . . . . . . . . . . . . . . . .4
pearl, in real cream sauce (*Birds Eye*), ½ cup . . . . . . . . . . . .60
**Onion, green** (scallion), raw, trimmed, chopped:
(*Dole*), ¼ cup . . . . . . . . . . . . . . . . . . . . . . . . . . . . . . . .10
½ cup . . . . . . . . . . . . . . . . . . . . . . . . . . . . . . . . . . . . .16
**Onion, pickled,** see "Onion, can or jar"
**Onion, Welsh,** 1 oz. . . . . . . . . . . . . . . . . . . . . . . . . . . . . .10
**Onion dip,** 2 tbsp.:
bold/spicy (*Heluva* Good Bodacious) . . . . . . . . . . . . . . . . . . .60
French (*Frito-Lay*) . . . . . . . . . . . . . . . . . . . . . . . . . . . . . .60
French (*Heluva* Good) . . . . . . . . . . . . . . . . . . . . . . . . . . . .60
French (*Marzetti* Veggie Dip) . . . . . . . . . . . . . . . . . . . . . .130
French (*Marzetti* Veggie Dip Light) . . . . . . . . . . . . . . . . . . .70
sour cream and (*Marzetti* Veggie Dip Fat Free) . . . . . . . . . . .35
**Onion dip mix,** 2 tbsp.*:
French (*McCormick*) . . . . . . . . . . . . . . . . . . . . . . . . . . . . .35
French (*Ruffles*) . . . . . . . . . . . . . . . . . . . . . . . . . . . . . . .70
spring (*McCormick*) . . . . . . . . . . . . . . . . . . . . . . . . . . . . .35
**Onion gravy,** zesty (*Heinz* Home Style), ¼ cup . . . . . . . . . . .25
**Onion gravy mix** (*McCormick*), ¼ cup* . . . . . . . . . . . . . . . .20
**Onion-flavor chips,** see "Snack chips and crisps"
**Onion oil** (*Watkins* Liquid Spice), 1 tsp. . . . . . . . . . . . . . . .40
**Onion powder** (*Tone's*), ¼ tsp. . . . . . . . . . . . . . . . . . . . . . .5
**Onion ring, canned** (*French's Taste Toppers*), 2 tbsp. . . . . . .45
**Onion ring, frozen:**
(*McKenzie's*), 3.25 oz. . . . . . . . . . . . . . . . . . . . . . . . . . .220
(*Mrs. Paul's*), 4 pcs., 2.9 oz. . . . . . . . . . . . . . . . . . . . . . .190
(*Ore-Ida Onion Ringers*), 6 pcs., 3.2 oz. . . . . . . . . . . . . . .220
(*Ore-Ida Vidalia O's*), 5 pcs., 3.2 oz. . . . . . . . . . . . . . . . .240
**Onion ring batter mix,** ¼ cup:
(*Don's Chuck Wagon/Vidalia Sweet*) . . . . . . . . . . . . . . . . . .100

**Onion ring batter, mix *(cont.)***
(*Golden Dipt* Fry Easy) . . . . . . . . . . . . . . . . . . . . . . . . . . .100
(*McCormick Produce Partners*) . . . . . . . . . . . . . . . . . . . .110
**Onion salt** (*McCormick*), ¼ tsp. . . . . . . . . . . . . . . . . . . . . . . .0
**Onion snack chips,** see "Snack chips and crisps"
**Orange,** fresh:
(*Dole*), 1 medium, 5.4 oz. . . . . . . . . . . . . . . . . . . . . . . . . .70
(*Frieda's* Blood/Cara Cara), 5 oz. . . . . . . . . . . . . . . . . . . . .70
(*Frieda's* Seville), 3 oz. . . . . . . . . . . . . . . . . . . . . . . . . . . .40
California:
navel, 2⅞" orange . . . . . . . . . . . . . . . . . . . . . . . . . . . .65
navel, sections w/out membrane, ½ cup . . . . . . . . . . . . .38
Valencia, 2⅝" orange . . . . . . . . . . . . . . . . . . . . . . . . . .59
Valencia, sections w/out membrane, ½ cup . . . . . . . . . . .44
Florida, 2⅝" orange . . . . . . . . . . . . . . . . . . . . . . . . . . . . . .65
Florida, sections w/out membrane, ½ cup . . . . . . . . . . . . . .42
**Orange, Mandarin,** see "Tangerine"
**Orange drink,** 8 fl. oz., except as noted:
(*Hawaiian Punch* Orange Ocean) . . . . . . . . . . . . . . . . . . .120
(*Snapple* Orangeade) . . . . . . . . . . . . . . . . . . . . . . . . . . . .120
(*Sunny Delight* Calcium) . . . . . . . . . . . . . . . . . . . . . . . . . .140
(*Turkey Hill* Orangeade) . . . . . . . . . . . . . . . . . . . . . . . . . .120
(*WhipperSnapple* Dream), 10 fl. oz. . . . . . . . . . . . . . . . . . .150
**Orange drink blends,** 8 fl. oz., except as noted:
apple, frozen* (*Cascadian Farm* Sunrise) . . . . . . . . . . . . .110
cranberry (*Tropicana Twister*) . . . . . . . . . . . . . . . . . . . . . .120
cranberry (*Tropicana Twister*), 11.5 fl. oz. . . . . . . . . . . . . .190
pineapple (*Tropicana*), 11.5 fl. oz. . . . . . . . . . . . . . . . . . . .180
pineapple apple (*Welch's*) . . . . . . . . . . . . . . . . . . . . . . . . .140
strawberry banana (*Dole*) . . . . . . . . . . . . . . . . . . . . . . . . .130
strawberry banana (*Dole*), 11.5 fl. oz. . . . . . . . . . . . . . . . . .180
strawberry banana (*Tropicana Twister*) . . . . . . . . . . . . . . . .130
strawberry banana (*Tropicana Twister*), 11.5 fl. oz. . . . . . . .190
**Orange juice,** 8 fl. oz., except as noted:
(*Dole*) . . . . . . . . . . . . . . . . . . . . . . . . . . . . . . . . . . . . . . .110
(*Dole*), 11.5 fl. oz. . . . . . . . . . . . . . . . . . . . . . . . . . . . . . .160
(*Hood*) . . . . . . . . . . . . . . . . . . . . . . . . . . . . . . . . . . . . . . .120
(*Langers*) . . . . . . . . . . . . . . . . . . . . . . . . . . . . . . . . . . . . .120
(*Minute Maid*) . . . . . . . . . . . . . . . . . . . . . . . . . . . . . . . . . .110
(*Nantucket Nectars*) . . . . . . . . . . . . . . . . . . . . . . . . . . . . .120

(*Season's Best* Calcium/Vitamin C/Pulp/Pulp Free) . . . . . . . 110
(*Tropicana Pure Premium*) . . . . . . . . . . . . . . . . . . . . . . 110
(*Turkey Hill*) . . . . . . . . . . . . . . . . . . . . . . . . . . . . . 100
fresh . . . . . . . . . . . . . . . . . . . . . . . . . . . . . . . . . . . 112
frozen* (*Cascadian Farm*) . . . . . . . . . . . . . . . . . . . . . . 120
frozen* (*Minute Maid* Calcium) . . . . . . . . . . . . . . . . . . . 120
frozen* (*Minute Maid* Original) . . . . . . . . . . . . . . . . . . . 110
**Orange juice blends,** 8 fl. oz.:
(*Tropicana* Ruby Red) . . . . . . . . . . . . . . . . . . . . . . . . 110
banana (*Tropicana*) . . . . . . . . . . . . . . . . . . . . . . . . . 140
guava (*Dole*) . . . . . . . . . . . . . . . . . . . . . . . . . . . . . 120
kiwi passion (*Tropicana Pure Tropics*) . . . . . . . . . . . . . . . 100
peach mango (*Dole*) . . . . . . . . . . . . . . . . . . . . . . . . . 120
peach mango (*Tropicana Pure Tropics*) . . . . . . . . . . . . . . . 110
pineapple (*Season's Best*) . . . . . . . . . . . . . . . . . . . . . 110
pineapple (*Tropicana* Calcium) . . . . . . . . . . . . . . . . . . . 130
pineapple (*Tropicana Pure Tropics*) . . . . . . . . . . . . . . . . . 120
strawberry (*Tropicana*) . . . . . . . . . . . . . . . . . . . . . . . 130
strawberry banana (*Dole*) . . . . . . . . . . . . . . . . . . . . . . 120
strawberry banana (*Tropicana Pure Tropics*) . . . . . . . . . . . . 110
tangerine (*Nantucket Nectars*) . . . . . . . . . . . . . . . . . . . 120
tangerine (*Tropicana*) . . . . . . . . . . . . . . . . . . . . . . . . 110
**Orange peel, candied** (*Seneca* Glacé), diced, 2 tbsp. . . . . . . 70
**Orange sauce,** Oriental (*Ka•Me* Mandarin), 2 tbsp. . . . . . . . . 80
**Oregano,** dried, 1 tsp. . . . . . . . . . . . . . . . . . . . . . . . . 3
**Oriental sauce,** see specific listings
**Oyster,** meat only, 4 oz., except as noted:
Eastern, farmed, raw . . . . . . . . . . . . . . . . . . . . . . . . . 67
Eastern, farmed, baked, broiled, or microwaved . . . . . . . . . . 90
Eastern, wild, raw, 1 lb. . . . . . . . . . . . . . . . . . . . . . . . 310
Eastern, wild, raw, 6 medium, 3 oz. . . . . . . . . . . . . . . . . . 57
Eastern, wild, baked, broiled, or microwaved . . . . . . . . . . . . 82
Eastern, wild, steamed or poached . . . . . . . . . . . . . . . . . . 155
Pacific, raw . . . . . . . . . . . . . . . . . . . . . . . . . . . . . . . 93
Pacific, raw, boiled or steamed, 1 medium . . . . . . . . . . . . . . 41
Pacific, boiled or steamed . . . . . . . . . . . . . . . . . . . . . . 185
**Oyster, canned,** 2 oz., except as noted:
whole (*Chicken of the Sea*) . . . . . . . . . . . . . . . . . . . . . 70
whole (*3 Diamonds*) . . . . . . . . . . . . . . . . . . . . . . . . . . 60
whole, boiled (*Crown Prince*), ⅓ cup . . . . . . . . . . . . . . . . 70

**Oyster, canned *(cont.)***
smoked (*Bumble Bee*) . . . . . . . . . . . . . . . . . . . . . . . . . . . . .120
smoked (*Chicken of the Sea*), 2.5 oz. . . . . . . . . . . . . . . . . . .140
smoked, medium (*Reese*) . . . . . . . . . . . . . . . . . . . . . . . . . .110
**Oyster sauce,** Asian (*Ka•Me*), 1 tbsp. . . . . . . . . . . . . . . . . . . .10

# P-Q

**FOOD AND MEASURE** | **CALORIES**

**Palm, hearts of,** in jars (*Haddon House*), 4.5 oz. . . . . . . . . .20
**Pancake, frozen,** 3 pcs., except as noted:
(*Aunt Jemima* Homestyle) . . . . . . . . . . . . . . . . . . . . . . . . .210
(*Aunt Jemima* Lowfat) . . . . . . . . . . . . . . . . . . . . . . . . . . . .170
(*Eggo*) . . . . . . . . . . . . . . . . . . . . . . . . . . . . . . . . . . . . . . .270
(*Hungry Jack* Original) . . . . . . . . . . . . . . . . . . . . . . . . . . .270
blueberry (*Hungry Jack*) . . . . . . . . . . . . . . . . . . . . . . . . . .250
blueberry or buttermilk (*Aunt Jemima*) . . . . . . . . . . . . . . . .210
buttermilk (*Hungry Jack*) . . . . . . . . . . . . . . . . . . . . . . . . . .270
mini (*Aunt Jemima*), 13 pcs. . . . . . . . . . . . . . . . . . . . . . . . .240
mini (*Hungry Jack*), 11 pcs. . . . . . . . . . . . . . . . . . . . . . . . . .270
**Pancake batter,** frozen, ½ cup:
(*Aunt Jemima* Homestyle) . . . . . . . . . . . . . . . . . . . . . . . . .260
blueberry (*Aunt Jemima*) . . . . . . . . . . . . . . . . . . . . . . . . . .290
buttermilk (*Aunt Jemima*) . . . . . . . . . . . . . . . . . . . . . . . . .270
**Pancake breakfast,** frozen, 1 pkg.:
buttermilk, w/bacon, home fries (*Great Starts*), 6.8 oz. . . . .450
w/sausage (*Great Starts*), 6 oz. . . . . . . . . . . . . . . . . . . . . . .490
**Pancake mix,** ⅓ cup dry, except as noted:
(*Aunt Jemima* Original) . . . . . . . . . . . . . . . . . . . . . . . . . . .150
(*Aunt Jemima* Complete) . . . . . . . . . . . . . . . . . . . . . . . . . .160
(*Betty Crocker* Original Complete), ⅓ cup or 3 cakes* . . . .200
(*Betty Crocker* Original Pouch), 3 cakes* . . . . . . . . . . . . . .250
(*Bisquick Shake 'N Pour* Original), 3 cakes* . . . . . . . . . . . .210
(*Hungry Jack* Extra Light) . . . . . . . . . . . . . . . . . . . . . . . . .160
(*Hungry Jack* Extra Light Complete/Original) . . . . . . . . . . .150
buckwheat (*Aunt Jemima*), ¼ cup . . . . . . . . . . . . . . . . . . . .100
buttermilk (*Aunt Jemima*), ¼ cup . . . . . . . . . . . . . . . . . . . .110
buttermilk (*Aunt Jemima* Complete) . . . . . . . . . . . . . . . . . .160
buttermilk (*Aunt Jemima* Complete Reduced Cal) . . . . . . . .130
buttermilk (*Betty Crocker* Complete Box), 3 cakes* . . . . . . .200
buttermilk (*Betty Crocker* Pouch), 3 cakes* . . . . . . . . . . . .210
buttermilk (*Bisquick Shake 'N Pour*), 3 cakes* . . . . . . . . . .200

**Pancake mix *(cont.)***
buttermilk (*Hungry Jack/Hungry Jack* Complete) . . . . . . . . .160
gluten-free or kamut (*Arrowhead Mills*), ¼ cup . . . . . . . . . . .130
whole wheat (*Aunt Jemima*), ¼ cup . . . . . . . . . . . . . . . . . . .120
**Pancake syrup** (see also "Maple syrup"), ¼ cup:
(*Aunt Jemima/Aunt Jemima* Country/Butter Rich) . . . . . . . .210
(*Aunt Jemima/Aunt Jemima* Country Rich Lite) . . . . . . . . . .100
(*Hungry Jack/Hungry Jack* Butter Flavor) . . . . . . . . . . . . . . .210
(*Hungry Jack* Lite/*Hungry Jack* Butter Flavor Lite) . . . . . . .100
butter flavor (*Aunt Jemima* Butterlite) . . . . . . . . . . . . . . . . . .105
cinnamon flavor (*Golden Griddle*) . . . . . . . . . . . . . . . . . . . . .240
**Papaya**, fresh:
(*Dole*), ½ medium, 4.9 oz. . . . . . . . . . . . . . . . . . . . . . . . . . .70
1 lb., 3½" × 5⅛" . . . . . . . . . . . . . . . . . . . . . . . . . . . . . . . . . .117
peeled, cubed, ½ cup . . . . . . . . . . . . . . . . . . . . . . . . . . . . . . .27
**Papaya, chilled,** in extra light syrup (*Sunfresh*), ½ cup . . . .70
**Papaya, dried** (*Sonoma*), 2 pcs., 2 oz. . . . . . . . . . . . . . . . . .200
**Papaya, frozen** (*Goya*), ⅓ pkg. . . . . . . . . . . . . . . . . . . . . . . .50
**Papaya juice blend** (*Ceres*), 5.25 fl. oz. . . . . . . . . . . . . . . . .87
**Papaya nectar,** see "Papaya drink"
**Paprika** (*McCormick*), ¼ tsp. . . . . . . . . . . . . . . . . . . . . . . . . .2
**Parsley,** fresh:
10 sprigs . . . . . . . . . . . . . . . . . . . . . . . . . . . . . . . . . . . . . . . . .4
chopped, ½ cup . . . . . . . . . . . . . . . . . . . . . . . . . . . . . . . . . . . .11
**Parsley, dried,** 1 tbsp. . . . . . . . . . . . . . . . . . . . . . . . . . . . . . . .4
**Parsnip,** fresh:
raw, sliced (*Frieda's*), 1 cup, 4.7 oz. . . . . . . . . . . . . . . . . . . .100
boiled, drained, 1 medium, 9" . . . . . . . . . . . . . . . . . . . . . . . .130
boiled, drained, sliced, ½ cup . . . . . . . . . . . . . . . . . . . . . . . . .63
**Passion fruit,** fresh:
(*Frieda's*), 5 oz. . . . . . . . . . . . . . . . . . . . . . . . . . . . . . . . . . .140
purple, 1 medium, .6 oz. . . . . . . . . . . . . . . . . . . . . . . . . . . . . .18
**Passion fruit, frozen,** chunks (*Goya*), ⅓ pkg. . . . . . . . . . . . .70
**Passion fruit juice,** blend (*Ceres*), 5.25 fl. oz. . . . . . . . . . . .87
**Passion fruit juice drink** (*Tropicana Twister*), 8 fl. oz. . . . .120
**Pasta,** dry (see also "Macaroni" and "Noodle"), 2 oz.:
all styles (*Delverde*) . . . . . . . . . . . . . . . . . . . . . . . . . . . . . . .200
all styles (*Mueller's* Classic/Italian/Micro Quick) . . . . . . . . .210
corn . . . . . . . . . . . . . . . . . . . . . . . . . . . . . . . . . . . . . . . . . . . . .202
spaghetti, plain . . . . . . . . . . . . . . . . . . . . . . . . . . . . . . . . . . . .210

spaghetti, protein-fortified .......................... 213
spaghetti, spinach .................................. 211
spaghetti, whole wheat ............................... 197
rice, brown (*Lundberg* Organic) ..................... 210
**Pasta, cooked,** 1 cup:
spaghetti, plain .................................... 197
spaghetti, protein-fortified .......................... 230
spaghetti, whole wheat ............................... 174
spinach ............................................. 182
**Pasta, frozen,** lasagna:
roll-ups (*Aunt Vi's*), 3 oz. ......................... 180
strips (*Aunt Vi's*), 4 oz. ........................... 210
**Pasta, refrigerated,** see specific pasta listings
**Pasta dish, frozen** (see also "Pasta entree, frozen" and specific pasta listings):
Alfredo (*Green Giant*), 9-oz. pkg. ................... 300
Alfredo (*Green Giant Pasta Accents*), 2 cups ........... 200
Alfredo, and vegetables (*Amy's* Skillet Meals), 1 cup ..... 220
cheddar (*Amy's* Skillet Meals Country), 1 cup ........... 250
cheddar, creamy (*Green Giant Pasta Accents*), 2⅓ cups ... 250
cheddar, white (*Birds Eye Pasta Secrets*), 2 cups ........ 240
cheese, 3 (*Birds Eye Pasta Secrets*), 2 cups ............ 230
cheese, 3 (*Green Giant*), 9-oz. pkg. ................... 270
cheese, 3 (*Green Giant Pasta Accents*), 2 cups .......... 300
garden herb (*Green Giant Pasta Accents*), 2 cups ........ 230
garlic (*Green Giant Pasta Accents*), 2 cups ............ 260
garlic, zesty (*Birds Eye Pasta Secrets*), 2 cups ......... 240
garlic, roasted (*Green Giant*), 9-oz. pkg. .............. 250
pesto, Italian (*Birds Eye Pasta Secrets*), 2⅓ cups ....... 240
primavera (*Birds Eye Pasta Secrets*), 2⅓ cups .......... 230
primavera (*Tree of Life EasyMeal*), 1 pkg.* w/tofu, oil ..... 460
ranch (*Birds Eye Pasta Secrets*), 6.6 oz. ............... 300
salad, w/vegetables (*Fitness Choice*), 4 oz. ............. 130
**Pasta dish, mix** (see also specific pasta listings):
Alfredo (*Annie's* Organic), ⅔ cup ..................... 270
Alfredo (*Bowl Appétit!*), 1 bowl ...................... 360
Alfredo, garlic (*Pasta Roni*), 1 cup* .................. 360
broccoli (*Pasta Roni*), 1 cup* ........................ 330
broccoli au gratin (*Pasta Roni*), 1 cup* ................ 280
cheddar, broccoli (*Annie's* Organic), ⅔ cup ............ 260

**Pasta dish, mix *(cont.)***
cheddar, zesty (*Lipton* Pasta & Sauce), 1 cup* . . . . . . . . . . .290
cheese, 4 (*Annie's* Organic), ⅔ cup . . . . . . . . . . . . . . . . . .260
cheese, nacho (*Knorr Forkfulls*), 1 bowl . . . . . . . . . . . . . . .370
cheese, triple or zesty (*Knorr Forkfulls*), 1 bowl . . . . . . . . .360
chicken (*Pasta Roni*), 1 cup* . . . . . . . . . . . . . . . . . . . . . . .310
chicken (*Pasta Roni* Homestyle), 1 cup* . . . . . . . . . . . . . . .230
chicken flavor, creamy (*Knorr Forkfulls*), 1 bowl . . . . . . . . .300
chicken flavor, quesadilla (*Knorr Forkfulls*), 1 bowl . . . . . . .340
chicken-flavored (*Bowl Appétit!*), 1 bowl . . . . . . . . . . . . . .260
chicken and garlic (*Pasta Roni* Low Fat), 1 cup* . . . . . . . . . .300
garlic, creamy (*Lipton* Pasta & Sauce), ½ pkg. . . . . . . . . . . .270
garlic, roasted, and olive oil w/sun-dried tomato
(*Lipton* Pasta & Sauce), 1 cup* . . . . . . . . . . . . . . . . . . .270
garlic and Parmesan (*Annie's* Organic), ⅔ cup . . . . . . . . . . .180
mushroom, creamy (*Lipton* Pasta & Sauce), 1 cup* . . . . . .320
Parmesano (*Pasta Roni*), 1 cup* . . . . . . . . . . . . . . . . . . . .390
pizza flavor (*Knorr Forkfulls*), 1 bowl . . . . . . . . . . . . . . . .330
Romanoff (*Pasta Roni*), 1 cup* . . . . . . . . . . . . . . . . . . . . .400
salad, Caesar (*Suddenly Salad*), 1 cup* . . . . . . . . . . . . . . .250
salad, Caesar (*Suddenly Salad* Lowfat), 1 cup* . . . . . . . . . .190
salad, classic (*Suddenly Salad*), 1 cup* . . . . . . . . . . . . . . .240
salad, classic (*Suddenly Salad* Lowfat), 1 cup* . . . . . . . . . .200
salad, garlic, roasted, Parmesan (*Suddenly Salad*),
¾ cup* . . . . . . . . . . . . . . . . . . . . . . . . . . . . . . . . . . . . .240
salad, Parmesan, creamy (*Suddenly Salad*) . . . . . . . . . . . .360
salad, ranch, bacon (*Suddenly Salad*), ¾ cup* . . . . . . . . . . .330
salad, ranch, bacon (*Suddenly Salad* Lowfat), ¾ cup* . . . .180
sour cream and chives (*Pasta Roni*) . . . . . . . . . . . . . . . . .320
Stroganoff (*Pasta Roni*), 1 cup* . . . . . . . . . . . . . . . . . . . .370
tomato (*Ragú Express* Traditional), ½ pkg.* . . . . . . . . . . . .190
tomato and basil (*Annie's* Organic), ⅔ cup . . . . . . . . . . . . .260
tomato, meat-flavored (*Ragú Express*), ½ pkg.* . . . . . . . . . .200
tomato, sweet, and garlic (*Ragú Express*), ½ pkg.* . . . . . .200
**Pasta entree, frozen** (see also "Pasta dishes, frozen,"
and specific pasta listings), 1 pkg., except as noted:
Alfredo:
w/grilled chicken (*Marie Callender's* Bowl), 10.5 oz. . . . .410
primavera (*Lean Cuisine Everyday Favorites*), 10 oz. . . .280
cheddar, w/beef, tomatoes (*Stouffer's*), 11 oz. . . . . . . . . . .500

cheese, 3 w/broccoli (*Cedarlane*), 9 oz. . . . . . . . . . . . . . . . .430
cheese, 3, w/red peppers (*Cascadian Farm*), 10 oz. . . . . . . . .340
marinara (*Cascadian Farm Veggie Bowl*), 9 oz. . . . . . . . . . . .180
and meatballs:
(*Country Skillet*), ¼ of 32-oz. pkg. . . . . . . . . . . . . . . . . .320
(*Marie Callender's* Skillet Meals), ½ of 24-oz. pkg. . . . . .570
(*Swanson Fun Feast*), 12 oz. . . . . . . . . . . . . . . . . . . . . . . .410
primavera (*Amy's*), 9.5 oz. . . . . . . . . . . . . . . . . . . . . . . . . .320
primavera (*Cascadian Farm Veggie Bowl*), 9 oz. . . . . . . . . .220
wheels and cheese (*Michelina's*), 8 oz. . . . . . . . . . . . . . . . .300
**Pasta flour,** see "Semolina flour"
**Pasta salad,** see "Pasta dish, mix"
**Pasta salad dressing mix,** vinaigrette (*McCormick*),
⅙ pkg. . . . . . . . . . . . . . . . . . . . . . . . . . . . . . . . . . . . . . . .15
**Pasta salad seasoning** (*McCormick*), ¼ pkg. . . . . . . . . . . . .25
**Pasta sauce,** can or jar, tomato (see also "Tomato sauce"
and specific sauce listings), ½ cup:
(*Aunt Millie's* Traditional) . . . . . . . . . . . . . . . . . . . . . . . . . .90
(*Emeril's Kicked Up Tomato*) . . . . . . . . . . . . . . . . . . . . . . . .70
(*Patsy's* Pizzaiola) . . . . . . . . . . . . . . . . . . . . . . . . . . . . . . .100
(*Prego* Traditional) . . . . . . . . . . . . . . . . . . . . . . . . . . . . . . .120
(*Progresso* Spaghetti) . . . . . . . . . . . . . . . . . . . . . . . . . . . .100
(*Ragú Old World Style* Traditional) . . . . . . . . . . . . . . . . . . .70
Amatriciana (*Patsy's*) . . . . . . . . . . . . . . . . . . . . . . . . . . . .120
balsamic, roasted onion (*Muir Glen*) . . . . . . . . . . . . . . . . . .50
basil (*Five Brothers*) . . . . . . . . . . . . . . . . . . . . . . . . . . . . . .70
basil (*Newman's Own* Bombolina) . . . . . . . . . . . . . . . . . . .100
basil (*Patsy's*) . . . . . . . . . . . . . . . . . . . . . . . . . . . . . . . . . . .90
basil (*Ragú* Light) . . . . . . . . . . . . . . . . . . . . . . . . . . . . . . . .50
basil and Italian cheese (*Ragú* Chunky Gardenstyle) . . . . . .110
beef, w/mushroom (*Ragú Robusto!*) . . . . . . . . . . . . . . . . . . .70
beef, sauteed, onion and garlic (*Ragú Robusto!*) . . . . . . . . .90
cheese, see "Cheese sauce, cooking"
w/cheese, 4 (*Classico* Di Parma) . . . . . . . . . . . . . . . . . . . . .80
w/cheese, 5 (*Five Brothers*) . . . . . . . . . . . . . . . . . . . . . . . . .90
w/cheese, 5 (*Newman's Own*) . . . . . . . . . . . . . . . . . . . . . . .90
w/cheese, 6 (*Ragú Robusto!*) . . . . . . . . . . . . . . . . . . . . . . . .80
fra diavolo (*Newman's Own* Hot & Spicy) . . . . . . . . . . . . . . .70
fra diavolo (*Patsy's*) . . . . . . . . . . . . . . . . . . . . . . . . . . . . .100
garden combination (*Ragú* Chunky Gardenstyle) . . . . . . . . .100

**Pasta sauce *(cont.)***
garden (*Ragú* Mama's Special) . . . . . . . . . . . . . . . . . . . . . . .110
garden combination (*Ragú* Chunky Gardenstyle) . . . . . . . . . .100
garlic, super (*Ragú* Chunky Gardenstyle) . . . . . . . . . . . . . . .100
garlic, roasted (*Classico* Di Sorrento) . . . . . . . . . . . . . . . . . . .60
garlic, roasted (*Emeril's Roasted Gaaahlic*) . . . . . . . . . . . . . . .70
garlic, roasted (*Ragú Robusto!*) . . . . . . . . . . . . . . . . . . . . . . .90
garlic, roasted, and peppers (*Newman's Own*) . . . . . . . . . . . .70
garlic, roasted, primavera (*Ragú* Light) . . . . . . . . . . . . . . . . . .45
garlic, roasted, and Vidalia onion (*Five Brothers*) . . . . . . . . . .80
garlic and basil (*Prego* Pasta Bake), ⅛ jar . . . . . . . . . . . . . . .80
garlic and onion (*Ragú* Chunky Gardenstyle) . . . . . . . . . . . . .110
green pepper and mushroom (*Del Monte*) . . . . . . . . . . . . . . .80
hamburger (*Prego*) . . . . . . . . . . . . . . . . . . . . . . . . . . . . . . .120
herb, 7 (*Ragú Robusto!*) . . . . . . . . . . . . . . . . . . . . . . . . . . . .80
marinara (*Newman's Own*) . . . . . . . . . . . . . . . . . . . . . . . . . . .60
marinara (*Patsy's*) . . . . . . . . . . . . . . . . . . . . . . . . . . . . . . . .100
marinara (*Progresso* Authentic) . . . . . . . . . . . . . . . . . . . . . . .100
marinara (*Ragú Old World Style*) . . . . . . . . . . . . . . . . . . . . . . .80
marinara, w/Burgundy (*Five Brothers*) . . . . . . . . . . . . . . . . . . .80
marinara, mushroom (*Newman's Own*) . . . . . . . . . . . . . . . . . . .60
marinara, w/pizza paste (*Aunt Millie's*) . . . . . . . . . . . . . . . . . .70
meat (*Aunt Millie's*) . . . . . . . . . . . . . . . . . . . . . . . . . . . . . . .100
meat (*Prego* Pasta Bake), ⅛ jar . . . . . . . . . . . . . . . . . . . . . . .120
meat (*Ragú Old World Style*) . . . . . . . . . . . . . . . . . . . . . . . . . .80
meat, Italian (*Ragú Robusto!* Classic) . . . . . . . . . . . . . . . . . . .90
meatball, mini (*Prego*) . . . . . . . . . . . . . . . . . . . . . . . . . . . . .160
mushroom (*Aunt Millie's*) . . . . . . . . . . . . . . . . . . . . . . . . . . . .90
mushroom (*Prego*) . . . . . . . . . . . . . . . . . . . . . . . . . . . . . . . .150
mushroom (*Ragú Old World Style*) . . . . . . . . . . . . . . . . . . . . . .70
mushroom, garlic (*Five Brothers*) . . . . . . . . . . . . . . . . . . . . . . .80
mushroom, garlic, and onion (*Prego* Pasta Bake), ⅛ jar . . . .90
mushroom, green pepper (*Ragú* Chunky Gardenstyle) . . . .100
mushroom, super chunky (*Ragú* Chunky Gardenstyle) . . . .110
onion, roasted (*Muir Glen*) . . . . . . . . . . . . . . . . . . . . . . . . . . .50
onion and garlic (*Prego*) . . . . . . . . . . . . . . . . . . . . . . . . . . . .120
onion and garlic, sauteed (*Aunt Millie's*) . . . . . . . . . . . . . . . .90
onion and garlic or mushroom, sauteed (*Ragú Robusto!*) . .90
onion and pepper (*Lydia's* Sugo Capricciosa) . . . . . . . . . . . .75
Parmesan and Romano (*Ragú Robusto!*) . . . . . . . . . . . . . . . .90

peppers and spice (*Newman's Own*) . . . . . . . . . . . . . . . . . . . .60
puttanesca (*Emeril's*) . . . . . . . . . . . . . . . . . . . . . . . . . . . .80
puttanesca (*Francesco Rinaldi*) . . . . . . . . . . . . . . . . . . . . .70
red pepper, spicy (*Classico* Di Roma Arrabbiata) . . . . . . . . . .60
red pepper, roasted (*Emeril's*) . . . . . . . . . . . . . . . . . . . . . .60
red pepper, roasted, and onion (*Classico* Di Salerno) . . . . . .60
red pepper, roasted, and onion (*Ragú* Chunky
Gardenstyle) . . . . . . . . . . . . . . . . . . . . . . . . . . . . . . . . .110
Romano, pecorino, and herb (*Classico* Di Palermo) . . . . . . .80
sausage, Italian, and garlic (*Prego*) . . . . . . . . . . . . . . . . . .120
sausage, Italian, w/peppers, onions (*Classico* d'Abruzzi) . . . .70
sausage, sweet, and cheese (*Ragú Robusto!*) . . . . . . . . . . .90
sausage-flavored (*Aunt Millie's*) . . . . . . . . . . . . . . . . . . . .100
spinach and cheese, Florentine (*Classico* Di Firenze) . . . . . . .80
tomato, chopped, olive oil and garlic (*Ragú Robusto!*) . . . .100
tomato, fire-roasted, and garlic (*Classico* Di Siena) . . . . . . . .60
tomato, spicy, and pesto (*Classico* Di Genoa) . . . . . . . . . . . .90
tomato, sun-dried (*Classico* Di Capri) . . . . . . . . . . . . . . . . . .80
tomato, sun-dried, and basil (*Ragú Chunky Gardenstyle*) . . .*110*
tomato and basil, see "basil," above
vegetable, summer, grilled (*Five Brothers*) . . . . . . . . . . . . . .80
vegetable, super (*Ragú* Chunky Gardenstyle) . . . . . . . . . . .100
vodka sauce (*Emeril's*) . . . . . . . . . . . . . . . . . . . . . . . . . .130
vodka sauce (*Patsy's*) . . . . . . . . . . . . . . . . . . . . . . . . . . .110
**Pasta sauce, refrigerated** (see also specific listings):
marinara (*Buitoni*), ½ cup . . . . . . . . . . . . . . . . . . . . . . . . .80
marinara, garlic, roasted (*Buitoni*), ½ cup . . . . . . . . . . . . . .60
tomato, herb Parmesan (*Buitoni*), ½ cup . . . . . . . . . . . . . .140
**Pasta sauce mix** (see also specific sauce listings):
(*Knorr* Parma Rosa), 2 tbsp. . . . . . . . . . . . . . . . . . . . . . . .60
(*McCormick* Pasta Rosa), ½ cup* . . . . . . . . . . . . . . . . . . . .40
(*Spatini* Spaghetti), ½ cup* . . . . . . . . . . . . . . . . . . . . . . . .20
garlic herb (*Knorr* Pasta Sauces), 2 tbsp. . . . . . . . . . . . . . .70
herb and garlic (*McCormick*), ½ cup* . . . . . . . . . . . . . . . . .20
Italian style (*McCormick* Spaghetti), ½ cup* . . . . . . . . . . . . .25
primavera (*McCormick*), ½ cup* . . . . . . . . . . . . . . . . . . . . .30
thick and zesty or mild (*McCormick* Spaghetti), ½ cup* . . . .25
**Pasta wrap,** see "Wraps, filled"
**Pastrami** (see also "Turkey pastrami"):
(*Boar's Head* Choice), 2 oz. . . . . . . . . . . . . . . . . . . . . . . .140

**Pastrami *(cont.)***
(*Boar's Head* First Cut), 2 oz. .......................... 90
(*Boar's Head* Red Round), 2 oz. .......................... 80
(*Boar's Head* Round), 2 oz. .......................... 70
(*Healthy Choice* Savory Selections), 6 slices, 1.9 oz. ....... 70
(*Healthy Deli*), 2 oz. .......................... 80
(*Hebrew National* Thin Sliced), 4 slices, 2 oz. ............ 90
(*Sara Lee*), 3 slices, 2.2 oz. .......................... 70
**Pâté, canned** (see also "Liverwurst"):
chicken liver, 1 tbsp. .......................... 26
goose liver, smoked, 1 tbsp. .......................... 60
**Pâté, refrigerated,** 2 oz.:
(*Boar's Head* Liverwurst) .......................... 150
(*Charcuterie de Bretagne* de Campagne) ............... 200
duck and pork mousse w/truffles (*Marcel & Henri*) ....... 240
glazed, w/truffles (*Tour Eiffel Campagnard Francaise*) ..... 210
**Pea pods,** see "Peas, edible pod"
**Peach,** fresh:
(*Dole*), 1 medium, 3.5 oz. .......................... 40
(*Frieda's* Donut/Late Season), 5 oz. .................. 60
2½" peach, 4 per lb. .......................... 37
sliced, ½ cup .......................... 37
**Peach, can or jar,** ½ cup, except as noted:
(*Del Monte Fruitrageous* Peachy Peach Pie), 4 oz. ........ 80
in juice (*Del Monte* Fruit Naturals) ................. 60
in juice (*Del Monte* Fruit Naturals Snack Cup), 4 oz. ....... 50
in juice (*Libby's*) .......................... 70
in extra light syrup (*Del Monte* Lite) .................. 60
in extra light syrup (*Del Monte* Lite Snack Cup), 4 oz. ...... 50
in light syrup:
- (*Del Monte Orchard Select*) .......................... 80
- banana berry (*Del Monte* Fruit-to-Go), 4 oz. ........... 70
- cinnamon (*Del Monte* Chunky Cut) .................. 80
- raspberry-flavored or spiced (*Del Monte*) ........... 80
- wild raspberry (*Del Monte Fruitrageous*), 4 oz. ........ 80

in heavy syrup (*Del Monte/Del Monte* Melba) ........... 100
in heavy syrup, diced (*Del Monte* Snack Cup), 4 oz. ....... 80
in heavy syrup, spiced, whole (*Del Monte*) ............ 100
**Peach, dried:**
(*Sun•Maid*), ¼ cup .......................... 100

(*Sunsweet*), 1.4 oz., about 3 pcs. . . . . . . . . . . . . . . . . . . . . .110
**Peach, frozen** (*Big Valley*), ⅔ cup . . . . . . . . . . . . . . . . . . . .50
**Peach butter** (*Smucker's*), 1 tbsp. . . . . . . . . . . . . . . . . . . . . .45
**Peach drink blends:**
(*Snapple* Summer Peach), 8 fl. oz. . . . . . . . . . . . . . . . . . . . . .120
mango (*WhipperSnapple*), 10 fl. oz. . . . . . . . . . . . . . . . . . . . .150
**Peach juice** (*Nantucket Nectars* Original), 8 fl. oz. . . . . . . .120
**Peach juice blends:**
(*Ceres*), 5.25 fl. oz. . . . . . . . . . . . . . . . . . . . . . . . . . . . . .87
mango, frozen* (*Cascadian Farm*), 8 fl. oz. . . . . . . . . . . . . .120
**Peach nectar:**
(*Goya*), 6 fl. oz. . . . . . . . . . . . . . . . . . . . . . . . . . . . . . .110
(*Libby's*), 5.5-fl.-oz. can . . . . . . . . . . . . . . . . . . . . . . . . . .90
(*Libby's*), 8 fl. oz. . . . . . . . . . . . . . . . . . . . . . . . . . . . . . .140
**Peach orange juice** (*Nantucket Nectars*),
8 fl. oz. . . . . . . . . . . . . . . . . . . . . . . . . . . . . . . . . . . . .130
**Peach and pear,** canned, in light syrup, wild berry
(*Del Monte* Fruit-to-Go Jumble), 4 oz. . . . . . . . . . . . . . . .80
**Peach salsa,** see "Salsa"
**Peanut,** shelled, 1 oz., except as noted:
(*Frito-Lay* Salted), 1.1 oz. . . . . . . . . . . . . . . . . . . . . . . . . .200
(*Planters* Cocktail/Salted) . . . . . . . . . . . . . . . . . . . . . . . . .170
dry-roasted (*Fisher*) . . . . . . . . . . . . . . . . . . . . . . . . . . . . .170
dry-roasted (*Planters*) . . . . . . . . . . . . . . . . . . . . . . . . . . . .160
dry-roasted (*Planters*), 1.75-oz. pkg. . . . . . . . . . . . . . . . . .290
dry-roasted, diced (*Blue Diamond*), ¼ cup . . . . . . . . . . . . .190
honey-roasted (*Fisher*) . . . . . . . . . . . . . . . . . . . . . . . . . . .170
honey-roasted (*Frito-Lay*), 1.1 oz. . . . . . . . . . . . . . . . . . . .180
honey-roasted (*Planters*) . . . . . . . . . . . . . . . . . . . . . . . . . .160
hot (*Frito-Lay*), 1.1 oz. . . . . . . . . . . . . . . . . . . . . . . . . . . .190
hot (*Planters* Heat) . . . . . . . . . . . . . . . . . . . . . . . . . . . . . .160
oil-roasted (*Fisher*) . . . . . . . . . . . . . . . . . . . . . . . . . . . . .170
roasted (*Planters*) . . . . . . . . . . . . . . . . . . . . . . . . . . . . . . .150
roasted, blanched (*Blue Diamond*), ¼ cup . . . . . . . . . . . . .200
**Peanut bake mix,** spicy (*A Taste of Thai*), ¼ pkt. . . . . . . . . .45
**Peanut butter,** 2 tbsp.:
(*Simply Jif*) . . . . . . . . . . . . . . . . . . . . . . . . . . . . . . . . . . .190
chunky or creamy (*Smucker's* Natural) . . . . . . . . . . . . . . . .200
chunky/crunchy:
(*Jif/Jif* Extra/Reduced Fat) . . . . . . . . . . . . . . . . . . . . . . .190

**Peanut butter, chunky/crunchy *(cont.)***
(*Peter Pan*) . . . . . . . . . . . . . . . . . . . . . . . . . . . . . . . . .190
(*Skippy/Skippy* Reduced Fat Spread) . . . . . . . . . . . . . . . .190
creamy/smooth:
(*Jif/Jif* Reduced Fat) . . . . . . . . . . . . . . . . . . . . . . . . . .190
(*Peter Pan*) . . . . . . . . . . . . . . . . . . . . . . . . . . . . . . . . .190
(*Skippy*) . . . . . . . . . . . . . . . . . . . . . . . . . . . . . . . . . . . .190
(*Smucker's* Natural Reduced Fat) . . . . . . . . . . . . . . . . . . .200
honey nut, roasted, chunky or creamy (*Skippy*) . . . . . . . . .190
**Peanut butter blend** (see also "Peanut butter and jelly"), 2 tbsp.:
apple cinnamon or berry (*Jif*) . . . . . . . . . . . . . . . . . . . . . .200
chocolate (*Jif* Silk) . . . . . . . . . . . . . . . . . . . . . . . . . . . . . .190
chocolate (*Skippy Doubly Delicious!*) . . . . . . . . . . . . . . . . .210
**Peanut butter topping** (*Smucker's Magic Shell*), 2 tbsp. . . .220
**Peanut butter and jelly:**
(*Goobers*), 3 tbsp. . . . . . . . . . . . . . . . . . . . . . . . . . . . . . . .230
w/crackers (*Smucker's Snackers*), 1 pkg. . . . . . . . . . . . . . .410
**Peanut butter and jelly sandwich,** grape or strawberry (*Smucker's Uncrustables*), 1 pc. . . . . . . . . . . . . . . . . . . . . . .200
**Peanut sauce, Thai:**
(*Annie Chun's*), 2 tbsp. . . . . . . . . . . . . . . . . . . . . . . . . . . .120
(*San-J* Thai), 2 tbsp. . . . . . . . . . . . . . . . . . . . . . . . . . . . . .70
satay (*A Taste of Thai*), *2 tbsp.* . . . . . . . . . . . . . . . . . . . . . .*50*
**Peanut sauce mix** (*A Taste of Thai*), ¼ pkt. . . . . . . . . . . . . .45
**Pear,** fresh, w/peel:
(*Dole*), 1 medium, 5.9 oz. . . . . . . . . . . . . . . . . . . . . . . . . . .100
Bartlett, 1 medium, approx. 2½ per lb. . . . . . . . . . . . . . . . . .98
1 large, approx. 2 per lb. . . . . . . . . . . . . . . . . . . . . . . . . . . .123
sliced, ½ cup . . . . . . . . . . . . . . . . . . . . . . . . . . . . . . . . . . . .49
**Pear, Asian:**
(*Frieda's*), 5 oz. . . . . . . . . . . . . . . . . . . . . . . . . . . . . . . . . . .60
1 medium, 2¼" × 2½" diam. . . . . . . . . . . . . . . . . . . . . . . . . . .51
**Pear, can or jar,** ½ cup, except as noted:
in juice (*Del Monte* Fruit Naturals) . . . . . . . . . . . . . . . . . . . .60
in juice (*Libby's Lite*) . . . . . . . . . . . . . . . . . . . . . . . . . . . . . . .60
in extra light syrup (*Del Monte* Lite) . . . . . . . . . . . . . . . . . . .60
in extra light syrup (*Del Monte* Lite Snack Cup), 4 oz. . . . . . .50
in light syrup, Bartlett (*Del Monte Orchard Select*) . . . . . . . .80
in light syrup, cinnamon flavor (*Del Monte*) . . . . . . . . . . . . .80

in heavy syrup (*Del Monte*) . . . . . . . . . . . . . . . . . . . . . . . .100
in heavy syrup, diced (*Del Monte* Snack Cup), 4 oz. . . . . . . .80
ginger flavor, natural (*Del Monte*) . . . . . . . . . . . . . . . . . . . .90
**Pear, dried:**
(*Sonoma* Organic), 4 pcs., 1.4 oz. . . . . . . . . . . . . . . . . . .140
halves, ½ cup . . . . . . . . . . . . . . . . . . . . . . . . . . . . . . . . .236
**Pear juice blend** (*Ceres*), 5.25 fl. oz. . . . . . . . . . . . . . . . .87
**Pear nectar:**
(*Goya*), 6 fl. oz. . . . . . . . . . . . . . . . . . . . . . . . . . . . . . .120
(*Libby's*), 5.5-fl.-oz. can . . . . . . . . . . . . . . . . . . . . . . . .100
(*Libby's*), 8 fl. oz. . . . . . . . . . . . . . . . . . . . . . . . . . . . . .150
**Peas,** see specific listings
**Peas, black-eyed,** see "Black-eyed peas"
**Peas, butter,** frozen (*Birds Eye* Southern), ½ cup . . . . . . . .110
**Peas, cream,** canned (*Bush's Best*), ½ cup . . . . . . . . . . . .110
**Peas, crowder, canned** (*Allens/East Texas Fair*), ½ cup . . .110
**Peas, crowder, frozen** (*Birds Eye*), ½ cup . . . . . . . . . . . . .120
**Peas, edible pod,** fresh:
raw (*Dole* Sugar), ½ cup, 2.5 oz. . . . . . . . . . . . . . . . . . . . .30
raw (*Frieda's* Snow/Sugar Snap), 3 oz. . . . . . . . . . . . . . . . .35
raw (*Mann's* Stringless Sugar Snap), 4 oz. . . . . . . . . . . . . .50
raw, w/sauce (*Frieda's* Snow), ½ cup . . . . . . . . . . . . . . . . .40
raw, w/sauce (*Frieda's* Sugar Snap), ½ cup . . . . . . . . . . . .35
boiled, drained, ½ cup . . . . . . . . . . . . . . . . . . . . . . . . . . .34
**Peas, edible pod, frozen:**
(*Cascadian Farm* Sugar Snap), ¾ cup . . . . . . . . . . . . . . . .35
(*Green Giant Select* Sugar Snap), ¾ cup . . . . . . . . . . . . . . .35
(*John Cope's* Sugar Snap), ⅔ cup . . . . . . . . . . . . . . . . . . .45
(*La Choy* Snow Pea), 3 oz., about 42 pods . . . . . . . . . . . . . .35
boiled, drained, ½ cup . . . . . . . . . . . . . . . . . . . . . . . . . . .42
stir-fry blend (*Birds Eye* Sugar Snap), ¾ cup . . . . . . . . . . .35
**Peas, field, canned,** (see also "Peas, crowder" and "Peas, purple hull"), ½ cup:
(*Glory Foods*) . . . . . . . . . . . . . . . . . . . . . . . . . . . . . . . . .80
w/snaps (*Glory Foods*) . . . . . . . . . . . . . . . . . . . . . . . . . . .70
w/bacon (*Trappey's*) . . . . . . . . . . . . . . . . . . . . . . . . . . . . .90
w/bacon and snaps (*Trappey's*) . . . . . . . . . . . . . . . . . . . .110
**Peas, field, frozen,** w/snaps (*McKenzie's*), ½ cup . . . . . .110
**Peas, green,** fresh:
raw, in pod, 1 lb. . . . . . . . . . . . . . . . . . . . . . . . . . . . . . . .140

**Peas, green *(cont.)***
raw, shelled, ½ cup . . . . . . . . . . . . . . . . . . . . . . . . . . . . .58
boiled, drained, ½ cup . . . . . . . . . . . . . . . . . . . . . . . . . . .67
**Peas, green, can or jar,** early or sweet, ½ cup:
(*Blue Boy*) . . . . . . . . . . . . . . . . . . . . . . . . . . . . . . . . . . .70
(*Del Monte*) . . . . . . . . . . . . . . . . . . . . . . . . . . . . . . . . .60
(*Greenleaf* Early June) . . . . . . . . . . . . . . . . . . . . . . . . .45
(*Libby's*) . . . . . . . . . . . . . . . . . . . . . . . . . . . . . . . . . . . .70
(*LeSueur*) . . . . . . . . . . . . . . . . . . . . . . . . . . . . . . . . . .60
(*Veg-All*) . . . . . . . . . . . . . . . . . . . . . . . . . . . . . . . . . . .60
**Peas, green, dried** (*Frieda's*), ⅓ cup, 3 oz. . . . . . . . . . . . .130
**Peas, green, frozen,** ⅔ cup, except as noted:
(*Birds Eye*), ½ cup . . . . . . . . . . . . . . . . . . . . . . . . . . . . .70
(*Greene's Farm* Garden) . . . . . . . . . . . . . . . . . . . . . . . .60
(*John Cope's/John Cope's* Tiny) . . . . . . . . . . . . . . . . . . .70
(*Richfood* Petite) . . . . . . . . . . . . . . . . . . . . . . . . . . . . . .70
(*Tree of Life* Organic) . . . . . . . . . . . . . . . . . . . . . . . . . .70
extra fine (*Bonduelle* Petite), 3 oz. . . . . . . . . . . . . . . . . . .68
garden (*Cascadian Farm*) . . . . . . . . . . . . . . . . . . . . . . . .70
sweet (*Green Giant*), ¾ cup . . . . . . . . . . . . . . . . . . . . . . .70
sweet, baby (*Birds Eye*) . . . . . . . . . . . . . . . . . . . . . . . . .70
sweet, baby (*Green Giant LeSueur*) . . . . . . . . . . . . . . . . .70
sweet, baby (*Green Giant Select LeSueur*) . . . . . . . . . . . . .60
tiny (*Seabrook Farms* Petite) . . . . . . . . . . . . . . . . . . . . . .70
**Peas, green, combinations, can or jar,** ½ cup:
and carrots (*Green Giant*) . . . . . . . . . . . . . . . . . . . . . . . .50
and carrots (*Libby's*) . . . . . . . . . . . . . . . . . . . . . . . . . . .60
and carrots (*Veg-All*) . . . . . . . . . . . . . . . . . . . . . . . . . . .60
and carrots, baby (*Bonduelle*) . . . . . . . . . . . . . . . . . . . . .45
w/mushrooms and onions (*LeSueur*) . . . . . . . . . . . . . . . . .60
w/pearl onions (*Green Giant*) . . . . . . . . . . . . . . . . . . . . . .60
**Peas, green, combinations, frozen:**
baby, blend (*Birds Eye* Tiny Tender), ¾ cup . . . . . . . . . . . .40
and carrots (*Cascadian Farm*), ⅔ cup . . . . . . . . . . . . . . . .50
and carrots (*John Cope's*), ½ cup . . . . . . . . . . . . . . . . . . .50
w/pearl onions (*Birds Eye*), ⅔ cup . . . . . . . . . . . . . . . . . .90
w/pearl onions (*Cascadian Farm*), ¾ cup . . . . . . . . . . . . . .60
w/pearl onions, baby peas (*Birds Eye*), ⅔ cup . . . . . . . . . .60
and potatoes w/cream (*Birds Eye*), ½ cup . . . . . . . . . . . . .90
**Peas, purple hull, canned** (*Bush's Best*), ½ cup . . . . . . . .110

**Peas, purple hull, frozen** (*McKenzie's*), ½ cup . . . . . . . . . . .110
**Peas, split,** see "Split peas"
**Peas, sugar snap or snow,** see "Peas, edible pod"
**Peas, sweet,** see "Peas, green"
**Peas, white acre,** canned (*East Texas Fair*), ½ cup . . . . . .100
**Peas and carrots or onions,** see "Peas, green, combinations"
**Pecan,** shelled:
(*Blue Diamond* Fancy Halves), ⅓ cup . . . . . . . . . . . . . . . . .220
(*Blue Diamond* Pieces), ¼ cup . . . . . . . . . . . . . . . . . . . . . . .210
(*Fisher*), 1 oz. . . . . . . . . . . . . . . . . . . . . . . . . . . . . . . . . .200
(*Planters*) . . . . . . . . . . . . . . . . . . . . . . . . . . . . . . . . . . . .190
(*Planters* Halves), 2-oz. pkg. . . . . . . . . . . . . . . . . . . . . . . .390
**Penne,** plain, see "Pasta"
**Penne dish, mix,** dry, except as noted:
w/black beans (*Marrakesh Express*), 1 cup* . . . . . . . . . . . . .170
Italian herb butter sauce (*Land O Lakes*), 2.5 oz. . . . . . . . . . .290
w/sausage-flavor tomato sauce (*Classico It's Pasta Anytime*), 15.25-oz. cont. . . . . . . . . . . . . . . . . . . . . . .540
tomato and mushroom sauce (*Classico It's Pasta Anytime*), 15.25-oz. cont. . . . . . . . . . . . . . . . . . . . . . .510
tomato, Parmesan (*Bowl Appétit!*), 1 bowl . . . . . . . . . . . . . .350
tomato, sun-dried, Parmesan sauce (*Knorr*), ½ cup . . . . . .270
**Penne entree,** frozen, 1 pkg.:
w/Italian sausage (*Michelina's*), 9 oz. . . . . . . . . . . . . . . . . .300
w/mushroom sauce (*Michelina's*), 8 oz. . . . . . . . . . . . . . . . .280
w/mushrooms (*Michelina's*), 8 oz. . . . . . . . . . . . . . . . . . . . .250
pollo (*Michelina's*), 8.5 oz. . . . . . . . . . . . . . . . . . . . . . . . . .290
primavera (*Michelina's*), 8.5 oz. . . . . . . . . . . . . . . . . . . . . .280
w/ tomato (*Lean Cuisine Everyday Favorites*), 10 oz. . . . . . .260
w/2 tomatoes, Italian sausage (*Budget Gourmet*), 8 oz. . . .270
vegetarian (*Yves* Veggie Penne), 10.5 oz. . . . . . . . . . . . . . .220
**Pepper,** seasoning:
black, whole, 1 tsp. . . . . . . . . . . . . . . . . . . . . . . . . . . . . . . .8
black, ground, 1 tsp. . . . . . . . . . . . . . . . . . . . . . . . . . . . . . .6
chili, 1 tsp. . . . . . . . . . . . . . . . . . . . . . . . . . . . . . . . . . . . . .9
red or cayenne, 1 tsp. . . . . . . . . . . . . . . . . . . . . . . . . . . . . .6
white, 1 tsp. . . . . . . . . . . . . . . . . . . . . . . . . . . . . . . . . . . . .7
**Pepper, banana,** hot or mild (*Vlasic*), 1 oz. . . . . . . . . . . . . .5
**Pepper, bell,** see "Pepper, sweet"
**Pepper, cherry,** hot (*Progresso*), 1 oz. . . . . . . . . . . . . . . . . .10

**Pepper, cherry, stuffed,** w/prosciutto and provolone
(*La Rosa D'Oro*), 2 oz. . . . . . . . . . . . . . . . . . . . . . . . . .60
**Pepper, chili,** fresh,
all varieties (*Frieda's* Cucina), 1-oz. pc. . . . . . . . . . . . . . . . . . .10
green or red, 1 medium, 1.6 oz. . . . . . . . . . . . . . . . . . . . . . .18
green or red, chopped, ½ cup . . . . . . . . . . . . . . . . . . . . . . .30
**Pepper, chili, can or jar:**
whole:
chipotle (*Herdez*), 3 pcs., 1 oz. . . . . . . . . . . . . . . . . . . . .30
chipotle in adobo sauce (*La Morena*), 2 pcs., 1 oz. . . . . .15
green (*Chi-Chi's*), ¾ pc. . . . . . . . . . . . . . . . . . . . . . . . .10
green (*Embasa*), 1 pc. . . . . . . . . . . . . . . . . . . . . . . . . . .15
poblano (*Herdez*), ½ pc., 1.2 oz. . . . . . . . . . . . . . . . . . . .10
yellow quero (*Corona Real* Chiles de Oro), 1 pc. . . . . . . . .6
chopped, chipotle in adobo sauce (*Embasa*), 2 tbsp. . . . . . .15
chopped, green (*Old El Paso*), 2 tbsp. . . . . . . . . . . . . . . . . . .5
diced, green (*Chi-Chi's*), 2 tbsp. . . . . . . . . . . . . . . . . . . . . .10
minced, red (*A Taste of Thai*), 2 tbsp. . . . . . . . . . . . . . . . . .40
**Pepper, green or red, sweet,** see "Pepper, sweet"
**Pepper, jalapeño,** can or jar:
(*La Victoria* Marinated/Pickled), 1.1 oz. . . . . . . . . . . . . . . . . .10
whole (*Chi-Chi's*), 2½ pcs. . . . . . . . . . . . . . . . . . . . . . . . .10
diced (*La Victoria*), 1.1 oz. . . . . . . . . . . . . . . . . . . . . . . . .10
sliced (*Hatch*), 2 tbsp. . . . . . . . . . . . . . . . . . . . . . . . . . . .5
sliced, nacho (*La Victoria*), 1.1 oz. . . . . . . . . . . . . . . . . . . .5
sliced, nacho, pickled (*La Costeña*), ¼ cup . . . . . . . . . . . . . .20
wheels (*Chi-Chi's*), 19 pcs., 1 oz. . . . . . . . . . . . . . . . . . . . .10
**Pepper, poblano,** see "Pepper, chili, can or jar"
**Pepper, roasted,** see "Pepper, sweet, in jars"
**Pepper, stuffed, entree,** frozen:
(*Stouffer's*), 10-oz. pkg. . . . . . . . . . . . . . . . . . . . . . . . . . .210
(*Stouffer's*), ½ of 15.5-oz. pkg. . . . . . . . . . . . . . . . . . . . . .180
(*Stouffer's Family Style Favorites*), ¼ of 32-oz. pkg. . . . . . .200
**Pepper, sweet,** fresh:
green or red, raw (*Dole*), 1 medium, 5.2 oz. . . . . . . . . . . . . .30
green or red, raw, chopped, ½ cup . . . . . . . . . . . . . . . . . . . .20
green or red, boiled, drained, 1 medium . . . . . . . . . . . . . . . .20
green or red, boiled, drained, chopped, ½ cup . . . . . . . . . . .19
yellow, raw, 1 large, 5" × 3" . . . . . . . . . . . . . . . . . . . . . . . .50
yellow, raw, 10 strips, 1.8 oz. . . . . . . . . . . . . . . . . . . . . . . .14

**Pepper, sweet, can or jars** (see also "Pimiento"):
roasted (*Frieda's*), 1-oz. pc. . . . . . . . . . . . . . . . . . . . . . . . . .35
roasted, fire (*Pompeian*), ½ cup . . . . . . . . . . . . . . . . . . . . .30
salad (*B&G*), 1 oz. . . . . . . . . . . . . . . . . . . . . . . . . . . . . . .10
salad, drained (*Progresso*), 2 tbsp. . . . . . . . . . . . . . . . . . . .15
**Pepper, sweet, frozen:**
chopped (*Seabrook Farms*), 1 oz. . . . . . . . . . . . . . . . . . . . . . . .6
green, diced (*Birds Eye* Southern), ¾ cup . . . . . . . . . . . . . . .20
stir-fry blend (*Birds Eye*), 3 oz. . . . . . . . . . . . . . . . . . . . . . . .25
**Pepper, Tabasco,** in vinegar (*Trappey's*), 1 oz. . . . . . . . . . . . .5
**Pepper, torrido** (*Trappey's* Santa Fe Grande),
1.3 oz. . . . . . . . . . . . . . . . . . . . . . . . . . . . . . . . . . . . . . .10
**Pepper dip,** red (*Victoria*), ¼ cup . . . . . . . . . . . . . . . . . . . . .50
**Pepper salad,** see "Pepper, sweet, can or jar"
**Pepper sauce,** see "Hot sauce," and specific listings
**Pepper steak,** see "Beef entree, frozen"
**Peppercorn sauce mix** (*Knorr* Classic), 2 tsp. . . . . . . . . . . .25
**Pepperoncini:**
(*Krinos*), ¼ cup . . . . . . . . . . . . . . . . . . . . . . . . . . . . . . . . .5
(*Progresso* Tuscan), 3 pcs., 1 oz. . . . . . . . . . . . . . . . . . . . . . .10
(*Trappey's* Tempero), 1 oz. . . . . . . . . . . . . . . . . . . . . . . . . . . .5
(*Zorba*), 5 pcs., 1.1 oz. . . . . . . . . . . . . . . . . . . . . . . . . . . . .15
**Pepperoni** (see also "Turkey pepperoni"):
(*Boar's Head*), 1 oz. . . . . . . . . . . . . . . . . . . . . . . . . . . . . .140
(*Boar's Head* Sandwich Style), 1 oz. . . . . . . . . . . . . . . . . . .130
(*Hormel* Chunk/Twin/Sliced), 1 oz. . . . . . . . . . . . . . . . . . . .140
(*Hormel Pillow Pack*), 14 slices, 1 oz. . . . . . . . . . . . . . . . . .140
(*Sara Lee*), 7 slices, 1.1 oz. . . . . . . . . . . . . . . . . . . . . . . . .140
(*Sara Lee* Sandwich), 7 slices, .9 oz. . . . . . . . . . . . . . . . . .120
**"Pepperoni," vegetarian,** frozen (*Yves* Pizza Slices),
1.7 oz. . . . . . . . . . . . . . . . . . . . . . . . . . . . . . . . . . . . . . .70
**Perch** (see also "Ocean perch"), meat only:
raw, 4 oz. . . . . . . . . . . . . . . . . . . . . . . . . . . . . . . . . . . . . .103
baked, broiled, or microwaved, 4 oz. . . . . . . . . . . . . . . . . . .133
**Persimmon,** fresh:
(*Frieda's* Fuyu/Hachiya/Sharon), 5 oz. . . . . . . . . . . . . . . . .100
Japanese, 1 medium . . . . . . . . . . . . . . . . . . . . . . . . . . . . . . .118
native, 1 medium, 1.1 oz. . . . . . . . . . . . . . . . . . . . . . . . . . . . .32
**Persimmon, dried** (*Sonoma*), 7 pcs., 1.4 oz. . . . . . . . . . . .140
**Pesto paste** (*Amore*), 2 tbsp. . . . . . . . . . . . . . . . . . . . . . . .110

**Pesto sauce,** in jars, ¼ cup, except as noted:
(*Pastene*) . . . . . . . . . . . . . . . . . . . . . . . . . . . . . . .231
(*Sacla Pasta Gusto* Genovese) . . . . . . . . . . . . . . . . .240
black (*Cora* Gourmet) . . . . . . . . . . . . . . . . . . . . . . .200
Genovese (*Italia in Talola*), 2 tbsp. . . . . . . . . . . . . . . . .160
green (*Cora* Gourmet) . . . . . . . . . . . . . . . . . . . . . . .140
red (*Cora* Gourmet), 2 tbsp. . . . . . . . . . . . . . . . . . . . .190
white (*Cora* Gourmet) . . . . . . . . . . . . . . . . . . . . . . .120
**Pesto sauce, refrigerated,** ¼ cup:
w/basil (*Buitoni*) . . . . . . . . . . . . . . . . . . . . . . . . . .290
w/basil (*Buitoni* Light) . . . . . . . . . . . . . . . . . . . . . .230
w/sun-dried tomato (*Buitoni*) . . . . . . . . . . . . . . . . . .190
**Pesto sauce mix,** dry:
(*Knorr* Pasta Sauces), 2 tsp. . . . . . . . . . . . . . . . . . . . .15
(*McCormick*), ¼ pkg. . . . . . . . . . . . . . . . . . . . . . . . . .10
creamy (*Knorr* Pasta Sauces), 1 tbsp. . . . . . . . . . . . . . . .25
**Pheasant,** raw:
meat w/skin, 4 oz. . . . . . . . . . . . . . . . . . . . . . . . . . .205
meat only, 4 oz. . . . . . . . . . . . . . . . . . . . . . . . . . . .151
meat only, ½ breast, 6.4 oz. . . . . . . . . . . . . . . . . . . . .243
meat only, 1 leg, 3.8 oz. . . . . . . . . . . . . . . . . . . . . . .143
**Phyllo,** see "Filo dough"
**Picante sauce** (see also "Salsa"), 2 tbsp.:
(*Chi-Chi's*) . . . . . . . . . . . . . . . . . . . . . . . . . . . . . .10
(*Pace*) . . . . . . . . . . . . . . . . . . . . . . . . . . . . . . . . .10
hot or medium (*Shotgun Willie's* Texas) . . . . . . . . . . . . .10
w/jalapeño (*La Victoria*) . . . . . . . . . . . . . . . . . . . . . .15
**Piccalilli,** see "Tomato relish"
**Pickle,** cucumber:
bread and butter (*B&G* Chips), 1 oz. . . . . . . . . . . . . . . . .30
bread and butter (*Cascadian Farm* Chips), 6 pcs., 1 oz. . . . . .25
bread and butter (*Mrs. Fanning's*), 3 pcs., 1 oz. . . . . . . . . .25
cold pack (*Hans Jurgen*), 1 oz. . . . . . . . . . . . . . . . . . . . .5
cornichons (*Italica*), 7 pcs., 1.1 oz. . . . . . . . . . . . . . . . . .0
dill (*Claussen*), ½ pc., 1 oz. . . . . . . . . . . . . . . . . . . . . .5
dill (*Del Monte*) 1½ pcs., 1 oz. . . . . . . . . . . . . . . . . . . . .5
dill, baby (*Cascadian Farm*), 1 oz. . . . . . . . . . . . . . . . . . .5
dill, hamburger chips (*B&G*), 6 pcs., 1 oz. . . . . . . . . . . . . .0
dill, hamburger chips (*Del Monte*), 5½ pcs., 1 oz. . . . . . . . . .5
dill, kosher (*B&G* Crunchy), 1 oz. . . . . . . . . . . . . . . . . . .0

dill, kosher (*Cascadian Farm*), ¾ pc., 1 oz. . . . . . . . . . . . . . . . .5
dill, kosher, chips (*B&G*), 4 pcs., 1 oz. . . . . . . . . . . . . . . . . . . . .0
dill, kosher, slices (*Cascadian Farm*), 2 slices, 1 oz. . . . . . . . .5
dill, kosher, tiny (*Del Monte*), 1½ pcs., 1 oz. . . . . . . . . . . . . .5
dill, slice (*Claussen* Super Slices for Burgers), .8-oz. slice . . .5
sweet, baby (*Cascadian Farm*), 1¾ pc., 1 oz. . . . . . . . . . . . .30
sweet, chips (*Del Monte*), 5 pcs., 1 oz. . . . . . . . . . . . . . . . . . .40
sweet, gherkin (*Vlasic*), 1 oz., about 3 pcs. . . . . . . . . . . . . . .35
sweet, gherkin or whole (*Del Monte*), 2 pcs., 1 oz. . . . . . . . .40
sweet, midget (*Del Monte*), 3 pcs., 1 oz. . . . . . . . . . . . . . . . .40

**Pickle loaf,** see "Lunch meat loaf"

**Pickle relish** (see also specific listings), cucumber, 1 tbsp.:
(*Crosse & Blackwell* Branston) . . . . . . . . . . . . . . . . . . . . . . .25
dill (*Cascadian Farm*) . . . . . . . . . . . . . . . . . . . . . . . . . . . . . .0
hamburger (*Del Monte*) . . . . . . . . . . . . . . . . . . . . . . . . . . .20
hamburger (*Heinz*) . . . . . . . . . . . . . . . . . . . . . . . . . . . . . .10
hot dog (*Del Monte*) . . . . . . . . . . . . . . . . . . . . . . . . . . . . .15
India (*Heinz*) . . . . . . . . . . . . . . . . . . . . . . . . . . . . . . . . . .20
sweet (*Cascadian Farm*) . . . . . . . . . . . . . . . . . . . . . . . . . .20
sweet (*Del Monte*) . . . . . . . . . . . . . . . . . . . . . . . . . . . . . .20
sweet (*Heinz*) . . . . . . . . . . . . . . . . . . . . . . . . . . . . . . . . .20

**Pie:**
apple (*Entenmann's* Homestyle), ⅙ pie . . . . . . . . . . . . . . . .370
apple (*Entenmann's* Ultimate), ⅛ pie . . . . . . . . . . . . . . . . .320
cherry (*Entenmann's*), ⅙ pie . . . . . . . . . . . . . . . . . . . . . . .360
coconut custard (*Entenmann's*), ⅕ pie . . . . . . . . . . . . . . .340
pumpkin (*Entenmann's*), ⅕ pie . . . . . . . . . . . . . . . . . . . . . .270
sweet potato (*Entenmann's*), ⅙ pie . . . . . . . . . . . . . . . . . .320

**Pie, frozen** (see also "Cobbler"):
apple (*Mountain Top*), ⅙ pie . . . . . . . . . . . . . . . . . . . . . . .340
apple (*Mountain Top* Old Fashioned), ⅛ pie . . . . . . . . . . . .350
apple (*Mrs. Smith's* Homestyle 9"), ⅛ pie . . . . . . . . . . . . . .340
apple (*Mrs. Smith's* Special Recipe 10"), 1/12 pie . . . . . . . . .330
apple (*Mrs. Smith's* Unbaked 9"), ⅛ pie . . . . . . . . . . . . . . .350
apple (*Sara Lee* Reduced Fat), ⅙ pie . . . . . . . . . . . . . . . . .290
apple, Dutch (*Mrs. Smith's* 9"), ⅛ pie . . . . . . . . . . . . . . . . .360
apple, Dutch (*Mrs. Smith's* 10"), ⅒ pie . . . . . . . . . . . . . . .320
apple, Dutch (*Sara Lee* Homestyle), ⅛ pie . . . . . . . . . . . . .350
apple crumb (*Mountain Top*), ⅙ pie . . . . . . . . . . . . . . . . . .320
berry banana cream (*Pet-Ritz*), ¼ pie . . . . . . . . . . . . . . . . .320

**Pie, frozen *(cont.)***
blueberry (*Mountain Top*), 1/6 pie .330
blueberry (*Mrs. Smith's* 9"), 1/8 pie .330
blueberry (*Sara Lee* Homestyle), 1/8 pie .360
blackberry (*Mountain Top*), 1/6 pie .330
Boston cream, see "Cake, frozen"
cappuccino (*Mrs. Smith's* 10"), 1/9 pie .300
cherry (*Mountain Top*), 1/6 pie .340
cherry (*Mountain Top* Old Fashioned), 1/8 pie .380
cherry (*Mrs. Smith's* 9"), 1/8 pie .320
cherry (*Mrs. Smith's* Special Recipe 10"), 1/12 pie .330
cherry (*Sara Lee* Homestyle), 1/8 pie .320
cherry–berry (*Mrs. Smith's* Special Recipe 10"), 1/12 pie .340
chocolate cream (*Mrs. Smith's* 8"), 1/3 pie .370
chocolate cream, mint (*Mrs. Smith's* 9"), 1/6 pie .390
chocolate silk (*Sara Lee* Supreme), 1/5 pie .500
coconut cream (*Sara Lee*), 1/5 pie .480
coconut custard (*Mrs. Smith's* 9"), 1/8 pie .260
cookies and cream (*Mrs. Smith's* 9"), 1/6 pie .360
French silk (*Mrs. Smith's* 10"), 1/9 pie .560
Key lime (*Mrs. Smith's* 10"), 1/9 pie .430
lemon cream (*Mrs. Smith's* 8"), 1/3 pie .440
lemon cream (*Pet-Ritz* Razz), 1/4 pie .320
lemon meringue (*Sara Lee* Homestyle), 1/6 pie .350
lemonade (*Mrs. Smith's*), 1/6 pie .370
mince (*Mountain Top*), 1/6 pie .350
mince (*Mrs. Smith's* 9"), 1/8 pie .380
mince (*Sara Lee* Homestyle), 1/8 pie .390
peach (*Mountain Top*), 1/6 pie .310
peach (*Mountain Top* Old Fashioned), 1/8 pie .360
peach (*Mrs. Smith's* 9"), 1/8 pie .320
peach (*Mrs. Smith's* Special Recipe 10"), 1/12 pie .300
peach (*Sara Lee* Homestyle), 1/8 pie .320
pecan (*Mrs. Smith's* 8"), 1/5 pie .560
pecan (*Mrs. Smith's* 10"), 1/8 pie .550
pecan (*Sara Lee* Homestyle), 1/8 pie .520
pumpkin (*Mountain Top*), 1/6 pie .250
pumpkin (*Mountain Top* Old Fashioned), 1/8 pie .250
pumpkin (*Sara Lee* Homestyle), 1/8 pie .260
pumpkin custard (*Mrs. Smith's* 9"), 1/8 pie .280

pumpkin custard (*Mrs. Smith's* 10"), 1/10 pie . . . . . . . . . . . .290
raspberry (*Mrs. Smith's* 9"), 1/8 pie . . . . . . . . . . . . . . . . . . . .330
raspberry (*Sara Lee* Homestyle), 1/8 pie . . . . . . . . . . . . . . . .380
S'mores cream (*Mrs. Smith's* 9"), 1/6 pie . . . . . . . . . . . . . . .410
strawberry–banana (*Mrs. Smith's* 9"), 1/6 pie . . . . . . . . . . . .380
sweet potato custard (*Mrs. Smith's* 9"), 1/8 pie . . . . . . . . . .340
**Pie, snack,** 1 pc.:
apple (*Drake's*), 4 oz. . . . . . . . . . . . . . . . . . . . . . . . . . . .400
apple (*Entenmann's*), 5 oz. . . . . . . . . . . . . . . . . . . . . . . . .370
apple (*Hostess*), 4.5 oz. . . . . . . . . . . . . . . . . . . . . . . . . .480
blueberry (*Entenmann's*), 5 oz. . . . . . . . . . . . . . . . . . . . . .440
blueberry (*Hostess*), 4.5 oz. . . . . . . . . . . . . . . . . . . . . . .480
cherry (*Drake's*), 4 oz. . . . . . . . . . . . . . . . . . . . . . . . . . .420
cherry (*Entenmann's*), 5 oz. . . . . . . . . . . . . . . . . . . . . . . .430
cherry (*Hostess*), 4.5 oz. . . . . . . . . . . . . . . . . . . . . . . . .470
lemon (*Entenmann's*), 5 oz. . . . . . . . . . . . . . . . . . . . . . . .430
lemon (*Hostess*), 4.5 oz. . . . . . . . . . . . . . . . . . . . . . . . . .500
peach (*Entenmann's*), 5 oz. . . . . . . . . . . . . . . . . . . . . . . .380
peach (*Hostess*), 4.5 oz. . . . . . . . . . . . . . . . . . . . . . . . . .480
pineapple (*Entenmann's*), 5 oz. . . . . . . . . . . . . . . . . . . . . .400
**Pie crust:**
chocolate cookie (*Oreo*), 1/6 crust . . . . . . . . . . . . . . . . . . .140
graham (*Honey Maid*), 1/6 crust . . . . . . . . . . . . . . . . . . . . .140
graham (*Ready Crust*), 1/8 crust . . . . . . . . . . . . . . . . . . . . .110
graham (*Ready Crust* Reduced Fat) . . . . . . . . . . . . . . . . . . . .90
graham (*Ready Crust* 2 Extra Servings), 1/10 crust . . . . . . . .130
graham, chocolate (*Ready Crust*), 1/8 crust . . . . . . . . . . . . .110
shortbread (*Ready Crust*), 1/8 crust . . . . . . . . . . . . . . . . . . .110
vanilla cookie (*Nilla*), 1/6 crust . . . . . . . . . . . . . . . . . . . . .140
**Pie crust, frozen or refrigerated,** 1/8 crust:
(*Mrs. Smith's* 18 oz.) . . . . . . . . . . . . . . . . . . . . . . . . . . . .100
(*Mrs. Smith's* 19.5 oz.) . . . . . . . . . . . . . . . . . . . . . . . . . .110
(*Pet-Ritz* 9") . . . . . . . . . . . . . . . . . . . . . . . . . . . . . . . . . .80
(*Pet-Ritz* Extra Large 9 5/8") . . . . . . . . . . . . . . . . . . . . . . .110
(*Pillsbury* All Ready) . . . . . . . . . . . . . . . . . . . . . . . . . . . . .120
deep dish, regular or all vegetable (*Pet-Ritz* 9") . . . . . . . . . .90
all vegetable (*Pet-Ritz* 9") . . . . . . . . . . . . . . . . . . . . . . . . .80
**Pie crust mix:**
(*Betty Crocker*), 1/8 of 9" crust . . . . . . . . . . . . . . . . . . . . .110
(*"Jiffy"*), 1/4 cup mix . . . . . . . . . . . . . . . . . . . . . . . . . . . .180

**Pie filling** (see also "Pastry filling,"), canned:
apple (*Lucky Leaf*), 3 oz. . . . . . . . . . . . . . . . . . . . . . . . . . . .90
apple (*Lucky Leaf* Lite), 3 oz. . . . . . . . . . . . . . . . . . . . . . . . .25
apricot (*Lucky Leaf*), 3 oz. . . . . . . . . . . . . . . . . . . . . . . . . . .90
berry, triple (*Crosse & Blackwell*), ⅓ cup . . . . . . . . . . . . . .120
blueberry (*Lucky Leaf*), 3 oz. . . . . . . . . . . . . . . . . . . . . . . . .90
blueberry (*Lucky Leaf* Premium), 3 oz. . . . . . . . . . . . . . . . .100
cherry (*Lucky Leaf*), 3 oz. . . . . . . . . . . . . . . . . . . . . . . . . . .100
cherry (*Lucky Leaf* Cherries Jubilee), 3 oz. . . . . . . . . . . . . . .80
cherry (*Lucky Leaf* Lite), 3 oz. . . . . . . . . . . . . . . . . . . . . . . .35
cherry blackberry (*Crosse & Blackwell*), ⅓ cup . . . . . . . . .100
lemon (*Lucky Leaf*), 3 oz. . . . . . . . . . . . . . . . . . . . . . . . . . .120
mince (*Crosse & Blackwell*), ¼ cup . . . . . . . . . . . . . . . . . .180
mince, w/brandy and rum (*Crosse & Blackwell*), ¼ cup . . .180
peach (*Lucky Leaf*), 3 oz. . . . . . . . . . . . . . . . . . . . . . . . . . . .80
pumpkin, mix (Libby's), ⅓ cup . . . . . . . . . . . . . . . . . . . . . . . .90
raisin (*Lucky Leaf*), 3 oz. . . . . . . . . . . . . . . . . . . . . . . . . . . .90
strawberry (*Lucky Leaf*), 3 oz. . . . . . . . . . . . . . . . . . . . . . . .80
**Pie glaze,** see "Strawberry pie glaze"
**Pie shell,** see "Pie crust"
**Pierogi,** frozen:
cheddar and potato (*Tofutti*), 4 pcs. . . . . . . . . . . . . . . . . . .185
cheese, American (*Mrs. T's*), 3 pcs. . . . . . . . . . . . . . . . . . .220
jalapeño cheddar (*Mrs. T's*), 3 pcs. . . . . . . . . . . . . . . . . . . .190
jalapeño cheddar, mini (*Mrs. T's 'Rogies*), 7 pcs. . . . . . . . .130
potato cheese, cheddar (*Mrs. T's*), 3 pcs. . . . . . . . . . . . . . .180
potato cheese, cheddar, mini (*Mrs. T's 'Rogies*), 7 pcs. . . . .130
potato onion (*Mrs. T's*), 3 pcs. . . . . . . . . . . . . . . . . . . . . . .180
potato roasted garlic (*Mrs. T's*), 3 pcs. . . . . . . . . . . . . . . .270
sauerkraut (*Mrs. T's*), 3 pcs. . . . . . . . . . . . . . . . . . . . . . . .170
**Pig's feet,** pickled, 1 oz. . . . . . . . . . . . . . . . . . . . . . . . . . . .58
**Pigeon peas,** fresh:
raw, ½ cup . . . . . . . . . . . . . . . . . . . . . . . . . . . . . . . . . . . . .105
boiled, drained, ½ cup . . . . . . . . . . . . . . . . . . . . . . . . . . . . .86
**Pigeon peas, dried,** mature:
(*Jack Rabbit*), ¼ cup . . . . . . . . . . . . . . . . . . . . . . . . . . . . . . .70
boiled, ½ cup . . . . . . . . . . . . . . . . . . . . . . . . . . . . . . . . . . . .102
**Pigeon peas, canned,** green (*Tupi*), ½ cup . . . . . . . . . . . . .70
**Pignolia nuts,** see "Pine nuts"

**Pike,** meat only:
northern, raw, 4 oz. . . . . . . . . . . . . . . . . . . . . . . . . . . .100
northern, baked, broiled, or microwaved, 4 oz. . . . . . . . . . .128
walleye, raw, 4 oz. . . . . . . . . . . . . . . . . . . . . . . . . . . . .105
walleye, baked, broiled, or microwaved, 4 oz. . . . . . . . . . . .135
**Pili nuts,** dried:
shelled, 1 oz. . . . . . . . . . . . . . . . . . . . . . . . . . . . . . . . .204
shelled, 1 cup . . . . . . . . . . . . . . . . . . . . . . . . . . . . . . .863
**Pimiento,** drained (*Roland*), ½ cup . . . . . . . . . . . . . . . . . .30
**Piña colada drink mixer:**
(*Goya*), ⅓ cup . . . . . . . . . . . . . . . . . . . . . . . . . . . . . . .120
(*Mr & Mrs T*), 4.5 fl. oz. . . . . . . . . . . . . . . . . . . . . . . . .180
frozen (*Bacardi*), 2 fl. oz. . . . . . . . . . . . . . . . . . . . . . . . .170
**Pine nuts,** dried:
raw (*Blue Diamond* Pine Nuts), ¼ cup . . . . . . . . . . . . . . . .190
pignolia (*Bazzini's Nut Club*), ¼ cup . . . . . . . . . . . . . . . . . .190
pignolia (*Krinos*), .5 oz. . . . . . . . . . . . . . . . . . . . . . . . . . .90
pignolia, 1 tbsp. . . . . . . . . . . . . . . . . . . . . . . . . . . . . . . . .51
pinyon, 1 oz. . . . . . . . . . . . . . . . . . . . . . . . . . . . . . . . . .178
pinyon, 10 kernels . . . . . . . . . . . . . . . . . . . . . . . . . . . . . . . .6
**Pineapple,** fresh:
(*Frieda's* Baby), 3 oz. . . . . . . . . . . . . . . . . . . . . . . . . . . . .70
(*Frieda's* South African Baby), 1 cup, 5 oz. . . . . . . . . . . . . .70
diced, ½ cup . . . . . . . . . . . . . . . . . . . . . . . . . . . . . . . . . . .39
sliced (*Dole*), 2 slices, 3" diam., 4 oz. . . . . . . . . . . . . . . . . .60
**Pineapple, candied,** all colors/styles (*Seneca* Glacé),
1 oz. . . . . . . . . . . . . . . . . . . . . . . . . . . . . . . . . . . . . . . .90
**Pineapple, can or jar,** ½ cup, except as noted:
in juice, all varieties, except sliced (*Del Monte*) . . . . . . . . . .70
in juice, crushed (*Dole*) . . . . . . . . . . . . . . . . . . . . . . . . . . .70
in juice, sliced (*Del Monte*), 4 oz., 2 slices . . . . . . . . . . . . .60
in juice, sliced (*Dole*), 4 oz., 2 slices . . . . . . . . . . . . . . . . . .60
in juice, tidbits (*Del Monte* Snack Cup), 4 oz. . . . . . . . . . . .50
in juice, tidbits or chunks (*Dole*) . . . . . . . . . . . . . . . . . . . . .60
in extra light syrup (*Sunfresh* Chilled) . . . . . . . . . . . . . . . . .80
in heavy syrup, all varieties, except sliced (*Dole*) . . . . . . . . .90
in heavy syrup, crushed or chunks (*Del Monte*) . . . . . . . . . .90
in heavy syrup (*Dole*), 2 slices . . . . . . . . . . . . . . . . . . . . . . .90
**Pineapple, dried** (*Setton Farm*), 1.4 oz. . . . . . . . . . . . . . . .140

**Pineapple, frozen,** sweetened, chunks, ½ cup . . . . . . . . . . .104
**Pineapple drink blends,** 8 fl. oz.:
coconut (*AriZona* Piña Colada) . . . . . . . . . . . . . . . . . . . . .140
grapefruit, pink (*Dole* Can) . . . . . . . . . . . . . . . . . . . . . . .130
guava nectar (*Goya*) . . . . . . . . . . . . . . . . . . . . . . . . . . .150
**Pineapple juice,** 8 fl. oz.:
(*Del Monte*) . . . . . . . . . . . . . . . . . . . . . . . . . . . . . . . .130
(*Del Monte* Not From Concentrate) . . . . . . . . . . . . . . . . . .110
(*Dole*) . . . . . . . . . . . . . . . . . . . . . . . . . . . . . . . . . . . .130
(*Dole* Can) . . . . . . . . . . . . . . . . . . . . . . . . . . . . . . . . .110
(*Dole* Can, Reconstituted) . . . . . . . . . . . . . . . . . . . . . . .120
**Pineapple juice blends,** 8 fl. oz., except as noted:
citrus (*Dole*) . . . . . . . . . . . . . . . . . . . . . . . . . . . . . . . .120
citrus (*Dole*), 11.5 fl. oz. . . . . . . . . . . . . . . . . . . . . . . .170
grapefruit (*Dole* Can), 6 fl. oz. . . . . . . . . . . . . . . . . . . . .100
orange (*Dole*) . . . . . . . . . . . . . . . . . . . . . . . . . . . . . . . .120
orange (*Dole*), 10 fl. oz. . . . . . . . . . . . . . . . . . . . . . . . .150
orange banana (*Dole*) . . . . . . . . . . . . . . . . . . . . . . . . . . .120
orange banana (*Dole*), 10 fl. oz. . . . . . . . . . . . . . . . . . . .150
orange banana (*Nantucket Nectars*) . . . . . . . . . . . . . . . . .140
orange strawberry (*Dole*) . . . . . . . . . . . . . . . . . . . . . . . .130
**Pineapple topping** (*Smucker's*), 2 tbsp. . . . . . . . . . . . . . . .110
**Pink beans,** boiled, ½ cup . . . . . . . . . . . . . . . . . . . . . . . .125
**Pinto beans:**
dry (*Arrowhead Mills*), ¼ cup . . . . . . . . . . . . . . . . . . . . . .150
boiled, ½ cup . . . . . . . . . . . . . . . . . . . . . . . . . . . . . . . . .117
**Pinto beans, canned** (see also "Chili beans" and "Refried beans"), ½ cup:
(*Bush's Best*) . . . . . . . . . . . . . . . . . . . . . . . . . . . . . . . .110
w/bacon (*Trappey's*) . . . . . . . . . . . . . . . . . . . . . . . . . . . .120
w/bacon and jalapeños (*Bush's Best*) . . . . . . . . . . . . . . . . .110
w/bacon and jalapeños (*Trappey's* Jalapinto) . . . . . . . . . . . .120
w/pork (*Bush's Best*) . . . . . . . . . . . . . . . . . . . . . . . . . . . .120
seasoned (*Glory Foods*) . . . . . . . . . . . . . . . . . . . . . . . . . . .90
**Pinto–great northern beans,** canned (*Bush's Best* Mixed Beans), ½ cup . . . . . . . . . . . . . . . . . . . . . . . . . . . . . . . .110
**Pipian,** in jars (*Doña Maria*), 2 tbsp. . . . . . . . . . . . . . . . . .250
**Pistachio nut,** shelled, except as noted:
raw (*Blue Diamond*), ¼ cup . . . . . . . . . . . . . . . . . . . . . . . .200
raw, ¼ cup . . . . . . . . . . . . . . . . . . . . . . . . . . . . . . . . . . . .176

dried, in shell (*River Queen*), ½ cup, 1 oz. edible . . . . . . . .170
dried, in shell (*Sunkist*), ½ cup, ¼ cup edible . . . . . . . . . .180
dry-roasted (*Planters*), ½ cup . . . . . . . . . . . . . . . . . . . . .160
roasted, in shell (*Setton Farms*), 1 oz. . . . . . . . . . . . . . . . .170
**Pita,** see "Bread"
**Pitanga,** 1 medium, .3 oz. . . . . . . . . . . . . . . . . . . . . . . . . .2
**Pizza,** frozen, 1 pie, except as noted:
artichoke heart (*Wolfgang Puck's*), ½ pie . . . . . . . . . . . . . .340
bacon burger (*Totino's* Crispy Crust Party Pizza), ½ pie . . .390
Canadian bacon (*Jeno's Crisp 'n Tasty*) . . . . . . . . . . . . . . . .440
Canadian bacon (*Totino's* Crisp Crust Party Pizza), ½ pie . .330
cheese (*Celeste* Large), ¼ pie . . . . . . . . . . . . . . . . . . . . . .300
cheese (*Celeste* for One) . . . . . . . . . . . . . . . . . . . . . . . . . .420
cheese (*Michelina's* Singles) . . . . . . . . . . . . . . . . . . . . . . .420
cheese (*Michelina's That'za Pizza!*) . . . . . . . . . . . . . . . . . .410
cheese (*Totino's* Family Size), ⅓ pie . . . . . . . . . . . . . . . . .370
cheese (*Totino's* Crisp Crust Party Pizza), ½ pie . . . . . . . . .320
cheese (*Wolfgang Puck's*), ¼ pie . . . . . . . . . . . . . . . . . . . .300
cheese, 4 (*Celeste* for One Original) . . . . . . . . . . . . . . . . . .470
cheese, 4 (*Celeste* Rising Crust), ⅙ pie . . . . . . . . . . . . . . .320
cheese, 4 (*Freschetta* 11.15 oz.), ½ pie . . . . . . . . . . . . . . .390
cheese, 4 (*Freschetta* 26.85 oz.), ⅕ pie . . . . . . . . . . . . . . .380
cheese, 4 (*Freschetta* Sauce Stuffed Crust), ⅕ pie . . . . . . .370
cheese, 4 (*Wolfgang Puck's*), ½ pie . . . . . . . . . . . . . . . . . .360
cheese, 4, zesty (*Celeste* for One) . . . . . . . . . . . . . . . . . . .470
"cheese," nondairy (*Amy's* Soy Cheeze), ⅓ pie . . . . . . . . . .280
chicken, barbecue (*Wolfgang Puck's*), ¼ pie . . . . . . . . . . . .370
chcken, roasted garlic rosemary (*Freschetta*), ⅓ pie . . . . . .260
chicken, Southwest (*Freschetta* Supreme), ½ pie . . . . . . . .340
chicken, zesty (*Celeste* for One Supreme) . . . . . . . . . . . . .380
combination (*Jeno's Crisp 'n Tasty*) . . . . . . . . . . . . . . . . . .500
combination (*Michelina's* Singles) . . . . . . . . . . . . . . . . . . .430
combination (*Totino's* Crispy Crust Party Pizza), ½ pie . . . .380
combination (*Totino's* Family Size), ¼ pie . . . . . . . . . . . . .310
deluxe (*Celeste* Large), ¼ pie . . . . . . . . . . . . . . . . . . . . . .340
deluxe (*Celeste* for One) . . . . . . . . . . . . . . . . . . . . . . . . . .470
deluxe (*Freschetta*), ⅙ pie . . . . . . . . . . . . . . . . . . . . . . . .350
deluxe (*Freschetta* Special), ⅙ pie . . . . . . . . . . . . . . . . . .350
ham and shrimp, Hawaiian style (*Contessa*), ⅓ pie . . . . . . .320
hamburger (*Jeno's Crisp 'n Tasty*) . . . . . . . . . . . . . . . . . . .500

**Pizza, frozen *(cont.)***
hamburger (*Totino's* Crisp Crust Party Pizza), ½ pie . . . . . .380
Margherita (*Freschetta*), ½ pie . . . . . . . . . . . . . . . . . . . . . .340
meat, 4 (*Freschetta*), ⅙ pie . . . . . . . . . . . . . . . . . . . . . . . .340
meat, 3 (*Celeste* Rising Crust), ⅙ pie . . . . . . . . . . . . . . . .340
meat, 3 (*Jeno's Crisp 'n Tasty*) . . . . . . . . . . . . . . . . . . . . .490
meat, 3 (*Totino's* Crisp Crust Party Pizza), ½ pie . . . . . . . . .360
mushroom and olive (*Amy's*), ⅓ pie . . . . . . . . . . . . . . . . . .250
mushroom and spinach (*Wolfgang Puck's*), ⅓ pie . . . . . . .230
nondairy (*Tofutti* Pizzaz), ⅓ pkg. . . . . . . . . . . . . . . . . . . . .175
pepperoni (*Banquet* Meal), 6.75-oz. pkg. . . . . . . . . . . . . . .480
pepperoni (*Celeste* Large), ¼ pie . . . . . . . . . . . . . . . . . . . .350
pepperoni (*Celeste* for One) . . . . . . . . . . . . . . . . . . . . . . . .470
pepperoni (*Celeste* Rising Crust), ⅙ pie . . . . . . . . . . . . . . .330
pepperoni (*Freschetta* 11.58 oz.), ½ pie . . . . . . . . . . . . . . .430
pepperoni (*Freschetta* 28.15 oz.), ⅙ pie . . . . . . . . . . . . . . .350
pepperoni (*Freschetta* Sauce Stuffed Crust), ⅕ pie . . . . . . .340
pepperoni (*Jeno's Crisp 'n Tasty*) . . . . . . . . . . . . . . . . . . . .510
pepperoni (*Michelina's* Singles) . . . . . . . . . . . . . . . . . . . . .440
pepperoni (*Totino's* Crisp Crust Party Pizza), ½ pie . . . . . . .380
pepperoni (*Totino's* Family Size), ⅓ pie . . . . . . . . . . . . . . . .420
pepperoni (*Wolfgang Puck's*), ¼ pie . . . . . . . . . . . . . . . . .360
pepperoni and mushroom (*Wolfgang Puck's*), ⅓ pie . . . . . .310
pesto, w/tomatoes and broccoli (*Amy's*), ⅓ pie . . . . . . . . . .300
sausage (*Celeste* for One) . . . . . . . . . . . . . . . . . . . . . . . . .480
sausage (*Freschetta*), ⅙ pie . . . . . . . . . . . . . . . . . . . . . . . .350
sausage (*Jeno's Crisp 'n Tasty*) . . . . . . . . . . . . . . . . . . . . .480
sausage (*Totino's* Crispy Crust Party Pizza), ½ pie . . . . . . .380
sausage (*Totino's* Family Size), ¼ pie . . . . . . . . . . . . . . . .300
sausage and herb (*Wolfgang Puck's*), ⅓ pie . . . . . . . . . . .350
sausage and mushroom (*Totino's* Crisp Crust Party Pizza),
 ½ pie . . . . . . . . . . . . . . . . . . . . . . . . . . . . . . . . . . . . . . . .360
sausage and pepperoni:
 (*Celeste* for One) . . . . . . . . . . . . . . . . . . . . . . . . . . . . . . .560
 (*Freschetta*), ⅕ pie . . . . . . . . . . . . . . . . . . . . . . . . . . . . .350
 (*Freschetta* Sauce Stuffed Crust), ⅕ pie . . . . . . . . . . . .390
 (*Totino's* Crisp Crust Party Pizza), ½ pie . . . . . . . . . . . .380
 (*Totino's* Crisp Crust Party Pizza Zesty Italiano),
  ½ pie . . . . . . . . . . . . . . . . . . . . . . . . . . . . . . . . . . . . . .390
shrimp, basil pesto (*Contessa*), ⅓ pie . . . . . . . . . . . . . . . .300

shrimp, roasted red pesto (*Contessa*), ⅓ pie . . . . . . . . . . .300
shrimp, roasted vegetables (*Contessa*), ⅓ pie . . . . . . . . . . .280
supreme (*Celeste* Rising Crust), ⅙ pie . . . . . . . . . . . . . . .360
supreme (*Celeste* Suprema for One) . . . . . . . . . . . . . . . . .530
supreme (*Freschetta* 12.9 oz.), ⅓ pie . . . . . . . . . . . . . . .290
supreme (*Freschetta* Sauce Stuffed Crust), ⅕ pie . . . . . . . .400
supreme (*Jeno's Crisp 'n Tasty*) . . . . . . . . . . . . . . . . . . .500
supreme (*Michelina's* Singles), 1 pie . . . . . . . . . . . . . . . .430
supreme (*Totino's* Crisp Crust Party Pizza), ½ pie . . . . . . . .380
supreme (*Wolfgang Puck's*), ½ of 12-oz. pie or ¼ of
24-oz. pie . . . . . . . . . . . . . . . . . . . . . . . . . . . . . . . . .400
vegetable (*Celeste* for One) . . . . . . . . . . . . . . . . . . . . . .430
vegetable (*Wolfgang Puck's*), ¼ pie . . . . . . . . . . . . . . . . .360
vegetable, combo (*Amy's*), ⅓ pie . . . . . . . . . . . . . . . . . . .250
vegetable, grilled (*Freschetta* Medley Sauce Stuffed Crust),
⅕ pie . . . . . . . . . . . . . . . . . . . . . . . . . . . . . . . . . . . .340
vegetable, grilled, cheeseless (*Wolfgang Puck's*), ⅓ pie . . .150
vegetable, primavera (*Freschetta*), ⅕ pie . . . . . . . . . . . . .350
vegetable, roasted (*Amy's*), ⅓ pie . . . . . . . . . . . . . . . . . .270
**Pizza, bagel,** frozen, mini, cheese, pepperoni/sausage and
pepperoni (*Ore-Ida Bagel Bites Hot Bites*), 4 pcs. . . . . . .200
**Pizza, French bread,** frozen, 1 pc.:
cheese (*Healthy Choice*) . . . . . . . . . . . . . . . . . . . . . . . .340
cheese (*Lean Cuisine*) . . . . . . . . . . . . . . . . . . . . . . . . . .310
cheese (*Stouffer's*) . . . . . . . . . . . . . . . . . . . . . . . . . . . .370
cheese, extra (*Stouffer's*) . . . . . . . . . . . . . . . . . . . . . . .400
cheese, 4, smothered (*Marie Callender's*) . . . . . . . . . . . . .530
cheese, 5 (*Stouffer's*) . . . . . . . . . . . . . . . . . . . . . . . . . .420
deluxe (*Lean Cuisine*) . . . . . . . . . . . . . . . . . . . . . . . . . .290
deluxe (*Stouffer's*) . . . . . . . . . . . . . . . . . . . . . . . . . . . .420
meat, 3, or sausage and pepperoni (*Stouffer's*) . . . . . . . . . .470
pepperoni (*Healthy Choice*) . . . . . . . . . . . . . . . . . . . . . .340
pepperoni (*Lean Cuisine*) . . . . . . . . . . . . . . . . . . . . . . . .300
pepperoni (*Marie Callender's*) . . . . . . . . . . . . . . . . . . . . .570
pepperoni (*Stouffer's*) . . . . . . . . . . . . . . . . . . . . . . . . . .390
pepperoni and mushroom (*Stouffer's*) . . . . . . . . . . . . . . . .440
sausage (*Healthy Choice*) . . . . . . . . . . . . . . . . . . . . . . . .320
sausage (*Stouffer's*) . . . . . . . . . . . . . . . . . . . . . . . . . . .420
sun-dried tomato (*Lean Cuisine*) . . . . . . . . . . . . . . . . . . .350
supreme (*Healthy Choice*) . . . . . . . . . . . . . . . . . . . . . . . .330

**Pizza, French bread, frozen *(cont.)***
supreme, super (*Marie Callender's*) . . . . . . . . . . . . . . . . . . .510
vegetable (*Healthy Choice*) . . . . . . . . . . . . . . . . . . . . . . . . . .280
vegetable, grilled (*Stouffer's*) . . . . . . . . . . . . . . . . . . . . . . .350
white (*Stouffer's*) . . . . . . . . . . . . . . . . . . . . . . . . . . . . . . . .470
**Pizza, stuffed/pocket,** frozen, 4.5-oz. pc., except as noted:
(*Hot Pockets Pizza Minis*), 7 pcs., 3.1 oz. . . . . . . . . . . . . . .280
cheese (*Amy's*) . . . . . . . . . . . . . . . . . . . . . . . . . . . . . . . . .300
cheese, double (*Hot Pockets Toaster Pizza*), 2.2 oz. . . . . . .170
cheese, 4 (*Hot Pockets*) . . . . . . . . . . . . . . . . . . . . . . . . . . .360
deluxe (*Lean Pockets*) . . . . . . . . . . . . . . . . . . . . . . . . . . . .290
pepperoni (*Croissant Pockets*) . . . . . . . . . . . . . . . . . . . . . .360
pepperoni (*Deli Stuffs*) . . . . . . . . . . . . . . . . . . . . . . . . . . .350
pepperoni (*Hot Pockets*) . . . . . . . . . . . . . . . . . . . . . . . . . .340
pepperoni (*Hot Pockets Toaster Pizza*), 2.2 oz. . . . . . . . . . .180
pepperoni/sausage (*Hot Pockets*) . . . . . . . . . . . . . . . . . . . .340
pepperoni/sausage (*Hot Pockets Toaster Pizza*), 2.2 oz. . . .170
sausage (*Hot Pockets*) . . . . . . . . . . . . . . . . . . . . . . . . . . . .370
supreme (*Croissant Pockets*) . . . . . . . . . . . . . . . . . . . . . . .350
vegetarian (*Amy's*) . . . . . . . . . . . . . . . . . . . . . . . . . . . . . .250
vegetarian, "cheese," soy (*Amy's* Cheeze) . . . . . . . . . . . . . .270
**Pizza burrito,** see "Burrito"
**Pizza crust,** refrigerated (*Pillsbury*), ⅕ crust . . . . . . . . . . .150
**Pizza crust mix,** ⅛ pkg., except as noted:
(*Betty Crocker*), ¼ crust . . . . . . . . . . . . . . . . . . . . . . . . . .160
(*Eagle Mills*) . . . . . . . . . . . . . . . . . . . . . . . . . . . . . . . . . . .160
white (*Watkins* Deep Dish) . . . . . . . . . . . . . . . . . . . . . . . . .180
whole wheat (*Watkins* Thin) . . . . . . . . . . . . . . . . . . . . . . . . .90
***Pizza Hut,*** 1 slice of medium pie, except as noted:
*The Edge,* 1 square:
  chicken supreme . . . . . . . . . . . . . . . . . . . . . . . . . . . . . . . .90
  *Meat Lover's* . . . . . . . . . . . . . . . . . . . . . . . . . . . . . . . . .160
  *Veggie Lover's* . . . . . . . . . . . . . . . . . . . . . . . . . . . . . . . .70
  The Works . . . . . . . . . . . . . . . . . . . . . . . . . . . . . . . . . . . .110
hand-tossed:
  beef . . . . . . . . . . . . . . . . . . . . . . . . . . . . . . . . . . . . . . . .330
  cheese . . . . . . . . . . . . . . . . . . . . . . . . . . . . . . . . . . . . . .240
  chicken supreme . . . . . . . . . . . . . . . . . . . . . . . . . . . . . . .230
  ham . . . . . . . . . . . . . . . . . . . . . . . . . . . . . . . . . . . . . . . .260
  *Meat Lover's* . . . . . . . . . . . . . . . . . . . . . . . . . . . . . . . . .320

pepperoni . . . . . . . . . . . . . . . . . . . . . . . . . . . . . .280
*Pepperoni Lover's* . . . . . . . . . . . . . . . . . . . . . . . .250
pork topping . . . . . . . . . . . . . . . . . . . . . . . . . . . .320
sausage, Italian . . . . . . . . . . . . . . . . . . . . . . . . . .340
super supreme . . . . . . . . . . . . . . . . . . . . . . . . . .290
supreme . . . . . . . . . . . . . . . . . . . . . . . . . . . . . . .270
*Veggie Lover's* . . . . . . . . . . . . . . . . . . . . . . . . . .220
*The Big New Yorker:*
beef . . . . . . . . . . . . . . . . . . . . . . . . . . . . . . . . . .480
cheese . . . . . . . . . . . . . . . . . . . . . . . . . . . . . . . .380
ham . . . . . . . . . . . . . . . . . . . . . . . . . . . . . . . . . .340
pepperoni . . . . . . . . . . . . . . . . . . . . . . . . . . . . . .370
pork topping . . . . . . . . . . . . . . . . . . . . . . . . . . . .470
sausage . . . . . . . . . . . . . . . . . . . . . . . . . . . . . . .570
supreme . . . . . . . . . . . . . . . . . . . . . . . . . . . . . . .450
*Veggie Lover's* . . . . . . . . . . . . . . . . . . . . . . . . . .450
pan pizza:
beef . . . . . . . . . . . . . . . . . . . . . . . . . . . . . . . . . .330
cheese . . . . . . . . . . . . . . . . . . . . . . . . . . . . . . . .290
chicken supreme . . . . . . . . . . . . . . . . . . . . . . . . .270
ham . . . . . . . . . . . . . . . . . . . . . . . . . . . . . . . . . .260
*Meat Lover's* . . . . . . . . . . . . . . . . . . . . . . . . . . . .360
pepperoni . . . . . . . . . . . . . . . . . . . . . . . . . . . . . .280
*Pepperoni Lover's* . . . . . . . . . . . . . . . . . . . . . . . .330
pork topping . . . . . . . . . . . . . . . . . . . . . . . . . . . .320
sausage, Italian . . . . . . . . . . . . . . . . . . . . . . . . . .340
super supreme . . . . . . . . . . . . . . . . . . . . . . . . . .340
supreme . . . . . . . . . . . . . . . . . . . . . . . . . . . . . . .320
*Veggie Lover's* . . . . . . . . . . . . . . . . . . . . . . . . . .270
*Personal Pan Pizza,* 1 pie:
beef . . . . . . . . . . . . . . . . . . . . . . . . . . . . . . . . . .710
cheese . . . . . . . . . . . . . . . . . . . . . . . . . . . . . . . .630
ham . . . . . . . . . . . . . . . . . . . . . . . . . . . . . . . . . .580
pepperoni . . . . . . . . . . . . . . . . . . . . . . . . . . . . . .620
pork topping . . . . . . . . . . . . . . . . . . . . . . . . . . . .700
sausage, Italian . . . . . . . . . . . . . . . . . . . . . . . . . .740
stuffed crust, 1 slice of large pie:
beef . . . . . . . . . . . . . . . . . . . . . . . . . . . . . . . . . .466
cheese . . . . . . . . . . . . . . . . . . . . . . . . . . . . . . . .445
chicken supreme . . . . . . . . . . . . . . . . . . . . . . . . .432

***Pizza Hut*, stuffed crust *(cont.)***

ham . . . . . . . . . . . . . . . . . . . . . . . . . . . . . . . . . .404
*Meat Lover's* . . . . . . . . . . . . . . . . . . . . . . . . . . . . .543
pepperoni . . . . . . . . . . . . . . . . . . . . . . . . . . . . . . .438
*Pepperoni Lover's* . . . . . . . . . . . . . . . . . . . . . . . . .525
pork topping . . . . . . . . . . . . . . . . . . . . . . . . . . . . .461
sausage, Italian . . . . . . . . . . . . . . . . . . . . . . . . . . .478
super supreme . . . . . . . . . . . . . . . . . . . . . . . . . . .505
supreme . . . . . . . . . . . . . . . . . . . . . . . . . . . . . . . .487
*Veggie Lover's* . . . . . . . . . . . . . . . . . . . . . . . . . . .421

Sicilian:

beef . . . . . . . . . . . . . . . . . . . . . . . . . . . . . . . . . . .260
cheese . . . . . . . . . . . . . . . . . . . . . . . . . . . . . . . . .290
chicken supreme . . . . . . . . . . . . . . . . . . . . . . . . . .270
ham . . . . . . . . . . . . . . . . . . . . . . . . . . . . . . . . . .257
*Meat Lover's* . . . . . . . . . . . . . . . . . . . . . . . . . . . . .350
pepperoni . . . . . . . . . . . . . . . . . . . . . . . . . . . . . . .280
*Pepperoni Lover's* . . . . . . . . . . . . . . . . . . . . . . . . .320
pork topping . . . . . . . . . . . . . . . . . . . . . . . . . . . . .320
sausage, Italian . . . . . . . . . . . . . . . . . . . . . . . . . . .333
super supreme . . . . . . . . . . . . . . . . . . . . . . . . . . .340
supreme . . . . . . . . . . . . . . . . . . . . . . . . . . . . . . . .310
*Veggie Lover's* . . . . . . . . . . . . . . . . . . . . . . . . . . .270

*Thin n' Crispy:*

beef . . . . . . . . . . . . . . . . . . . . . . . . . . . . . . . . . . .270
cheese . . . . . . . . . . . . . . . . . . . . . . . . . . . . . . . . .200
chicken supreme . . . . . . . . . . . . . . . . . . . . . . . . . .200
ham . . . . . . . . . . . . . . . . . . . . . . . . . . . . . . . . . .170
*Meat Lover's* . . . . . . . . . . . . . . . . . . . . . . . . . . . . .310
pepperoni . . . . . . . . . . . . . . . . . . . . . . . . . . . . . . .190
*Pepperoni Lover's* . . . . . . . . . . . . . . . . . . . . . . . . .250
pork topping . . . . . . . . . . . . . . . . . . . . . . . . . . . . .270
sausage, Italian . . . . . . . . . . . . . . . . . . . . . . . . . . .290
super supreme . . . . . . . . . . . . . . . . . . . . . . . . . . .280
supreme . . . . . . . . . . . . . . . . . . . . . . . . . . . . . . . .250
*Veggie Lover's* . . . . . . . . . . . . . . . . . . . . . . . . . . .190

appetizers:

Buffalo wings, hot, 4 pcs. . . . . . . . . . . . . . . . . . . .210
Buffalo wings, mild, 5 pcs. . . . . . . . . . . . . . . . . . .200
garlic bread, 1 slice . . . . . . . . . . . . . . . . . . . . . . .150

bread stick, 1 pc. . . . . . . . . . . . . . . . . . . . . . . . . . . .130
bread stick dipping sauce . . . . . . . . . . . . . . . . . . . . . . .30
pasta, 1 serving:
*Cavatini* . . . . . . . . . . . . . . . . . . . . . . . . . . . . . . . .480
*Cavatini Supreme* . . . . . . . . . . . . . . . . . . . . . . . . . .560
spaghetti, w/marinara . . . . . . . . . . . . . . . . . . . . . . . .490
spaghetti, w/meat sauce . . . . . . . . . . . . . . . . . . . . . .600
spaghetti, w/meatballs . . . . . . . . . . . . . . . . . . . . . . .850
sandwiches, 1 pc:
ham & cheese . . . . . . . . . . . . . . . . . . . . . . . . . . . . .550
supreme . . . . . . . . . . . . . . . . . . . . . . . . . . . . . . . . .640
dessert pizza, apple or cherry, 1 pc. . . . . . . . . . . . . . . . . . .250
**Pizza pocket,** see "Pizza, stuffed/pocket"
**Pizza rolls,** see "Pizza snack"
**Pizza sauce** (see also "Pasta sauce"), ¼ cup:
(*Progresso*) . . . . . . . . . . . . . . . . . . . . . . . . . . . . . . .20
(*Ragú*) . . . . . . . . . . . . . . . . . . . . . . . . . . . . . . . . . . .25
(*Ragú Pizza Quick* Traditional) . . . . . . . . . . . . . . . . . . . .40
garlic and basil (*Ragú Pizza Quick*) . . . . . . . . . . . . . . . . .40
pepperoni (*Ragú Pizza Quick*) . . . . . . . . . . . . . . . . . . . . .50
**Pizza snack** (see also "Nacho snack"), frozen, 6 pcs.:
cheese (*Amy's*) . . . . . . . . . . . . . . . . . . . . . . . . . . . . .180
cheese (*Michelina's* Rolls) . . . . . . . . . . . . . . . . . . . . . .230
cheese (*Totino's Pizza Rolls*) . . . . . . . . . . . . . . . . . . . .210
cheese, nacho, or hamburger (*Michelina's* Rolls) . . . . . . . .220
combination (*Michelina's* Rolls) . . . . . . . . . . . . . . . . . . .230
combination (*Totino's Pizza Rolls*) . . . . . . . . . . . . . . . . .230
hamburger (*Totino's Pizza Rolls*) . . . . . . . . . . . . . . . . . .210
meat, 4 (*Michelina's* Rolls) . . . . . . . . . . . . . . . . . . . . . .230
meat, 3 (*Totino's Pizza Rolls*) . . . . . . . . . . . . . . . . . . . .220
pepperoni (*Michelina's* Rolls) . . . . . . . . . . . . . . . . . . . .240
pepperoni (*Totino's Pizza Rolls*) . . . . . . . . . . . . . . . . . .230
pepperoni, sausage, or supreme (*Totino's Pizza Rolls*) . . . .220
**Plantain:**
raw (*Frieda's*), 3 oz. . . . . . . . . . . . . . . . . . . . . . . . . . .100
raw, 1 large, 9.7 oz. . . . . . . . . . . . . . . . . . . . . . . . . . .218
raw, sliced, ½ cup . . . . . . . . . . . . . . . . . . . . . . . . . . . . .91
cooked, sliced, ½ cup . . . . . . . . . . . . . . . . . . . . . . . . . .89
**Plantain, frozen:**
baked, ripe (*Goya* Plátanos Maduros Horneados), 3 oz. . . . .237

**Plantain, frozen *(cont.)***
fried (*Latin Fiesta*), 4 pcs. .......................210
fried (*Goya* Plátanos Tostones), 4 pcs. ...............210
**Plum,** fresh:
(*Dole*), 2 medium ..........................80
Japanese or hybrid, 2⅛" fruit ....................36
sliced, ½ cup ..............................46
**Plum, canned,** purple:
in juice, 1 plum w/liquid ......................27
in juice, pitted, 1 cup .......................146
in light syrup, 1 plum w/liquid ..................29
in light syrup, pitted, 1 cup ...................159
in heavy syrup, 1 plum w/liquid ..................41
in heavy syrup, pitted, 1 cup ...................230
**Plum, dried:**
(*Dole*), ¼ cup ............................110
dehydrated, ½ cup ..........................224
w/pits (*Sunsweet*), 1.4 oz., 3 large or 6 medium ........100
w/pits, ½ cup .............................193
pitted (*Sunsweet Lemon/Orange Essence*), 1.4 oz., 5 pcs. . .100
pitted, 10 pcs. ............................201
pitted, bite size (*Sunsweet*), 1.4 oz., 7 pcs. ...........100
stewed, w/pits, unsweetened, ½ cup ...............113
**Plum, dried, canned,** in heavy syrup:
pitted, ½ cup .............................123
5 pcs., w/2 tbsp. liquid ......................90
**Plum sauce** (*Ka•Me*), 2 tbsp. ....................70
**Plum–passion fruit, dried** (*Sunsweet Fruitlings*), 1.4 oz.,
⅓ cup ................................110
**Poi,** ½ cup ..............................134
**Pocket sandwich,** see specific listings
**Poke greens,** canned (*Allens*), ½ cup ...............35
**Pokeberry shoots:**
raw, ½ cup ...............................18
boiled, drained, ½ cup .......................16
**Polenta,** dry (*Bellino* Instant), ¼ cup ..............140
**Polenta, canned** (*Greene's Farm*), ½ cup .............80
**Polenta, refrigerated,** 2 slices, ½", except as noted:
plain (*Frieda's*), 4 oz. ......................100
plain (*San Gennaro*) ........................70

basil and garlic (*San Gennaro*) . . . . . . . . . . . . . . . . . . . . . . . .71
sun-dried tomato (*San Gennaro*) . . . . . . . . . . . . . . . . . . . . . .74
**Polish sausage** (see also "Kielbasa"), 1 link:
fresh, grilled (*Johnsonville*), 3 oz. . . . . . . . . . . . . . . . . . . . . .290
precooked (*Johnsonville*), 2.7 oz. . . . . . . . . . . . . . . . . . . . . .240
**Pollock,** meat only, 4 oz.:
Atlantic, raw . . . . . . . . . . . . . . . . . . . . . . . . . . . . . . . . . . .104
Atlantic, baked, broiled, or microwaved . . . . . . . . . . . . . . . .134
walleye, raw . . . . . . . . . . . . . . . . . . . . . . . . . . . . . . . . . . .91
walleye, baked, broiled, or microwaved . . . . . . . . . . . . . . . .128
**Pomegranate:**
(*Frieda's*), 5 oz. . . . . . . . . . . . . . . . . . . . . . . . . . . . . . . .100
w/peel, 9.7-oz. fruit . . . . . . . . . . . . . . . . . . . . . . . . . . . . .104
**Pompano,** Florida, meat only:
raw, 4 oz. . . . . . . . . . . . . . . . . . . . . . . . . . . . . . . . . . . . .186
baked, broiled, or microwaved, 4 oz. . . . . . . . . . . . . . . . . . .239
**Popcorn,** unpopped, except as noted:
(*Jolly Time* Sugar Corn), 3 cups* . . . . . . . . . . . . . . . . . . . .120
(*Pop•Secret* Homestyle), 3 tbsp. . . . . . . . . . . . . . . . . . . . . .170
(*Pop Weaver* Premium Hybrid), 1 oz. . . . . . . . . . . . . . . . . . .100
(*Pop Weaver Naks Paks* Coconut Oil), 3 tbsp. . . . . . . . . . . . .140
(*Pop Weaver Naks Paks* Safflower Oil), 3 tbsp. . . . . . . . . . . .150
butter/butter flavor:
(*America's Best*), 5 cups* . . . . . . . . . . . . . . . . . . . . . . . .90
(*B. K. Heuermann's Exclusive*), 2 tbsp. . . . . . . . . . . . . . . .140
(*B. K. Heuermann's Exclusive* Intense Taste), 2 tbsp. . . .160
(*B. K. Heuermann's Exclusive* Low Fat), 2 tbsp. . . . . . . .120
(*Healthy Choice*), 3 tbsp. . . . . . . . . . . . . . . . . . . . . . . . .120
(*Jolly Time Blast O Butter*), 3½ cups* . . . . . . . . . . . . . .150
(*Jolly Time Blast O Butter* Light), 4 cups* . . . . . . . . . . .130
(*Jolly Time Butter•Licious*), 4 cups* . . . . . . . . . . . . . . .140
(*Jolly Time Butter•Licious* Light), 5 cups* . . . . . . . . . . .120
(*Jolly Time Healthy Pop*), 5 cups* . . . . . . . . . . . . . . . . . .90
(*Newman's Own*), 3½ cups* . . . . . . . . . . . . . . . . . . . . . .170
(*Newman's Own* Butter Boom), 3½ cups* . . . . . . . . . . . .170
(*Newman's Own* Light), 3½ cups* . . . . . . . . . . . . . . . . .110
(*Pop•Secret* Extra Butter), 3 tbsp. . . . . . . . . . . . . . . . . .180
(*Pop•Secret* Light), 3 tbsp. . . . . . . . . . . . . . . . . . . . . . .140
(*Pop•Secret* Light Snack Size), ¼ cup . . . . . . . . . . . . . .160
(*Pop•Secret* 94% Fat Free), 3 tbsp. . . . . . . . . . . . . . . . .120

**Popcorn, butter/butter flavor *(cont.)***
(*Pop•Secret Land O Lakes*/Rev it Up), 3 tbsp. . . . . . . . . .180
(*Pop•Secret Jumbo Pop*), 3 tbsp. . . . . . . . . . . . . . . . . . .170
(*Pop Weaver* Microwave), ⅓ bag, 1.2 oz. . . . . . . . . . . .140
(*Pop Weaver* Microwave Light), ⅓ bag, 1.2 oz. . . . . . . .115
white, buttery (*Jolly Time*), 4 cups* . . . . . . . . . . . . . . . .150
cheddar (*Jolly Time*), 3 cups* . . . . . . . . . . . . . . . . . . . . . .160
crispy (*Jolly Time* Light), 5 cups* . . . . . . . . . . . . . . . . . . .120
natural flavor:
(*B. K. Heuermann's Exclusive*) . . . . . . . . . . . . . . . . . . . .120
(*Healthy Choice*), 3 tbsp. . . . . . . . . . . . . . . . . . . . . . . . .120
(*Newman's Own*), 3½ cups* . . . . . . . . . . . . . . . . . . . . . .170
(*Pop•Secret*), 3 tbsp. . . . . . . . . . . . . . . . . . . . . . . . . . . .170
(*Pop•Secret* 94% Fat Free), 3 tbsp. . . . . . . . . . . . . . . . .120
(*Pop•Secret* 94% Fat Free), 6 cups* . . . . . . . . . . . . . . .110
(*Pop Weaver* Microwave), ⅓ bag, 1.2 oz. . . . . . . . . . . .140
white, crispy (*Jolly Time*), 4 cups* . . . . . . . . . . . . . . . . . . .150
white/yellow (*Jolly Time*), 5 cups air-popped . . . . . . . . . . .100
**Popcorn, popped:**
(*Bachman*), 1 oz. . . . . . . . . . . . . . . . . . . . . . . . . . . . . . . .140
(*Bachman* Lite), 1 oz. . . . . . . . . . . . . . . . . . . . . . . . . . . . .110
(*Bearitos* No Oil), 5 cups, 1.1 oz. . . . . . . . . . . . . . . . . . . .110
(*Bearitos* No Oil/Salt), 4¼ cups, 1.1 oz. . . . . . . . . . . . . . .120
(*Herr's*), 1 oz., 3 cups . . . . . . . . . . . . . . . . . . . . . . . . . . .140
(*Weight Watchers*), 1 pkg. . . . . . . . . . . . . . . . . . . . . . . . . .100
butter (*Bearitos* Buttery), 2½ cups, 1.1 oz. . . . . . . . . . . . . .170
butter (*Bearitos* Buttery Lite), 3½ cups, 1.1 oz. . . . . . . . . .140
butter (*Chester's*), 3 cups . . . . . . . . . . . . . . . . . . . . . . . . .170
butter (*Snyder's*), ⅝ oz. . . . . . . . . . . . . . . . . . . . . . . . . . .110
butter (*Utz*), 2 cups . . . . . . . . . . . . . . . . . . . . . . . . . . . . .170
caramel (*Bearitos* Fat Free), 1 cup, 1.1 oz. . . . . . . . . . . . .120
caramel (*Cracker Jack* Fat Free), ¾ cup . . . . . . . . . . . . . .110
caramel (*Utz* Cluster), 1 oz. . . . . . . . . . . . . . . . . . . . . . . . .142
caramel, w/peanuts (*Cracker Jack*), ½ cup . . . . . . . . . . . . .120
cheddar, white (*Bearitos*), 2⅓ cups, 1.1 oz. . . . . . . . . . . . .170
cheddar, white (*Chester's*), 3 cups . . . . . . . . . . . . . . . . . . .200
cheddar, white (*Smartfood*), 1¾ cups . . . . . . . . . . . . . . . .160
cheddar, white (*Smartfood* Reduced Fat), 3 cups . . . . . . . .140
cheddar, white (*Utz*), 2 cups . . . . . . . . . . . . . . . . . . . . . . .150
cheese (*Bachman*), 1 oz. . . . . . . . . . . . . . . . . . . . . . . . . . .150

cheese (*Utz*), 2 cups . . . . . . . . . . . . . . . . . . . . . . . . . . .150
cheese (*Utz* Hulless Puff'n Corn), 2 cups . . . . . . . . . . . . . .160
toffee, butter (*Cracker Jack* Fat Free), ¾ cup . . . . . . . . . . . .110
**Popcorn cakes:**
all varieties (*Hain* Mini), .5 oz. . . . . . . . . . . . . . . . . . . . . .50
plain (*Hain*), .3-oz. pc. . . . . . . . . . . . . . . . . . . . . . . . . . . .35
butter (*Hain*), .3-oz. pc. . . . . . . . . . . . . . . . . . . . . . . . . . .50
**Poppy seed,** 1 tsp. . . . . . . . . . . . . . . . . . . . . . . . . . . . . .15
**Porgy,** see "Scup"
**Pork** (see also "Ham" and "Pork, refrigerated"), meat only,
4 oz., except as noted:
loin, whole, braised, lean w/fat . . . . . . . . . . . . . . . . . . . . .271
loin, whole, braised, lean only . . . . . . . . . . . . . . . . . . . . . .231
loin, whole, broiled, lean w/fat . . . . . . . . . . . . . . . . . . . . . .274
loin, whole, broiled, lean only . . . . . . . . . . . . . . . . . . . . . . .238
loin, whole, roasted, lean w/fat . . . . . . . . . . . . . . . . . . . . .281
loin, whole, roasted, lean only . . . . . . . . . . . . . . . . . . . . . .237
loin, blade, chop, bone-in, braised or roasted, lean w/fat . . .366
loin, blade, chop, bone-in, braised, lean only . . . . . . . . . . .255
loin, blade, roast, bone-in, broiled, lean w/fat . . . . . . . . . . .363
loin, blade, chop, bone-in, broiled, lean only . . . . . . . . . . . .265
loin, blade, chop, bone-in, pan-fried, lean only . . . . . . . . . .273
loin, blade, roast, bone-in, roasted, lean only . . . . . . . . . . .280
loin, center, chop, bone-in, braised, lean w/fat . . . . . . . . . .280
loin, center, chop, bone-in, braised or broiled, lean only . . .229
loin, center, chop, bone-in, broiled, lean w/fat . . . . . . . . . . .272
loin, center, roast, bone-in, roasted, lean w/fat . . . . . . . . . .265
loin, center, roast, bone-in, roasted, lean only . . . . . . . . . . .226
loin, center rib, chop, bone-in, braised, lean w/fat . . . . . . . .284
loin, center rib, chop, bone-in, braised, lean only . . . . . . . .234
loin, center rib, chop, bone-in, broiled, lean w/fat . . . . . . . .298
loin, center rib, chop, bone-in, broiled, lean only . . . . . . . . .248
loin, center rib, roast, bone-in, roasted, lean w/fat . . . . . . . .289
loin, center rib, roast, bone-in, roasted, lean only . . . . . . . .253
loin, sirloin, chop, bone-in, braised, lean w/fat . . . . . . . . . .278
loin, sirloin, chop, bone-in, braised, lean only . . . . . . . . . . .223
loin, sirloin, chop, bone-in, broiled, lean w/fat . . . . . . . . . . .294
loin, sirloin, chop, bone-in, broiled, lean only . . . . . . . . . . .242
loin, sirloin, roast, bone-in, roasted, lean w/fat . . . . . . . . . .296
loin, sirloin, roast, bone-in, roasted, lean only . . . . . . . . . . .245

**Pork** ***(cont.)***
loin, tenderloin, roasted, lean only . . . . . . . . . . . . . . . . . . . .186
loin, top loin, chop, boneless, braised, lean w/fat . . . . . . . .264
loin, top loin, chop, boneless, braised, lean only . . . . . . . . .229
loin, top loin, chop, boneless, broiled, lean w/fat . . . . . . . . .260
loin, top loin, chop, boneless, broiled, lean only . . . . . . . . .230
loin, top loin, roast, boneless, roasted, lean w/fat . . . . . . .256
loin, top loin, roast, boneless, roasted, lean only . . . . . . . . .220
shoulder, whole, roasted, lean w/fat . . . . . . . . . . . . . . . . . .331
shoulder, whole, roasted, lean w/fat, diced, 1 cup . . . . . . .394
shoulder, whole, roasted, lean only . . . . . . . . . . . . . . . . . . .261
shoulder, whole, roasted, lean only, diced, 1 cup . . . . . . . . .311
shoulder, arm, picnic, braised, lean w/fat . . . . . . . . . . . . . .373
shoulder, arm, picnic, braised, lean w/fat, diced, 1 cup . . . .444
shoulder, arm, picnic, braised, lean only . . . . . . . . . . . . . . .281
shoulder, arm, picnic, roasted, lean w/fat . . . . . . . . . . . . . .359
shoulder, arm, picnic, roasted, lean w/fat, diced, 1 cup . . . .428
shoulder, arm, picnic, roasted, lean only . . . . . . . . . . . . . . .259
shoulder, Boston blade, steak, braised, lean w/fat . . . . . . . .362
shoulder, Boston blade, steak, braised, lean only . . . . . . . .310
shoulder, Boston blade, steak, broiled, lean w/fat . . . . . . . .294
shoulder, Boston blade, steak, broiled, lean only . . . . . . . . .257
shoulder, Boston blade, roast, roasted, lean w/fat . . . . . . . .305
shoulder, Boston blade, roast, roasted, lean only . . . . . . . .263
spareribs, braised, lean w/fat . . . . . . . . . . . . . . . . . . . . . . .450
**Pork, ground,** raw (*Johnsonville*), 4 oz. . . . . . . . . . . . . . . .340
**Pork, refrigerated,** 4 oz., except as noted:
blade steak (*Armour*) . . . . . . . . . . . . . . . . . . . . . . . . . . . . .200
blade steak, loin (*Armour*) . . . . . . . . . . . . . . . . . . . . . . . . .210
boneless roast (*Always Tender* Chef's Prime) . . . . . . . . . . .160
bottom round (*Armour*) . . . . . . . . . . . . . . . . . . . . . . . . . . . .120
chops, center cut or loin (*Always Tender*) . . . . . . . . . . . . . .190
chops, loin (*Armour*) . . . . . . . . . . . . . . . . . . . . . . . . . . . . . .210
chops, loin, boneless (*Armour*) . . . . . . . . . . . . . . . . . . . . . .160
chops, loin, center cut (*Armour*) . . . . . . . . . . . . . . . . . . . . .190
chops, loin, center cut, boneless (*Always Tender*) . . . . . . . .160
chops, rib, center cut (*Armour*) . . . . . . . . . . . . . . . . . . . . . .210
chops, rib, center cut, boneless, thin (*Armour*) . . . . . . . . . .160
chops, sirloin, boneless (*Armour*) . . . . . . . . . . . . . . . . . . . .150
cubed steak or kabob cubes (*Armour*) . . . . . . . . . . . . . . . . .160

loin, boneless (*Armour*) . . . . . . . . . . . . . . . . . . . . . . . . . .150
loin back ribs (*Armour*) . . . . . . . . . . . . . . . . . . . . . . . . . .250
loin half, onion and garlic (*Armour*) . . . . . . . . . . . . . . . . . .170
loin ribs, country style (*Armour*) . . . . . . . . . . . . . . . . . . . .210
loin roast, center cut (*Armour*) . . . . . . . . . . . . . . . . . . . . .190
loin filet and roast:
(*Always Tender* Original) . . . . . . . . . . . . . . . . . . . . . . .130
honey mustard (*Always Tender*) . . . . . . . . . . . . . . . . . .140
lemon garlic (*Always Tender*) . . . . . . . . . . . . . . . . . . . .130
mesquite barbecue (*Always Tender*) . . . . . . . . . . . . . . .130
salsa (*Always Tender*) . . . . . . . . . . . . . . . . . . . . . . . . . .140
roast (*Armour*) . . . . . . . . . . . . . . . . . . . . . . . . . . . . . . . .300
roast, au jus (*Always Tender*), 5 oz. . . . . . . . . . . . . . . . . .180
roast, Italian style (*Armour*) . . . . . . . . . . . . . . . . . . . . . . .150
roast, onion and garlic or porketta style (*Armour*) . . . . . . .190
roast, teriyaki (*Armour*) . . . . . . . . . . . . . . . . . . . . . . . . . .160
shoulder butt roast, smoked (*Boar's Head*), 3 oz. . . . . . . . .170
shoulder butt steak (*Armour*) . . . . . . . . . . . . . . . . . . . . . .200
shoulder roast (*Always Tender* Country Roast) . . . . . . . . . .200
shoulder roast (*Armour*) . . . . . . . . . . . . . . . . . . . . . . . . . .200
shoulder roast, boneless (*Armour*) . . . . . . . . . . . . . . . . . .160
shoulder roast, onion garlic (*Always Tender*) . . . . . . . . . . .200
sirloin, boneless (*Armour*) . . . . . . . . . . . . . . . . . . . . . . . .150
spareribs (*Always Tender* Country style) . . . . . . . . . . . . . .260
spareribs (*Always Tender* Ribs) . . . . . . . . . . . . . . . . . . . . .240
spareribs (*Always Tender* Spareribs/Special
Trim Ribs) . . . . . . . . . . . . . . . . . . . . . . . . . . . . . . . . . . .280
spareribs (*Armour* for Barbecue) . . . . . . . . . . . . . . . . . . . .220
spareribs (*Armour* St. Louis Style) . . . . . . . . . . . . . . . . . . .260
tenderloin (*Armour*) . . . . . . . . . . . . . . . . . . . . . . . . . . . . .110
tenderloin, lemon pepper, garden herb, or peppercorn
(*Armour*) . . . . . . . . . . . . . . . . . . . . . . . . . . . . . . . . . . .120
tenderloin, mesquite and green chili (*Armour*) . . . . . . . . . .100
tenderloin, peppercorn (*Always Tender*) . . . . . . . . . . . . . . .130
tenderloin, teriyaki (*Always Tender*) . . . . . . . . . . . . . . . . .140
tenderloin, teriyaki (*Armour*) . . . . . . . . . . . . . . . . . . . . . .110
**Pork dinner,** frozen, 1 pkg.:
rib-shape (*Swanson Traditional Favorites*), 10.5 oz. . . . . . . .470
riblet (*Banquet Extra Helping*), 15.25 oz. . . . . . . . . . . . . . . .720
and roast potato (*Stouffer's* HomeStyle), 15⅜ oz. . . . . . . .510

**Pork entree, frozen,** 1 pkg., except as noted:
chop, country-fried (*Marie Callender's*), 15 oz. . . . . . . . . . .540
country-breaded, and cheddar bacon potato (*Healthy Choice* Duo), 8 oz. . . . . . . . . . . . . . . . . . . . . . . . . . . . .280
country-fried (*Banquet*), 10.25 oz. . . . . . . . . . . . . . . . . . . . .430
cutlet, breaded (*Stouffer's* HomeStyle), 10 oz. . . . . . . . . . .370
fried rice (*Yu Sing*), 8.5 oz. . . . . . . . . . . . . . . . . . . . . . . .450
fried rice, and shrimp (*Yu Sing*), 8 oz. . . . . . . . . . . . . . . . .400
honey-roasted (*Lean Cuisine Café Classics*), 9.5 oz. . . . . . .240
rib patty, w/barbecue sauce (*Banquet* Family), 1 patty w/sauce . . . . . . . . . . . . . . . . . . . . . . . . . . . . . . . . . . .110
riblet, boneless (*Banquet*), 10 oz. . . . . . . . . . . . . . . . . . . . .400
**Pork entree mix,** chops, w/herb stuffing (*Campbell's Supper Bakes*), ⅙ pkg.* . . . . . . . . . . . . . . . . . . . . . . . .380
**Pork gravy,** in jars, ¼ cup:
(*Franco-American* Roast Pork) . . . . . . . . . . . . . . . . . . . . . . .45
(*Heinz* Homestyle) . . . . . . . . . . . . . . . . . . . . . . . . . . . . . . . .25
**Pork gravy mix** (*McCormick*), ¼ cup* . . . . . . . . . . . . . . . . .20
**Pork lunch meat** (see also "Ham"), 2 oz.:
(*Healthy Deli*) . . . . . . . . . . . . . . . . . . . . . . . . . . . . . . . . . . .70
seasoned (*Boar's Head*) . . . . . . . . . . . . . . . . . . . . . . . . . . . .80
roast, sirloin (*Black Bear*) . . . . . . . . . . . . . . . . . . . . . . . . . .70
**Pork rind snack,** ½ oz.:
(*Baken-ets*) . . . . . . . . . . . . . . . . . . . . . . . . . . . . . . . . . . . . .80
(*Baken-ets* Cracklins) . . . . . . . . . . . . . . . . . . . . . . . . . . . . . .90
(*Utz/Utz* Barbecue) . . . . . . . . . . . . . . . . . . . . . . . . . . . . . . .80
barbecue (*Baken-ets*) . . . . . . . . . . . . . . . . . . . . . . . . . . . . . .70
hot and spicy (*Baken-ets/Baken-ets* Cracklins) . . . . . . . . . . .80
**Pork sandwich,** frozen, barbecued, 1 pc.:
(*Hormel Quick Meal*) . . . . . . . . . . . . . . . . . . . . . . . . . . . . .360
rib-shaped (*Hormel Quick Meal*) . . . . . . . . . . . . . . . . . . . . .430
**Pork seasoning mix:**
chops (*McCormick Bag'n Season*), ⅙ pkg. . . . . . . . . . . . . . .15
tenderloin (*McCormick Bag'n Season*), ⅛ pkg. . . . . . . . . . . .15
**Pot roast,** see "Beef dinner" and "Beef entree"
**Potato,** fresh:
raw (*Dole*), 1 medium, 5.2 oz. . . . . . . . . . . . . . . . . . . . . . .100
raw (*Frieda's* Baby/Fingerling/Red/Purple/Yukon Gold/ Yellow Finnish), ½ cup, 3 oz. . . . . . . . . . . . . . . . . . . . . . .70

raw (*Frieda's* Fingerling Bag), 4 pcs., 5.2 oz. . . . . . . . . . . . . .100
raw, unpeeled, 1 lb. . . . . . . . . . . . . . . . . . . . . . . . . . . . . .269
raw, peeled, 2½" potato . . . . . . . . . . . . . . . . . . . . . . . . . .88
baked, in skin, 2⅓" × 4¾" . . . . . . . . . . . . . . . . . . . . . . .220
baked, w/out skin, 2⅓" × 4¾", 7.1 oz. . . . . . . . . . . . . . . .145
baked, w/out skin, ½ cup . . . . . . . . . . . . . . . . . . . . . . . . .57
boiled in skin, peeled, 2½" diam., 4.8 oz. . . . . . . . . . . . . .118
boiled in skin, peeled, ½ cup . . . . . . . . . . . . . . . . . . . . . .68
boiled w/out skin, 2½" potato . . . . . . . . . . . . . . . . . . . . .116
boiled w/out skin, ½ cup . . . . . . . . . . . . . . . . . . . . . . . . .67
microwaved in skin, 2½" diam, 7.1 oz. . . . . . . . . . . . . . . .212
microwaved in skin, peeled, ½ cup . . . . . . . . . . . . . . . . . .78

**Potato, can or jar:**

drained, 1.2-oz. potato . . . . . . . . . . . . . . . . . . . . . . . . . .21
sliced, new (*Del Monte*), ⅔ cup . . . . . . . . . . . . . . . . . . . .60
whole, new (*Del Monte*), 2 medium w/liquid . . . . . . . . . . . .60
whole, white (*Libby's*), ⅔ cup . . . . . . . . . . . . . . . . . . . . .80

**Potato, frozen** (see also "Potato dish, frozen"):

whole (*Birds Eye* Southern), 3 pcs. . . . . . . . . . . . . . . . . . .50
whole (*Bonduelle* Parisian), 3 oz., about 10 . . . . . . . . . . . .80
whole, baby (*Birds Eye* Gourmet), 4 oz., about 7 pcs. . . . . .100
whole, baby blend (*Birds Eye* Gourmet), 2.6 oz. . . . . . . . . .45
fried or french-fried, 3 oz., except as noted:
(*Cascadian Farm* Oven French Fries) . . . . . . . . . . . . . . .130
(*Crispy Classics* Crinkle Cut/French Fries) . . . . . . . . . . .170
(*Inland Valley* Crinkle Cut 32 oz.) . . . . . . . . . . . . . . . . .150
(*Inland Valley* French Fries) . . . . . . . . . . . . . . . . . . . . .130
(*Inland Valley* Steak Fries) . . . . . . . . . . . . . . . . . . . . . .110
(*Inland Valley CrissCut Fries*) . . . . . . . . . . . . . . . . . . . .160
(*Inland Valley Fajita Fries*) . . . . . . . . . . . . . . . . . . . . . .170
(*Inland Valley Long Branch Fries*) . . . . . . . . . . . . . . . . .160
(*Ore-Ida* Country French Fries) . . . . . . . . . . . . . . . . . . .120
(*Ore-Ida* Deep Fries) . . . . . . . . . . . . . . . . . . . . . . . . . .140
(*Ore-Ida* Shoestrings) . . . . . . . . . . . . . . . . . . . . . . . . .150
(*Ore-Ida* Steak Fries) . . . . . . . . . . . . . . . . . . . . . . . . . .110
(*Ore-Ida Crispers!*) . . . . . . . . . . . . . . . . . . . . . . . . . . .210
(*Ore-Ida Crispy Crunchies/Fast Food Fries*) . . . . . . . . . .160
(*Ore-Ida Golden Fries*) . . . . . . . . . . . . . . . . . . . . . . . . .120
(*Ore-Ida Pixie Crinkles*) . . . . . . . . . . . . . . . . . . . . . . . .130

**Potato, frozen, fried or french-fried** ***(cont.)***
(*Ore-Ida Zesty*) . . . . . . . . . . . . . . . . . . . . . . . . . . . . .150
(*Pacific Valley* Crinkle Cut) . . . . . . . . . . . . . . . . . . . . . .70
seasoned (*Inland Valley CrissCut Fries*) . . . . . . . . . . . . .190
hash brown (*Cascadian Farm*), 1 cup . . . . . . . . . . . . . . . . . .70
hash brown (*Inland Valley Home Browns*), 1 patty . . . . . . .130
hash brown (*Inland Valley Simply Shreds*), 1 cup . . . . . . . . .70
hash brown (*Ore-Ida* Toaster), 2 pcs., 3.6 oz. . . . . . . . . . . .220
hash brown (*Ore-Ida Golden Patties*), 2.2-oz. pc. . . . . . . . .130
hash brown, shredded (*Pacific Valley*), 1 cup . . . . . . . . . . . .60
hash brown, Southern style (*Inland Valley*), ⅔ cup . . . . . . .70
mashed (*Inland Valley*), ⅔ cup . . . . . . . . . . . . . . . . . . . . .160
mashed (*Inland Valley* Portionable), 8 pcs. . . . . . . . . . . . . .150
mashed (*Ore-Ida*), ⅔ cup, and ⅓ cup 2% milk . . . . . . . . . .160
mashed, garlic, roasted (*Inland Valley*), ⅔ cup . . . . . . . . . .150
O'Brien (*Inland Valley Simply Shreds O'Brien*), 1 cup . . . . . .60
and onions, in sauce (*Birds Eye Simply Grillin'*), 4.5 oz. . . .180
w/peppers, onions (*Cascadian Farm* Country), ¾ cup . . . . . .60
puffs (*Cascadian Farm Spud Puppies*), 3 oz. . . . . . . . . . . . .150
puffs (*Inland Valley Tater Puffs*), 3 oz. . . . . . . . . . . . . . . .160
puffs (*Tater Tots*), 9 pcs., 3 oz. . . . . . . . . . . . . . . . . . . . .170
puffs, mini (*Tater Tots*), 19 pcs., 3 oz. . . . . . . . . . . . . . . .180
puffs, onion (*Tater Tots*), 9 pcs., 3 oz. . . . . . . . . . . . . . . .150
roasted, and broccoli (*Birds Eye*), ⅔ cup . . . . . . . . . . . . . .100
roasted, red (*Cascadian Farm*), 1¼ cups . . . . . . . . . . . . . .110
roasted, wedges (*Pacific Valley*) . . . . . . . . . . . . . . . . . . . .120
**Potato mix,** see "Potato dish, mix"
**Potato, sweet,** see "Sweet potato"
**Potato chips and crisps,** 1 oz., except as noted:
(*Bachman*) . . . . . . . . . . . . . . . . . . . . . . . . . . . . . . . . . . .160
(*Bachman* Wavy) . . . . . . . . . . . . . . . . . . . . . . . . . . . . . .150
(*Grandma Utz's/Utz* Homestyle) . . . . . . . . . . . . . . . . . . . .140
(*Herr's/Herr's* Ripple) . . . . . . . . . . . . . . . . . . . . . . . . . . .140
(*Lay's* Baked) . . . . . . . . . . . . . . . . . . . . . . . . . . . . . . . . .110
(*Lay's* Classic/Limon/Wavy) . . . . . . . . . . . . . . . . . . . . . .150
(*Lay's/Ruffles WOW*) . . . . . . . . . . . . . . . . . . . . . . . . . . . . .75
(*Munchos*) . . . . . . . . . . . . . . . . . . . . . . . . . . . . . . . . . . .160
(*Ruffles* Baked) . . . . . . . . . . . . . . . . . . . . . . . . . . . . . . .120
(*Ruffles/Ruffles The Works!*) . . . . . . . . . . . . . . . . . . . . . .160
(*Snyder's*) . . . . . . . . . . . . . . . . . . . . . . . . . . . . . . . . . . .140

(*Snyder's* Ripple/Unsalted) . . . . . . . . . . . . . . . . . . . . . . . .140
(*Terra* Yukon Gold) . . . . . . . . . . . . . . . . . . . . . . . . . . . .130
(*Terra Blues/Terra Red Bliss*) . . . . . . . . . . . . . . . . . . . . .140
(*Utz/Utz* Kettle Classics/Ripple/Wavy/No Salt) . . . . . . . . . . .150
barbecue (*Bachman*) . . . . . . . . . . . . . . . . . . . . . . . . . . .150
barbecue (*Lay's KC Masterpiece* Baked) . . . . . . . . . . . . . . .120
barbecue (*Lay's/Ruffles KC Masterpiece*) . . . . . . . . . . . . . .150
barbecue (*Snyder's*) . . . . . . . . . . . . . . . . . . . . . . . . . . .150
barbecue (*Snyder's* Rib) . . . . . . . . . . . . . . . . . . . . . . . . .140
barbecue (*Utz* Carolina/Kettle Classics) . . . . . . . . . . . . . . .150
barbecue (*Utz* Homestyle) . . . . . . . . . . . . . . . . . . . . . . .140
barbecue, cheddar (*Ruffles Flavor Rush*) . . . . . . . . . . . . . .160
barbecue, mesquite (*Lay's* Homestyle) . . . . . . . . . . . . . . . .140
Buffalo style (*Ruffles*) . . . . . . . . . . . . . . . . . . . . . . . . . .160
cheddar (*Lay's* Cracker Barrel) . . . . . . . . . . . . . . . . . . . .150
cheddar/salsa (*Ruffles Flavor Rush* Ultimate) . . . . . . . . . . .160
cheddar/sour cream (*Ruffles*) . . . . . . . . . . . . . . . . . . . . .160
cheddar/sour cream (*Ruffles* Baked) . . . . . . . . . . . . . . . . .120
cheddar/sour cream (*Ruffles WOW*) . . . . . . . . . . . . . . . . . . .75
cheddar/sour cream (*Utz*) . . . . . . . . . . . . . . . . . . . . . . . .160
chili, green, and lime (*Snyder's*) . . . . . . . . . . . . . . . . . . .150
chili, habañero (*Kettle Chips*) . . . . . . . . . . . . . . . . . . . . .140
crab (*Utz*) . . . . . . . . . . . . . . . . . . . . . . . . . . . . . . . . .150
crab, spicy (*Snyder's* Chesapeake Bay) . . . . . . . . . . . . . . .140
dill, kosher (*Snyder's*) . . . . . . . . . . . . . . . . . . . . . . . . .140
grilled steak and onion (*Snyder's*) . . . . . . . . . . . . . . . . . .140
hot (*Bachman*) . . . . . . . . . . . . . . . . . . . . . . . . . . . . . . .150
hot (*Utz* Red Hot) . . . . . . . . . . . . . . . . . . . . . . . . . . . . .150
hot, Buffalo or jalapeño (*Snyder's*) . . . . . . . . . . . . . . . . . .150
ketchup (*Herr's Heinz*) . . . . . . . . . . . . . . . . . . . . . . . . . .150
mustard and honey (*Kettle* Crisps) . . . . . . . . . . . . . . . . . .110
onion, French (*Kettle* Crisps) . . . . . . . . . . . . . . . . . . . . .110
ranch (*Lay's* Wavy) . . . . . . . . . . . . . . . . . . . . . . . . . . . .150
salt and vinegar (*Lay's*) . . . . . . . . . . . . . . . . . . . . . . . . .150
salt and vinegar (*Snyder's*) . . . . . . . . . . . . . . . . . . . . . . .140
salt and vinegar (*Utz*) . . . . . . . . . . . . . . . . . . . . . . . . . .150
sour cream/onion (*Bachman*) . . . . . . . . . . . . . . . . . . . . . .150
sour cream/onion (*Lay's*) . . . . . . . . . . . . . . . . . . . . . . . .160
sour cream/onion (*Lay's* Baked) . . . . . . . . . . . . . . . . . . . .120
sour cream/onion (*Snyder's*) . . . . . . . . . . . . . . . . . . . . . .150

**Potato chips and crisps *(cont.)***
sour cream/onion, zesty (*Ruffles Flavor Rush*) . . . . . . . . . . .150
sticks (*Butterfield*), ⅔ cup, 1 oz. . . . . . . . . . . . . . . . . . . . . . .150
sticks (*Butterfield* 1.7 oz.), 1 cup . . . . . . . . . . . . . . . . . . . . .250
sticks (*French's*), 1 cup . . . . . . . . . . . . . . . . . . . . . . . . . . .250
sticks, hot (*Chester's* Fries Flamin') . . . . . . . . . . . . . . . . . .150
sweet potato, see "Sweet potato chips"
taco (*Snyder's* Fiesta) . . . . . . . . . . . . . . . . . . . . . . . . . . . .150
vinegar (*Bachman*) . . . . . . . . . . . . . . . . . . . . . . . . . . . . . .150
yogurt–green onion (*Terra* Yukon Gold) . . . . . . . . . . . . . . . .130
**Potato chips/dip kit,** 1 kit:
onion dip (*Ruffles*) . . . . . . . . . . . . . . . . . . . . . . . . . . . . . .460
ranch dip (*Ruffles*) . . . . . . . . . . . . . . . . . . . . . . . . . . . . . .470
**Potato dish, frozen** (see also "Potato, frozen"):
au gratin (*Cascadian Farm*), ⅔ cup . . . . . . . . . . . . . . . . . . .110
au gratin (*Stouffer's* Side Dish), ½ cup . . . . . . . . . . . . . . . .130
au gratin, ham and broccoli (*Banquet* Family), ⅔ cup . . . . .210
baked, twice, butter flavor (*Ore-Ida*), 1 pc. . . . . . . . . . . . . .160
cheddar (*Lean Cuisine Everyday Favorites*), 10⅜ oz. . . . . . .260
cheddar broccoli (*Healthy Choice* Solos), 10.5-oz. pkg. . . . .280
cheddar broccoli (*Michelina's*), 9.5 oz. . . . . . . . . . . . . . . . .380
mashed, w/beef gravy (*Larry's*), 4.5-oz. tray . . . . . . . . . . . .160
mashed, w/chicken gravy (*Larry's*), 4.5-oz. tray . . . . . . . . . .170
pancake, see "Potato pancake"
pie, cheesy and broccoli w/ham (*Banquet*), 7-oz. pkg. . . . . .410
roasted, w/broccoli (*Lean Cuisine Everyday Favorites*),
  10.25-oz. pkg. . . . . . . . . . . . . . . . . . . . . . . . . . . . . . . . . .240
roasted, w/broccoli, cheese sauce (*Green Giant*), ¾ cup . . .120
roasted, w/garlic and herbs (*Green Giant*), 1¼ cups . . . . . .270
roasted, w/ham (*Healthy Choice* Bowl), 8.5-oz. pkg. . . . . . .210
scalloped (*Stouffer's Family Style Favorite*), ½ cup . . . . . . .140
scalloped (*Stouffer's* Side Dish 11½ oz.), ½ cup . . . . . . . . .170
skins (*Inland Valley* Munch Skins Meals), ⅔ cup, 5 oz. . . . .150
stuffed, bacon and cheese (*Larry's*), 1 pc. . . . . . . . . . . . . . .200
stuffed, bacon and cheese or cheddar (*Oh Boy!*), 1 pc. . . . .130
stuffed, broccoli and cheese (*Larry's*), 1 pc. . . . . . . . . . . . .190
stuffed, sour cream and chive (*Oh Boy!*), 1 pc. . . . . . . . . . .110
**Potato dish, mix,** ½ cup*, except as noted:
au gratin or julienne (*Betty Crocker*) . . . . . . . . . . . . . . . . .150

bacon and cheddar, twice baked (*Betty Crocker*),
  ⅔ cup* . . . . . . . . . . 210
bacon and cheese (*Knorr* Skillet Potatoes), ½ cup . . . . . . . 110
broccoli au gratin (*Betty Crocker*) . . . . . . . . . . 150
cheddar and bacon or 3 cheese (*Betty Crocker*) . . . . . . . . . 150
chicken/vegetable (*Betty Crocker*), ⅔ cup* . . . . . . . . . . 160
hash brown (*Betty Crocker*) . . . . . . . . . . 190
mashed:
  (*Betty Crocker Potato Buds*), ⅔ cup* . . . . . . . . . . 160
  (*Idahoan* Complete) . . . . . . . . . . 110
  butter, creamy or and herb (*Betty Crocker*) . . . . . . . . . . 160
  butter and herb (*Bowl Appétit!*), 1 bowl . . . . . . . . . . 210
  butter and herb or roasted garlic (*Idahoan*) . . . . . . . . . . 110
  cheddar and bacon or 4 cheese (*Betty Crocker*) . . . . . . . 150
  cheese, 4 (*Idahoan*) . . . . . . . . . . 100
  cheesy (*Bowl Appétit!*), 1 bowl . . . . . . . . . . 270
  cheesy broccoli (*Bowl Appétit!*), 1 bowl . . . . . . . . . . 260
  chicken and herb (*Betty Crocker*) . . . . . . . . . . 150
  garlic, roasted (*Betty Crocker*) . . . . . . . . . . 150
  and gravy, beef or chicken (*Betty Crocker*), ¾ cup* . . . . 170
  sour cream/chive (*Betty Crocker*) . . . . . . . . . . 150
  sour cream/chive (*Bowl Appétit!*), 1 bowl . . . . . . . . . . 210
ranch or scalloped (*Betty Crocker*), ½ cup* . . . . . . . . . . 160
scalloped (*Betty Crocker* 8.25 oz.), ½ cup* . . . . . . . . . . 150
scalloped, cheesy (*Betty Crocker*) . . . . . . . . . . 150
sour cream/chive (*Betty Crocker*) . . . . . . . . . . 160
**Potato entree, frozen,** see "Potato dish, frozen"
**Potato flour,** 1 cup . . . . . . . . . . 628
**Potato knish,** refrigerated (*Joshua's Coney Island*),
  1 pc. . . . . . . . . . . 380
**Potato pancake,** frozen:
(*Inland Valley*), 2-oz. cake . . . . . . . . . . 120
(*Kineret* Latkas), 1.5-oz. cake . . . . . . . . . . 80
(*King Kold*), 2 cakes, 2 oz. . . . . . . . . . . 190
(*Ratner's*), 1.5-oz. cake . . . . . . . . . . 110
(*Tofutti*), 1.3-oz. cake . . . . . . . . . . 71
mini (*Kineret* Latkas), 10 pcs., 3 oz. . . . . . . . . . . 220
**Potato salad,** refrigerated:
(*Blue Ridge Farms*), ½ cup . . . . . . . . . . 180

**Potato salad, refrigerated *(cont.)***
(*Chef's Express*), 4 oz. . . . . . . . . . . . . . . . . . . . . . . . . . . .260
red skin (*Blue Ridge Farms*), 4 oz., about ½ cup . . . . . . . . .190
**Potato seasoning,** ⅙ pkt., except as noted:
fries, oven (*McCormick Produce Partners*), ⅕ pkt. . . . . . . . .30
roasted, cheddar (*McCormick Produce Partners*) . . . . . . . . .35
roasted, herb or onion (*McCormick Produce Partners*) . . . . .30
**Potato sticks,** see "Potato chips and crisps"
**Poultry,** see specific listings
**Poultry seasoning,** 1 tsp. . . . . . . . . . . . . . . . . . . . . . . . . . .5
**Pout, ocean,** meat only:
raw, 4 oz. . . . . . . . . . . . . . . . . . . . . . . . . . . . . . . . . . . . .90
baked, broiled, or microwaved, 4 oz. . . . . . . . . . . . . . . . . . .116
**Praline sauce** (*Trader Vic's*), 2 tbsp. . . . . . . . . . . . . . . . . .120
**Preserves,** see "Chutney" and "Jam and preserves"
**Pretzels,** 1 oz., except as noted:
(*Goldfish*), 43 pcs., 1.1 oz. . . . . . . . . . . . . . . . . . . . . . . . .120
(*Snyder's* Homestyle/Olde Tyme/Specials) . . . . . . . . . . . . .120
cheese, cheddar (*Rold Gold* Tiny Twists) . . . . . . . . . . . . . . .110
cheese, mini (*Snyder's*) . . . . . . . . . . . . . . . . . . . . . . . . . . . .140
hard (*Snyder's* Unsalted/Pump and Onion) . . . . . . . . . . . . .100
honey mustard (*Rold Gold* Tiny Twists) . . . . . . . . . . . . . . .110
mini (*Bachman* Petite) . . . . . . . . . . . . . . . . . . . . . . . . . . . .100
mini (*Snyder's/Snyder's* Organic/Unsalted) . . . . . . . . . . . . .110
nibblers (*Snyder's* No Salt/Fat Free/Sourdough) . . . . . . . . .120
nibblers, garlic, honey mustard, or savory (*Snyder's*) . . . . .130
pieces, ranch, cheddar, caramel, or BBQ (*Snyder's*) . . . . . .130
pieces, honey mustard onion or jalapeño (*Snyder's*) . . . . . .140
pizza flavor (*Combos* Pizzaria) . . . . . . . . . . . . . . . . . . . . . .130
pizza flavor, pepperoni (*Combo*) . . . . . . . . . . . . . . . . . . . . .140
rods (*Bachman*), 1.1 oz. . . . . . . . . . . . . . . . . . . . . . . . . . . .110
rods (*Rold Gold*) . . . . . . . . . . . . . . . . . . . . . . . . . . . . . . . .110
rods or snaps (*Snyder's*) . . . . . . . . . . . . . . . . . . . . . . . . . .120
sourdough (*Bachman*) . . . . . . . . . . . . . . . . . . . . . . . . . . . .110
sourdough (*Rold Gold* Specials) . . . . . . . . . . . . . . . . . . . . .110
sourdough, hard (*Rold Gold*) . . . . . . . . . . . . . . . . . . . . . . .100
sourdough, hard (*Snyder's*) . . . . . . . . . . . . . . . . . . . . . . . .100
sticks (*Bachman* Stix) . . . . . . . . . . . . . . . . . . . . . . . . . . . .100
sticks (*Rold Gold*) . . . . . . . . . . . . . . . . . . . . . . . . . . . . . . .100
sticks (*Snyder's* Dipping) . . . . . . . . . . . . . . . . . . . . . . . . . .100

sticks (*Snyder's* Olde Tyme) . . . . . . . . . . . . . . . . . . . . . . . .110
sticks, butter, tiny (*Snyder's*) . . . . . . . . . . . . . . . . . . . . . . .120
sticks, honey wheat (*Snyder's* Organic) . . . . . . . . . . . . . . .130
sticks, oat bran (*Snyder's* Organic) . . . . . . . . . . . . . . . . . .120
thins (*Bachman* Thin 'n Right), 1.1 oz. . . . . . . . . . . . . . . .120
thins (*Rold Gold* Fat Free) . . . . . . . . . . . . . . . . . . . . . . . .100
thins (*Snyder's*) . . . . . . . . . . . . . . . . . . . . . . . . . . . . . . .110
twists (*Bachman*) . . . . . . . . . . . . . . . . . . . . . . . . . . . . . .100
twists (*Rold Gold* Thin/Tiny) . . . . . . . . . . . . . . . . . . . . . .110
**Pretzels, soft:**
(*SuperPretzel*), 2.25-oz. pc. . . . . . . . . . . . . . . . . . . . . . .180
bites (*SuperPretzel*), 5 pcs., 1.9 oz. . . . . . . . . . . . . . . . .140
cheese-filled (*SuperPretzel SoftStix*), 2 pcs., 1.8 oz. . . . . . .140
**Pretzel dip,** honey mustard:
(*Nance's*), 2 tbsp. . . . . . . . . . . . . . . . . . . . . . . . . . . . . . .90
(*Snyder's*), 1 oz. . . . . . . . . . . . . . . . . . . . . . . . . . . . . . . .70
**Prickly pear**
(*Frieda's* Cactus Pear), 5 oz. . . . . . . . . . . . . . . . . . . . . . . .60
1 medium, 4.8 oz. . . . . . . . . . . . . . . . . . . . . . . . . . . . . . . .42
**Prosciutto:**
(*Black Bear* di Parma), 1 oz. . . . . . . . . . . . . . . . . . . . . . . .80
(*Citterio/Citterio Fresco*), 2 slices, 1.1 oz. . . . . . . . . . . . . .70
(*Primissimo* Proscuitti), 2 oz. . . . . . . . . . . . . . . . . . . . . . .120
**Prune,** see "Plum, dried"
**Prune juice,** 8 fl. oz.:
(*Langers*) . . . . . . . . . . . . . . . . . . . . . . . . . . . . . . . . . . . .180
(*Sunsweet*) . . . . . . . . . . . . . . . . . . . . . . . . . . . . . . . . . . .170
**Pudding,** ready-to-eat, 4-oz. cup:
all flavors (*Jell-O Free*) . . . . . . . . . . . . . . . . . . . . . . . . . .100
all flavors, except tapioca (*Jell-O*) . . . . . . . . . . . . . . . . . .160
banana (*Kozy Shack*) . . . . . . . . . . . . . . . . . . . . . . . . . . . . .130
butterscotch (*Swiss Miss*) . . . . . . . . . . . . . . . . . . . . . . . . .160
chocolate (*Kozy Shack*) . . . . . . . . . . . . . . . . . . . . . . . . . . .140
chocolate (*Swiss Miss*) . . . . . . . . . . . . . . . . . . . . . . . . . . .160
chocolate (*Swiss Miss* Fat Free) . . . . . . . . . . . . . . . . . . . . .90
chocolate cream pie (*Swiss Miss*) . . . . . . . . . . . . . . . . . . .170
chocolate–vanilla swirl (*Swiss Miss*) . . . . . . . . . . . . . . . . .160
lemon meringue pie (*Swiss Miss*) . . . . . . . . . . . . . . . . . . . .150
rice, see "Rice pudding"
tapioca (*Jell-O*) . . . . . . . . . . . . . . . . . . . . . . . . . . . . . . . .140

**Pudding,** ready-to-eat ***(cont.)***
tapioca (*Swiss Miss*) . . . . . . . . . . . . . . . . . . . . . . . . . . .140
tapioca or vanilla (*Kozy Shack*) . . . . . . . . . . . . . . . . . . . . .130
vanilla (*Swiss Miss*) . . . . . . . . . . . . . . . . . . . . . . . . . . .160
**Pudding, nondairy,** 1 cont.:
all varieties (*Imagine*) . . . . . . . . . . . . . . . . . . . . . . . . . .140
tofu, almond, or vanilla (*Azumaya Tofu Spoonables/Nasoya Tofu Temptations*) . . . . . . . . . . . . . . . . . . . . . . . . . .120
tofu, chocolate (*Azumaya Tofu Spoonables/Nasoya Tofu Temptations*) . . . . . . . . . . . . . . . . . . . . . . . . . . . .170
**Pudding and pie filling mix,** ½ cup*
all flavors (*Jell-O* Fat Free Instant) . . . . . . . . . . . . . . . . .140
all flavors (*Jell-O* Sugar Free) . . . . . . . . . . . . . . . . . . . . .130
all flavors, except chocolate and chocolate fudge (*Jell-O* Fat/Sugar Free Instant) . . . . . . . . . . . . . . . . . . . . . . . .70
banana cream (*Jell-O*) . . . . . . . . . . . . . . . . . . . . . . . . .140
banana cream (*Jell-O* Instant) . . . . . . . . . . . . . . . . . . . . .150
butterscotch (*Jell-O*) . . . . . . . . . . . . . . . . . . . . . . . . . .160
butterscotch (*Jell-O* Instant) . . . . . . . . . . . . . . . . . . . . .150
chocolate or chocolate fudge (*Jell-O* Instant) . . . . . . . . . . .160
chocolate or chocolate fudge (*Jell-O* Fat/Sugar Free Instant) . . . . . . . . . . . . . . . . . . . . . . . . . . . . . .80
chocolate, chocolate fudge, or milk chocolate (*Jell-O*) . . . .150
coconut cream (*Jell-O*) . . . . . . . . . . . . . . . . . . . . . . . .150
coconut cream (*Jell-O* Instant) . . . . . . . . . . . . . . . . . . . .160
custard (*Jell-O Americana*) . . . . . . . . . . . . . . . . . . . . . .140
flan (*Jell-O*) . . . . . . . . . . . . . . . . . . . . . . . . . . . . . . .140
lemon (*Jell-O*) . . . . . . . . . . . . . . . . . . . . . . . . . . . . .140
lemon (*Jell-O* Instant) . . . . . . . . . . . . . . . . . . . . . . . . .150
pistachio (*Jell-O* Instant) . . . . . . . . . . . . . . . . . . . . . . .160
rice, see "Rice pudding mix"
tapioca (*Jell-O Americana*) . . . . . . . . . . . . . . . . . . . . . .130
vanilla (*Jell-O*) . . . . . . . . . . . . . . . . . . . . . . . . . . . . .140
vanilla (*Jell-O* Instant) . . . . . . . . . . . . . . . . . . . . . . . .150
vanilla, French (*Jell-O* Instant) . . . . . . . . . . . . . . . . . . .160
**Pudding, plum** (*Crosse & Blackwell*), ⅓ pkg. . . . . . . . . . . .410
**Pummelo:**
(*Frieda's*), 5 oz. . . . . . . . . . . . . . . . . . . . . . . . . . . . . .50
1 medium, 5½" diam., 1⅓ lb. . . . . . . . . . . . . . . . . . . . . .231
sections, ½ cup . . . . . . . . . . . . . . . . . . . . . . . . . . . . . .36

**Pumpkin,** fresh:
(*Frieda's* Mini), ¾ cup, 3 oz. . . . . . . . . . . . . . . . . . . . . . . . .20
pulp, boiled, drained, mashed, ½ cup . . . . . . . . . . . . . . . . . .24
**Pumpkin, canned** (*Libby's* Solid Pack), ½ cup . . . . . . . . . . .40
**Pumpkin pie spice,** 1 tsp. . . . . . . . . . . . . . . . . . . . . . . . . .6
**Pumpkin seed:**
roasted, in shell, 1 oz. or 85 seeds . . . . . . . . . . . . . . . . . .127
roasted, shelled, 1 oz. . . . . . . . . . . . . . . . . . . . . . . . . . .148
dried, shelled, 1 oz. or 142 kernels . . . . . . . . . . . . . . . . . .154
**Punch,** see "Fruit punch" and specific fruit listings
**Purslane,** boiled, drained, ½ cup . . . . . . . . . . . . . . . . . . . .10
**Quail,** raw:
meat w/skin, 1 quail, 3.8 oz. (4.3 oz. w/bone) . . . . . . . . . . .210
meat w/skin, 4 oz. . . . . . . . . . . . . . . . . . . . . . . . . . . . . .218
meat only, 1 quail, 3.2 oz. (4.3 oz. w/bone and skin) . . . . . .123
breast meat only, 1 breast, 2 oz. . . . . . . . . . . . . . . . . . . . . .69
**Quesadilla,** frozen (*Cedarlane*), 3 pcs. . . . . . . . . . . . . . . .250
**Quince:**
(*Frieda's*), 5 oz. . . . . . . . . . . . . . . . . . . . . . . . . . . . . . . .80
1 medium, 5.3 oz. . . . . . . . . . . . . . . . . . . . . . . . . . . . . . .52
peeled, seeded, 1 oz. . . . . . . . . . . . . . . . . . . . . . . . . . . . .16
**Quinoa,** dry:
(*Eden*), ¼ cup . . . . . . . . . . . . . . . . . . . . . . . . . . . . . . . .170
(*Frieda's*), ⅓ cup . . . . . . . . . . . . . . . . . . . . . . . . . . . . . .170
**Quinoa seeds** (*Arrowhead Mills*), ¼ cup . . . . . . . . . . . . . . .140

# R

**FOOD AND MEASURE** **CALORIES**

**Rabbit,** domesticated, meat only:
roasted, 4 oz. . . . . . . . . . . . . . . . . . . . . . . . . . . . . . . . . . . .223
stewed, 4 oz. . . . . . . . . . . . . . . . . . . . . . . . . . . . . . . . . . . .234
stewed, diced, 1 cup . . . . . . . . . . . . . . . . . . . . . . . . . . . . . .288
**Radiatore pasta dish, frozen,** and vegetables (*Birds Eye*),
1 cup . . . . . . . . . . . . . . . . . . . . . . . . . . . . . . . . . . . . . . . .200
**Radiatore pasta dish, mix:**
basil and herb (*Near East*), 1 cup* . . . . . . . . . . . . . . . . . . .240
w/beans, mixed (*Marrakesh Express*), 1 cup* . . . . . . . . . . .200
cheddar, mild (*Lipton* Pasta & Sauce), ½ pkg. . . . . . . . . . .210
**Radicchio,** fresh:
(*Frieda's*), 2 cups, 3 oz. . . . . . . . . . . . . . . . . . . . . . . . . . . .20
1 medium leaf, .3 oz. . . . . . . . . . . . . . . . . . . . . . . . . . . . . . .2
shredded, ½ cup . . . . . . . . . . . . . . . . . . . . . . . . . . . . . . . . . .5
**Radish:**
(*Dole*), 7 medium, 3 oz. . . . . . . . . . . . . . . . . . . . . . . . . . . . .15
10 medium, ¾"–1" . . . . . . . . . . . . . . . . . . . . . . . . . . . . . . . . .7
sliced, ½ cup . . . . . . . . . . . . . . . . . . . . . . . . . . . . . . . . . . . .10
**Radish, black** (*Frieda's*), ¾ cup, 3 oz. . . . . . . . . . . . . . . . . .15
**Radish, Chinese** (*Frieda's* Lo Bok), ⅔ cup,
3 oz. . . . . . . . . . . . . . . . . . . . . . . . . . . . . . . . . . . . . . . . . . . .25
**Radish, Oriental:**
(*Frieda's* Daikon), ½ cup, 1.1 oz. . . . . . . . . . . . . . . . . . . . . .15
(*Frieda's* Korean), ⅔ cup, 3 oz. . . . . . . . . . . . . . . . . . . . . . .15
raw, 1 medium, 7" . . . . . . . . . . . . . . . . . . . . . . . . . . . . . . . . .62
raw, sliced, ½ cup . . . . . . . . . . . . . . . . . . . . . . . . . . . . . . . . .8
boiled, drained, sliced, ½ cup . . . . . . . . . . . . . . . . . . . . . . . .13
**Radish, white-icicle,** 1 medium, .6 oz. . . . . . . . . . . . . . . . . .2
**Raisin sauce** (*Chelten House*), 2 tbsp. . . . . . . . . . . . . . . . . .60
**Raisins,** ¼ cup, except as noted:
seeded, not packed . . . . . . . . . . . . . . . . . . . . . . . . . . . . . . .107
seedless (*Dole* California/*Dole Cinnaraisins*) . . . . . . . . . . . .130
seedless (*Sun•Maid*) . . . . . . . . . . . . . . . . . . . . . . . . . . . . . .130
golden (*Dole*) . . . . . . . . . . . . . . . . . . . . . . . . . . . . . . . . . . .130

golden, not packed . . . . . . . . . . . . . . . . . . . . . . . . . . . . .110
chocolate-coated, see "Candy"
**Raisins, baking,** chocolate-coated (*Nestlé*), 1⅓ tbsp. . . . . . .70
**Raisins and cherries,** dried (*Sun•Maid Fast Fruit*),
¼ cup, 1.4 oz. . . . . . . . . . . . . . . . . . . . . . . . . . . . . . . .130
**Ranch dip,** 2 tbsp:
(*Marie's*) . . . . . . . . . . . . . . . . . . . . . . . . . . . . . . . . . . .150
(*Marzetti* Veggie Dip) . . . . . . . . . . . . . . . . . . . . . . . . . . .130
(*Marzetti* Veggie Dip Fat Free) . . . . . . . . . . . . . . . . . . . . .35
(*Marzetti* Veggie Dip Light) . . . . . . . . . . . . . . . . . . . . . . .80
bacon (*Marzetti* Veggie Dip) . . . . . . . . . . . . . . . . . . . . . .120
roasted garlic or Southwestern (*Marzetti* Veggie Dip) . . . . .140
**Ranch dip mix,** 2 tbsp.*:
(*McCormick*) . . . . . . . . . . . . . . . . . . . . . . . . . . . . . . . . . .35
(*Ruffles*) . . . . . . . . . . . . . . . . . . . . . . . . . . . . . . . . . . . .70
**Rapini,** see "Broccoli rabe"
**Raspberry,** fresh:
(*Dole*), 1 cup . . . . . . . . . . . . . . . . . . . . . . . . . . . . . . . . .50
½ cup . . . . . . . . . . . . . . . . . . . . . . . . . . . . . . . . . . . . . . .31
**Raspberry, frozen:**
(*Big Valley*), ⅔ cup . . . . . . . . . . . . . . . . . . . . . . . . . . . . .60
(*Birds Eye*), 5 oz. . . . . . . . . . . . . . . . . . . . . . . . . . . . . . .90
(*Cascadian Farm*), 1 cup . . . . . . . . . . . . . . . . . . . . . . . . .60
(*Tree of Life*), ⅔ cup . . . . . . . . . . . . . . . . . . . . . . . . . . .50
in syrup (*Big Valley* Tub), ⅔ cup . . . . . . . . . . . . . . . . . . .150
**Raspberry drink,** blue (*Tropicana Twister*), 8 fl. oz. . . . . . .120
**Raspberry juice blends:**
(*Dole* Country), 8 fl. oz. . . . . . . . . . . . . . . . . . . . . . . . . .140
(*Dole* Country), 10 fl. oz. . . . . . . . . . . . . . . . . . . . . . . . .180
kiwi (*Dole*), 8 fl. oz. . . . . . . . . . . . . . . . . . . . . . . . . . . . .140
**Raspberry syrup** (*Maple Grove Farms*), ¼ cup . . . . . . . . . .210
**Raspberry topping** (*Smucker's Plate Scrapers*), 2 tbsp. . . .100
**Raspberry–tamarind dipping sauce** (*Helen's Tropical Exotics*), 2 tbsp. . . . . . . . . . . . . . . . . . . . . . . . . . . . . . . .50
**Ravioli** (see also "Ravioli entree"), frozen or refrigerated:
cheese (*Celentano*), 4 pcs., 4.3 oz. . . . . . . . . . . . . . . . . .260
cheese (*Celentano* Low Fat), 4.2 oz. . . . . . . . . . . . . . . . . .280
cheese, 4 (*Buitoni*), 1⅓ cups . . . . . . . . . . . . . . . . . . . . . .380
cheese, 4 (*Buitoni* Light), 1 cup . . . . . . . . . . . . . . . . . . . .230
cheese, 3, mini (*Buitoni*), 1 cup . . . . . . . . . . . . . . . . . . . .260

**Ravioli** ***(cont.)***
cheese, mini (*Celentano*), 12 pcs., 4 oz. . . . . . . . . . . . . . . . .260
chicken, Parmesan (*Buitoni*), 1¼ cups . . . . . . . . . . . . . . . . .310
chicken, roast, and garlic (*Buitoni*), 1¼ cups . . . . . . . . . . .330
gorgonzola (*Buitoni*), 1¼ cups . . . . . . . . . . . . . . . . . . . . .360
meat (*Celentano*), 4 pcs., 4.3 oz. . . . . . . . . . . . . . . . . . . . .270
vegetable, garden (*Buitoni*), 1 cup . . . . . . . . . . . . . . . . . . .250
**Ravioli entree, can or pkg.,** 1 cup, except as noted:
beef (*Chef Boyardee*) . . . . . . . . . . . . . . . . . . . . . . . . . . . .230
beef (*Chef Boyardee*), 7-oz. can . . . . . . . . . . . . . . . . . . . . .170
beef (*Chef Boyardee* Micro Cup), 7.5-oz. cont. . . . . . . . . . . .190
beef (*Chef Boyardee* Overstuffed) . . . . . . . . . . . . . . . . . . . .280
beef (*Chef Boyardee* 99% Fat Free) . . . . . . . . . . . . . . . . . . .210
beef (*Chef Boyardee Junior* Micro Cup), 1 cont. . . . . . . . . . .210
beef (*Dinty Moore American Classics*), 1 bowl . . . . . . . . . . .300
beef, mini (*Chef Boyardee*) . . . . . . . . . . . . . . . . . . . . . . . . .240
cheese (*Chef Boyardee* 99% Fat Free) . . . . . . . . . . . . . . . . .210
w/tomato sauce (*Hormel* Microcup) . . . . . . . . . . . . . . . . . . .220
**Ravioli entree, frozen,** 1 pkg., except as noted:
(*Amy's*), 8 oz. . . . . . . . . . . . . . . . . . . . . . . . . . . . . . . . . .340
cheese:
  (*Healthy Choice* Solos), 9 oz. . . . . . . . . . . . . . . . . . . . . .260
  (*Lean Cuisine Everyday Favorites*), 8.5 oz. . . . . . . . . . . .260
  (*Michelina's* Jumbo), 11 oz. . . . . . . . . . . . . . . . . . . . . . .400
  (*Stouffer's*), 10⅝ oz. . . . . . . . . . . . . . . . . . . . . . . . . . . .230
  Alfredo, and broccoli (*Michelina's*), 8 oz. . . . . . . . . . . . .390
  4 (*Wolfgang Puck's*), 13 oz. . . . . . . . . . . . . . . . . . . . . . .330
  w/sauce (*Master Choice*), 1 cup . . . . . . . . . . . . . . . . . . . .280
  3 (*Marie Callender's*), 16 oz. . . . . . . . . . . . . . . . . . . . . . .610
  and tomato sauce (*Freezer Queen* Meal), 7.75 oz. . . . . .350
meat, w/pomodoro sauce (*Michelina's*), 8 oz. . . . . . . . . . . .310
mushroom and spinach (*Wolfgang Puck's*), 13 oz. . . . . . . .260
sweet potato (*Wolfgang Puck's*), 13 oz. . . . . . . . . . . . . . . .360
**Red bean** (see also "Kidney beans"), canned, ½ cup:
(*Bush's Best*) . . . . . . . . . . . . . . . . . . . . . . . . . . . . . . . . . .110
(*Westbrae Natural* Fat Free) . . . . . . . . . . . . . . . . . . . . . . . .90
**Red kuri squash** (*Frieda's*), ¾ cup, 3 oz. . . . . . . . . . . . . . . .30
**Red snapper,** see "Snapper"
**Redfish,** see "Ocean perch"

**Refried beans, canned,** ½ cup:
(*Bearitos* Fat Free) . . . . . . . . . . . . . . . . . . . . . . . . . . . .110
(*Old El Paso*) . . . . . . . . . . . . . . . . . . . . . . . . . . . . . . . . .100
(*Ortega*) . . . . . . . . . . . . . . . . . . . . . . . . . . . . . . . . . . . . .150
(*Rosarita* Traditional) . . . . . . . . . . . . . . . . . . . . . . . . . . .100
black bean (*Bearitos* Fat Free) . . . . . . . . . . . . . . . . . . . .110
black bean (*Bearitos* Low Fat) . . . . . . . . . . . . . . . . . . . .130
black bean (*La Costeña*) . . . . . . . . . . . . . . . . . . . . . . . . .180
black bean spicy (*Greene's Farm*) . . . . . . . . . . . . . . . . . . .80
w/cheese (*Old El Paso*) . . . . . . . . . . . . . . . . . . . . . . . . . .130
w/green chilies (*Bearitos* Fat Free) . . . . . . . . . . . . . . . . .100
pinto bean (*Bearitos* Low Fat) . . . . . . . . . . . . . . . . . . . . .140
pinto bean (*La Costeña*) . . . . . . . . . . . . . . . . . . . . . . . . . .160
pinto bean (*La Sierra*) . . . . . . . . . . . . . . . . . . . . . . . . . . .150
w/sausage (*Old El Paso*) . . . . . . . . . . . . . . . . . . . . . . . . . .200
spicy (*Greene's Farm*) . . . . . . . . . . . . . . . . . . . . . . . . . . .100
spicy (*Old El Paso* Fat Free) . . . . . . . . . . . . . . . . . . . . . .100
spicy, jalapeño (*Rosarita*) . . . . . . . . . . . . . . . . . . . . . . . .100
vegetarian (*Hain*) . . . . . . . . . . . . . . . . . . . . . . . . . . . . . . . .90
vegetarian (*Old El Paso*) . . . . . . . . . . . . . . . . . . . . . . . . .100
**Relish,** see "Pickle relish" and specific listings
**Remoulade sauce,** in jars (*Zatarain's*), ¼ cup . . . . . . . . . . .80
**Rhubarb,** fresh:
(*Frieda's*), ⅔ cup, 3 oz. . . . . . . . . . . . . . . . . . . . . . . . . . . .20
diced, ½ cup . . . . . . . . . . . . . . . . . . . . . . . . . . . . . . . . . . . .13
**Rhubarb, frozen,** cooked, sweetened, ½ cup . . . . . . . . . . .139
**Rib sauce** (*Texas Best* Original), 2 tbsp. . . . . . . . . . . . . . . . .50
**Rice** (see also "Wild rice"), ¼ cup dry, except as noted:
arborio, white (*Frieda's* Risotto) . . . . . . . . . . . . . . . . . . .160
basmati, brown (*Lundberg* Organic) . . . . . . . . . . . . . . . . . .160
basmati, brown (*Texmati*) . . . . . . . . . . . . . . . . . . . . . . . . .170
basmati, white (*Lundberg Nutra-Farmed*/Organic) . . . . . . . .180
basmati, white (*Texmati*) . . . . . . . . . . . . . . . . . . . . . . . . . .150
blend (*Lundberg Black Japonica/Jubilee*) . . . . . . . . . . . . . .170
blend (*Lundberg Countrywild/Wild Blend*) . . . . . . . . . . . . .150
blend (*Texmati Royal Blend*), ⅓ cup . . . . . . . . . . . . . . . . . .160
blend, brown and wild (*Lundberg* Organic) . . . . . . . . . . . . .150
brown (*Lundberg Christmas/Wehani*) . . . . . . . . . . . . . . . . .170
brown (*S&W*) . . . . . . . . . . . . . . . . . . . . . . . . . . . . . . . . . . .150

**Rice *(cont.)***
brown (*Uncle Ben's* Original) . . . . . . . . . . . . . . . . . . . . . . . .170
brown, instant (*Uncle Ben's*), ½ cup, 1 cup* . . . . . . . . . . .190
brown, long-grain (*Carolina/Mahatma*) . . . . . . . . . . . . . . . .150
brown, long or short grain (*Lundberg*) . . . . . . . . . . . . . . . .170
cracked (*Gourmet House*) . . . . . . . . . . . . . . . . . . . . . . . . . .170
gold, parboiled (*Carolina/Mahatma*) . . . . . . . . . . . . . . . . . .160
glutinous or sweet . . . . . . . . . . . . . . . . . . . . . . . . . . . . . . . .171
Indian style or jasmine (*Texmati Kasmati/Jasmati*) . . . . . . .150
jasmine, white (*Mahatma* Thai) . . . . . . . . . . . . . . . . . . . . . .160
sushi (*Rice Select Sushi*) . . . . . . . . . . . . . . . . . . . . . . . . . .190
white, long grain:
(*Carolina/Mahatma*) . . . . . . . . . . . . . . . . . . . . . . . . . . .150
(*River/Water Maid*) . . . . . . . . . . . . . . . . . . . . . . . . . . . .160
(*S&W*) . . . . . . . . . . . . . . . . . . . . . . . . . . . . . . . . . . . . . .150
instant (*Carolina/Mahatma*) . . . . . . . . . . . . . . . . . . . . . .160
instant (*Uncle Ben's*), ½ cup, 1 cup* . . . . . . . . . . . . . . .190
parboiled (*Uncle Ben's Converted* Original), ⅓ cup* . . . .170
white, short grain (*Goya* Valencia) . . . . . . . . . . . . . . . . . . .150
**Rice and beans,** see "Rice dish"
**Rice beverage,** 8 fl. oz.:
(*Rice Dream*) . . . . . . . . . . . . . . . . . . . . . . . . . . . . . . . . . . .120
carob (*Rice Dream*) . . . . . . . . . . . . . . . . . . . . . . . . . . . . . .150
chocolate (*Rice Dream*) . . . . . . . . . . . . . . . . . . . . . . . . . . .170
vanilla (*Rice Dream*) . . . . . . . . . . . . . . . . . . . . . . . . . . . . .130
**Rice cake** (see also "Popcorn cake"):
all varieties, baked (*Hain Ringers*), 37 pcs., 1 oz. . . . . . . . .110
apple cinnamon (*Quaker* Crispy Mini's), 8 pcs. . . . . . . . . . . .60
banana nut (*Mother's*), 1 pc. . . . . . . . . . . . . . . . . . . . . . . . .50
banana nut (*Quaker* Crispy Mini's), 8 pcs. . . . . . . . . . . . . . . .65
barbecue flavor (*Quaker* Crispy Mini's), 10 pcs. . . . . . . . . . .70
butter flavor, corn grain (*Mother's* Unsalted), 1 pc. . . . . . . . .35
caramel corn (*Quaker* Crispy Mini's), 7 pcs. . . . . . . . . . . . . .60
cheese, cheddar or nacho (*Quaker* Crispy Mini's),
9 pcs. . . . . . . . . . . . . . . . . . . . . . . . . . . . . . . . . . . . . . . . .70
chocolate (*Quaker* Crispy Mini's), 7 pcs. . . . . . . . . . . . . . . .60
honey nut (*Quaker* Crispy Mini's), 8 pcs. . . . . . . . . . . . . . . .60
ranch (*Quaker* Crispy Mini's), 10 pcs. . . . . . . . . . . . . . . . . . .75
sour cream and onion (*Quaker* Crispy Mini's), 10 pcs. . . . . .70
**Rice chips** brown (*Eden*), 50 pcs., 1.1 oz. . . . . . . . . . . . . .150

**Rice dish, canned,** 1 cup:
fried (*La Choy*) .290
Spanish (*Old El Paso*) .140
**Rice dish, frozen,** 1 pkg., except as noted:
and beans:
Santa Fe (*Lean Cuisine Everyday Favorites*), 10⅜ oz. .300
Southwestern (*Healthy Choice* Solo), 10 oz. .250
Spanish, w/chicken (*Ortega*), 10.25 oz. .400
broccoli, in cheese sauce, w/pasta (*Freezer Queen* Family Side Dish), 1 cup .190
cheesy, and chicken (*Healthy Choice* Solo), 9 oz. .230
risotto, cheese and mushroom (*Wolfgang Puck's*), 11 oz. .520
Spanish, and chicken (*Michelina's*), 8 oz. .290
Szechuan (*Cascadian Farm Veggie Bowl*), 9 oz. .210
teriyaki (*Cascadian Farm Veggie Bowl*), 9 oz. .270
w/vegetables, stir-fry (*Budget Gourmet*), 8 oz. .350
w/vegetables, teriyaki stir-fry (*Amy's* Skillet Meals), 1 cup .320
w/vegetables, Thai stir-fry (*Amy's*), 9.5 oz. .270
w/vegetables, wild-rice pilaf (*Budget Gourmet*), 8 oz. .340
**Rice dish, mix,** 1 cup*, except as noted:
Alfredo broccoli (*Lipton* Rice & Sauce) .320
almond, toasted, pilaf (*Near East*) .230
and beans, black (*Carolina/Mahatma*) .200
and beans, black, Mediterranean, pilaf (*Near East*) .260
and beans, red (*Carolina/Mahatma*) .190
and beans, red (*Success*) .240
and beans, smoky (*Chef's Originals* Cowboy), ¼ cup .180
beef (*Lipton* Rice & Sauce) .270
beef (*Mahatma*) .200
beef (*Rice-A-Roni*) .310
beef (*Rice-A-Roni* ⅓ Less Salt) .280
beef (*Success*) .190
beef and mushroom (*Rice-A-Roni*) .290
biryani (*Neera's*) .132
broccoli (*Rice-A-Roni*) .270
broccoli au gratin (*Rice-A-Roni*) .370
broccoli au gratin (*Rice-A-Roni* ⅓ Less Salt) .320

**Rice dish, mix *(cont.)***

broccoli au gratin risotto (*Knorr* Italian) . . . . . . . . . . . . . . .260
broccoli and cheese (*Mahatma*) . . . . . . . . . . . . . . . . . . . . . .200
broccoli and cheese (*Success*) . . . . . . . . . . . . . . . . . . . . . . .210
brown and wild (*Success*) . . . . . . . . . . . . . . . . . . . . . . . . .190
Cajun style (*Lipton* Rice & Sauce) . . . . . . . . . . . . . . . . . . .270
Cajun style, w/beans (*Lipton* Rice & Sauce) . . . . . . . . . . . .310
cheddar, white, and herbs (*Rice-A-Roni*) . . . . . . . . . . . . . .340
cheddar broccoli (*Bowl Appétit!*), 1 bowl . . . . . . . . . . . . . .290
cheddar broccoli (*Lipton* Rice & Sauce) . . . . . . . . . . . . . . .280
cheese, 4 (*Rice-A-Roni*) . . . . . . . . . . . . . . . . . . . . . . . . . .280
cheese, nacho (*Mahatma*) . . . . . . . . . . . . . . . . . . . . . . . . .250
cheese, 3, risotto (*Marrakesh Express*) . . . . . . . . . . . . . . . .200
chicken (*Carolina/Mahatma*) . . . . . . . . . . . . . . . . . . . . . . .190
chicken (*Lipton* Rice & Sauce) . . . . . . . . . . . . . . . . . . . . . .280
chicken (*Rice-A-Roni*) . . . . . . . . . . . . . . . . . . . . . . . . . . .310
chicken (*Rice-A-Roni* Low Fat) . . . . . . . . . . . . . . . . . . . . .210
chicken (*Rice-A-Roni* ⅓ Less Salt) . . . . . . . . . . . . . . . . . . .280
chicken (*Success* Classic) . . . . . . . . . . . . . . . . . . . . . . . . .150
chicken, broccoli (*Rice-A-Roni*) . . . . . . . . . . . . . . . . . . . . .230
chicken, Cajun (*Rice-A-Roni*) . . . . . . . . . . . . . . . . . . . . . .250
chicken, creamy (*Lipton* Rice & Sauce) . . . . . . . . . . . . . . .290
chicken, garlic (*Rice-A-Roni*) . . . . . . . . . . . . . . . . . . . . . .260
chicken, grilled (*Success*) . . . . . . . . . . . . . . . . . . . . . . . . .190
chicken, herb-roasted (*Rice-A-Roni*) . . . . . . . . . . . . . . . . .260
chicken, roasted (*Lipton* Rice & Sauce) . . . . . . . . . . . . . . .260
chicken, roasted, and garlic pilaf (*Near East*) . . . . . . . . . . .220
chicken, Southwestern (*Lipton* Rice & Sauce) . . . . . . . . . . .260
chicken and herb (*Uncle Ben's Natural Select*) . . . . . . . . . .200
chicken w/mushrooms (*Rice-A-Roni*) . . . . . . . . . . . . . . . . .360
chicken Parmesan risotto (*Lipton* Rice & Sauce) . . . . . . . . .270
chicken pilaf (*Near East*) . . . . . . . . . . . . . . . . . . . . . . . . .210
chicken teriyaki (*Rice-A-Roni*) . . . . . . . . . . . . . . . . . . . . .260
chicken and vegetables (*Rice-A-Roni*) . . . . . . . . . . . . . . . .290
chili (*Lundberg One-Step*) . . . . . . . . . . . . . . . . . . . . . . . . .180
curry (*Lundberg One-Step*) . . . . . . . . . . . . . . . . . . . . . . . .160
curry pilaf (*Near East*) . . . . . . . . . . . . . . . . . . . . . . . . . . .220
dirty rice, Jamaican style (*Neera's*) . . . . . . . . . . . . . . . . . .175
fried (*Rice-A-Roni*) . . . . . . . . . . . . . . . . . . . . . . . . . . . . .320
fried (*Rice-A-Roni* ⅓ Less Salt) . . . . . . . . . . . . . . . . . . . . .260

garlic basil (*Lundberg One-Step*) . . . . . . . . . . . . . . . . . . . .160
garlic basil (*A Taste of Thai*), ¾ cup* . . . . . . . . . . . . . . . . .160
garlic and butter (*Uncle Ben's Natural Select*) . . . . . . . . . . .200
garlic and herb (*Near East*) . . . . . . . . . . . . . . . . . . . . . . . .220
golden (*A Taste of Thai*), ¾ cup* . . . . . . . . . . . . . . . . . . . .180
jambalaya (*Mahatma*) . . . . . . . . . . . . . . . . . . . . . . . . . . . .190
long grain and wild (*Carolina/Mahatma/Success*) . . . . . . . .190
long grain and wild (*Rice-A-Roni* Original) . . . . . . . . . . . . .240
long grain and wild (*Uncle Ben's* Original) . . . . . . . . . . . . . .190
long grain and wild pilaf (*Near East*) . . . . . . . . . . . . . . . . .220
Mexican (*Chef's Originals* Sonoran), ¼ cup . . . . . . . . . . . .180
Mexican (*Rice-A-Roni*) . . . . . . . . . . . . . . . . . . . . . . . . . . .250
mushroom (*Lipton* Rice & Sauce) . . . . . . . . . . . . . . . . . . . .270
mushroom, wild, and herb pilaf (*Near East*) . . . . . . . . . . . .220
Oriental stir-fry (*Lipton* Rice & Sauce) . . . . . . . . . . . . . . . .270
pilaf (see also specific listings):
 (*Carolina/Mahatma* Classic) . . . . . . . . . . . . . . . . . . . . . .190
 (*Near East*) . . . . . . . . . . . . . . . . . . . . . . . . . . . . . . . . . .220
 (*Rice-A-Roni*) . . . . . . . . . . . . . . . . . . . . . . . . . . . . . . . .310
 brown rice (*Near East*) . . . . . . . . . . . . . . . . . . . . . . . . . .210
risotto (see also specific listings):
 garlic and herb (*Chef's Originals*), ¼ cup . . . . . . . . . . . .130
 garlic primavera (*Marrakesh Express*) . . . . . . . . . . . . . . .210
 Milanese (*Knorr* Italian), ⅓ cup . . . . . . . . . . . . . . . . . . . .260
 Milanese, w/saffron (*Marrakesh Express*) . . . . . . . . . . . .220
 Milanese, porcini, or tomato (*Alessi*), ⅓ cup . . . . . . . . .190
 onion herb (*Knorr* Italian), ⅓ cup . . . . . . . . . . . . . . . . . .300
 sun-dried tomato (*Marrakesh Express*) . . . . . . . . . . . . . . .200
 vegetable primavera (*Knorr* Italian), ⅓ cup . . . . . . . . . .280
saffron, see "yellow," below
salsa style (*Lipton* Rice & Sauce) . . . . . . . . . . . . . . . . . . . .220
scampi style (*Lipton* Rice & Sauce) . . . . . . . . . . . . . . . . . .270
Spanish (*Carolina/Mahatma*) . . . . . . . . . . . . . . . . . . . . . . .180
Spanish (*Rice-A-Roni*) . . . . . . . . . . . . . . . . . . . . . . . . . . .300
Spanish (*Success*) . . . . . . . . . . . . . . . . . . . . . . . . . . . . . .190
Spanish pilaf (*Near East*) . . . . . . . . . . . . . . . . . . . . . . . . .310
Stroganoff (*Rice-A-Roni*) . . . . . . . . . . . . . . . . . . . . . . . . .360
teriyaki (*Lipton* Rice & Sauce) . . . . . . . . . . . . . . . . . . . . . .270
vegetable garden (*Rice-A-Roni*) . . . . . . . . . . . . . . . . . . . . .240
vegetable, roasted, and chicken pilaf (*Near East*) . . . . . . . .220

**Rice dish, mix *(cont.)***
wild rice (*Lipton* Rice & Sauce) . . . . . . . . . . . . . . . . . . . . .280
yellow (*Success*) . . . . . . . . . . . . . . . . . . . . . . . . . . . . .150
yellow, saffron (*Carolina/Mahatma*) . . . . . . . . . . . . . . . . . .190
yellow, saffron, spicy (*Mahatma*) . . . . . . . . . . . . . . . . . . .180
**Rice entree, frozen,** see "Rice dish, frozen"
**Rice flour,** ¼ cup, except as noted:
brown (*Hodgson Mill*), scant ¼ cup . . . . . . . . . . . . . . . . . .110
brown (*Lundberg* Organic) . . . . . . . . . . . . . . . . . . . . . . .110
brown (*Lundberg Nutra-Farmed*) . . . . . . . . . . . . . . . . . . . .120
white (*Arrowhead Mills*) . . . . . . . . . . . . . . . . . . . . . . . .130
**Rice pudding,** ready-to-eat (*Kozy Shack*), ½ cup . . . . . . . .140
**Rice pudding mix:**
(*Watkins*), 1½ tbsp. . . . . . . . . . . . . . . . . . . . . . . . . . .50
all varieties (*Lundberg* Elegant), ½ cup . . . . . . . . . . . . . . . .70
cinnamon and raisin (*Uncle Ben's*), 1.5 oz., ½ cup* . . . . . .160
**Rice puffs** (*Eden* Arare), 30 pcs., 1.1 oz. . . . . . . . . . . . . .110
**Rice seasoning:**
Mexican (*Lawry's*), 1½ tbsp. . . . . . . . . . . . . . . . . . . . . . .40
Spanish (*Bearitos*), 1 tsp. . . . . . . . . . . . . . . . . . . . . . . .10
**Rigatoni pasta dish, mix,** 1 cup*:
cheddar, white, and broccoli sauce (*Pasta Roni*) . . . . . . . . .320
herb and butter (*Pasta Roni*) . . . . . . . . . . . . . . . . . . . . .350
**Rigatoni pasta entree,** frozen, 1 pkg.:
w/broccoli and chicken (*Healthy Choice* Medley), 9 oz. . . . .280
w/broccoli, chicken, cream sauce (*Budget Gourmet*),
8 oz. . . . . . . . . . . . . . . . . . . . . . . . . . . . . . . . . . .260
cheese, stuffed (*Michelina's*), 8.5 oz. . . . . . . . . . . . . . . . .300
w/meatballs (*Lean Cuisine Hearty Portions*), 15⅜ oz. . . . . .440
pomodoro (*Michelina's*), 8 oz. . . . . . . . . . . . . . . . . . . . .220
risotto Parmigiano (*Michelina's*), 8 oz. . . . . . . . . . . . . . . .450
**Risotto,** see "Rice dishes, mix" and "Rice entree"
**Rockfish,** meat only:
raw, 4 oz. . . . . . . . . . . . . . . . . . . . . . . . . . . . . . . . .107
baked, broiled, or microwaved, 4 oz. . . . . . . . . . . . . . . . . .137
**Roe** (see also "Caviar"):
raw, 1 tbsp. . . . . . . . . . . . . . . . . . . . . . . . . . . . . . . . .20
baked, broiled, or microwaved, 4 oz. . . . . . . . . . . . . . . . . .231
**Roletti pasta dish,** frozen, and vegetables (*Birds Eye*),
1 cup . . . . . . . . . . . . . . . . . . . . . . . . . . . . . . . . . .190

**Roll** (see also "Biscuit"), 1 roll, except as noted:
(*Rhodes* Fat Free) . . . . . . . . . . . . . . . . . . . . . . . . . .85
deli (*Wonder*) . . . . . . . . . . . . . . . . . . . . . . . . . . . .180
dinner (*Wonder*) . . . . . . . . . . . . . . . . . . . . . . . . . .100
dinner, all varieties (*Awrey's*), 2 rolls, 1.6 oz. . . . . . . . . . . .120
dinner, brown-and-serve (*Stroehmann*) . . . . . . . . . . . . . . . . .80
dinner, finger, poppy or sesame (*Pepperidge Farm*),
3 rolls . . . . . . . . . . . . . . . . . . . . . . . . . . . . . . .150
dinner, soft (*Pepperidge Farm*) . . . . . . . . . . . . . . . . . . . . .90
dinner, wheat, sweet, soft (*Pepperidge Farm*) . . . . . . . . . . . .100
egg, twist (*Levy's* Old Country) . . . . . . . . . . . . . . . . . . . .170
hamburger (*Arnold*) . . . . . . . . . . . . . . . . . . . . . . . . . .140
hamburger (*Martin's* Sliced) . . . . . . . . . . . . . . . . . . . . . .100
hamburger (*Pepperidge Farm*) . . . . . . . . . . . . . . . . . . . . .120
hamburger (*Wonder*) . . . . . . . . . . . . . . . . . . . . . . . . . .110
hoagie (*Awrey's*) . . . . . . . . . . . . . . . . . . . . . . . . . . . .230
hoagie (*Martin's* Seeded) . . . . . . . . . . . . . . . . . . . . . . .270
hoagie (*Martin's* Unseeded) . . . . . . . . . . . . . . . . . . . . . .260
hot dog (*Arnold*) . . . . . . . . . . . . . . . . . . . . . . . . . . . .120
hot dog, potato (*Arnold*) . . . . . . . . . . . . . . . . . . . . . . .130
hot dog, potato (*Martin's* Long Roll) . . . . . . . . . . . . . . . . .150
kaiser (*Awrey's*) . . . . . . . . . . . . . . . . . . . . . . . . . . . .190
kaiser (*Levy's* Old Country) . . . . . . . . . . . . . . . . . . . . . .170
onion (*Levy's* Old Country) . . . . . . . . . . . . . . . . . . . . . .160
potato (*Martin's*) . . . . . . . . . . . . . . . . . . . . . . . . . . .100
sandwich (*Martin's*) . . . . . . . . . . . . . . . . . . . . . . . . . .150
sandwich (*Pepperidge Farm* Hearty) . . . . . . . . . . . . . . . . . .210
sandwich, potato, golden (*Pepperidge Farm*) . . . . . . . . . . . . .220
sandwich, potato, sesame (*Arnold*) . . . . . . . . . . . . . . . . . .170
sandwich, sesame (*Arnold*) . . . . . . . . . . . . . . . . . . . . . . .140
sandwich, sesame (*Marty's* Large) . . . . . . . . . . . . . . . . . . .190
sandwich, sesame (*Pepperidge Farm*) . . . . . . . . . . . . . . . . .130
sandwich, wheat, country (*Pepperidge Farm*) . . . . . . . . . . . . .210
sub (*Levy's* Old Country) . . . . . . . . . . . . . . . . . . . . . . . .140
wheat or cracked wheat (*Rhodes*) . . . . . . . . . . . . . . . . . . .140
white (*Rhodes*) . . . . . . . . . . . . . . . . . . . . . . . . . . . . . .95
**Roll, mix,** hot (*Pillsbury* Specialty), ¼ cup mix . . . . . . . . .110
**Roll, refrigerated** (see also "Biscuit, refrigerated"),
1 pc.:
crescent (*Grands!* Quick), 2.5 oz. . . . . . . . . . . . . . . . . . . .270

**Roll, refrigerated *(cont.)***
crescent (*Pillsbury*), 1 oz. . . . . . . . . . . . . . . . . . . . . . . . . .110
crescent (*Pillsbury* Reduced Fat), 1 oz. . . . . . . . . . . . . . . . . .100
dinner (*Pillsbury* Traditional Tube), 1.4 oz. . . . . . . . . . . . . .110
dinner, French (*Pillsbury Home Baked Classics*), 1.4 oz. . . .110
**Roll, sweet,** see "Bun, sweet"
**Romaine,** see "Lettuce" and "Salad blend"
**Roseapple,** 1 oz. . . . . . . . . . . . . . . . . . . . . . . . . . . . . . . . .7
**Roselle,** 1 oz., ½ cup . . . . . . . . . . . . . . . . . . . . . . . . . . . .14
**Rosemary,** dried, 1 tsp. . . . . . . . . . . . . . . . . . . . . . . . . . . .4
**Rotini dish, mix:**
cheese, 3 (*Bowl Appétit!*), 1 bowl . . . . . . . . . . . . . . . . . . .360
cheese, 3 (*Lipton* Pasta & Sauce), ½ pkg. . . . . . . . . . . . . .240
w/cheese sauce, four (*Near East* Meal Cup), 1 pkg. . . . . . . .200
chicken and broccoli (*Near East* Meal Cup), 1 pkg. . . . . . . .190
chicken and broccoli (*Nile Spice* Cup), 1 pkg. . . . . . . . . . . .190
w/mushroom sauce (*Knorr* Side Dish), ⅔ cup . . . . . . . . . .260
4-cheese (*Knorr* Side Dish), ⅓ cup . . . . . . . . . . . . . . . . . .130
**Roughy, orange,** meat only:
raw, 4 oz. . . . . . . . . . . . . . . . . . . . . . . . . . . . . . . . . . . . . .78
baked, broiled, or microwaved, 4 oz. . . . . . . . . . . . . . . . . .101
**Rutabaga,** fresh, ½ cup:
boiled, drained, cubed . . . . . . . . . . . . . . . . . . . . . . . . . . . .33
boiled, drained, mashed . . . . . . . . . . . . . . . . . . . . . . . . . . .47
**Rye,** whole-grain, ½ cup . . . . . . . . . . . . . . . . . . . . . . . . . .284
**Rye flakes,** rolled (*Arrowhead Mills*), ⅓ cup . . . . . . . . . . . .110
**Rye flour:**
(*Hodgson Mill* Organic/Whole Grain), ¼ cup . . . . . . . . . . . . .90
medium (*Pillsbury*), ¼ cup . . . . . . . . . . . . . . . . . . . . . . . .100

# S

| FOOD AND MEASURE | CALORIES |
|---|---|
| **Sablefish,** meat only: | |
| raw, 4 oz. | 222 |
| baked, broiled, or microwaved, 4 oz. | 284 |
| smoked, 4 oz. | 291 |
| **Saffron,** 1 tsp. | 2 |
| **Sage,** ground, 1 tsp. | 2 |
| **Salad blend** (see also "Lettuce" and "Salad kit"), fresh, 3 oz., except as noted: | |
| (*Dole* Very Veggie) | 20 |
| (*Fresh Express Fancy Field Greens/Greener European*) | 15 |
| (*Fresh Express Riviera*) | 10 |
| (*Fresh Express Veggie Lover's/*Royal Blend) | 20 |
| (*Ready Pac* Classic/Harvest Crisp/Hearty Green Salad) | 10 |
| (*Ready Pac* Organic Country Garden) | 15 |
| (*Ready Pac* Spring Mix) | 35 |
| Aspen (*Ready Pac* Organic), 4.5-oz. pkg. | 25 |
| Caesar (*Ready Pac*) | 15 |
| coleslaw (*Dole* Classic) | 25 |
| coleslaw, w/broccoli (*Mann's*), 4 oz. | 35 |
| coleslaw, w/carrots (*Fresh Express* 3-Color) | 20 |
| European, French, Italian, or Mediterranean (*Dole*) | 15 |
| iceberg, carrots, red cabbage, romaine (*Fresh Express*) | 15 |
| mesclun (*Ready Pac*), 4.5-oz. pkg. | 35 |
| **Salad kit,** w/dressing, fresh, 3.5 oz.: | |
| (*Dole* All American Toss) | 50 |
| Caesar (*Dole/Dole* Family/Creamy Garlic) | 170 |
| Caesar (*Fresh Express*) | 160 |
| Caesar (*Fresh Express* Light) | 100 |
| Caesar (*Fresh Express* Supreme) | 150 |
| Caesar, w/light dressing (*Dole*) | 100 |
| cheese, triple (*Dole* Toss) | 80 |
| coleslaw (*Fresh Express*) | 120 |
| Greek marinade (*Dole* Classic) | 100 |
| Mediterranean marinade (*Dole*) | 90 |

**Salad kit *(cont.)***
Oriental or ranch (*Fresh Express*) . . . . . . . . . . . . . . . . . . . . .140
ranch (*Fresh Express* Light) . . . . . . . . . . . . . . . . . . . . . . . .100
Romano (*Dole*) . . . . . . . . . . . . . . . . . . . . . . . . . . . . . . .150
sunflower ranch (*Dole*) . . . . . . . . . . . . . . . . . . . . . . . . . .170
taco (*Fresh Express Taco Fiesta*) . . . . . . . . . . . . . . . . . . . .110
**Salad dressing,** 2 tbsp.:
bacon and tomato (*Henri's*) . . . . . . . . . . . . . . . . . . . . . . .130
balsamic vinaigrette (*Cardini's*) . . . . . . . . . . . . . . . . . . . . .150
balsamic vinaigrette (*Marzetti*) . . . . . . . . . . . . . . . . . . . . .100
balsamic vinaigrette (*Newman's Own*) . . . . . . . . . . . . . . . . . .90
balsamic vinaigrette (*Pfeiffer*) . . . . . . . . . . . . . . . . . . . . .100
blue cheese (*Marzetti* Light) . . . . . . . . . . . . . . . . . . . . . . . .90
blue cheese (*Marzetti* Low Fat) . . . . . . . . . . . . . . . . . . . . . .45
blue cheese (*Ott's* Famous Original) . . . . . . . . . . . . . . . . . . .80
blue cheese (*Ott's* Famous Reduced Calorie) . . . . . . . . . . . . .60
blue cheese, chunky (*Hellmann's/Best Foods*) . . . . . . . . . . .130
blue cheese, chunky (*Marie's*) . . . . . . . . . . . . . . . . . . . . . .170
blue cheese, honey French (*Marzetti*) . . . . . . . . . . . . . . . . .160
Caesar (*Cardini's* "The Original Caesar Dressing") . . . . . . . .160
Caesar (*Hellmann's/Best Foods* Fat Free) . . . . . . . . . . . . . . .30
Caesar (*Marzetti*) . . . . . . . . . . . . . . . . . . . . . . . . . . . . . .120
Caesar (*Marzetti* Light) . . . . . . . . . . . . . . . . . . . . . . . . . . .70
Caesar (*Newman's Own*) . . . . . . . . . . . . . . . . . . . . . . . . . .150
Caesar (*Randall's* Real) . . . . . . . . . . . . . . . . . . . . . . . . . .130
Caesar, creamy (*Hellmann's/Best Foods*) . . . . . . . . . . . . . . .160
Caesar, creamy (*Ott's*) . . . . . . . . . . . . . . . . . . . . . . . . . . .110
Caesar, creamy (*Wish-Bone Just 2 Good!*) . . . . . . . . . . . . . . .40
Caesar ranch (*Henri's*) . . . . . . . . . . . . . . . . . . . . . . . . . . .140
carrot ginger, sesame (*Randall's*) . . . . . . . . . . . . . . . . . . . . .45
champagne (*Girard's*) . . . . . . . . . . . . . . . . . . . . . . . . . . . .150
coleslaw, see "slaw," below
cucumber, creamy (*Henri's*) . . . . . . . . . . . . . . . . . . . . . . . . .90
Dijon lime (*Newman's Own* Parisienne) . . . . . . . . . . . . . . . .120
dill, creamy (*Nasoya Vegi-Dressing*) . . . . . . . . . . . . . . . . . . .70
feta, Greek, vinaigrette (*Girard's*) . . . . . . . . . . . . . . . . . . .100
French (*Henri's* Original) . . . . . . . . . . . . . . . . . . . . . . . . . .120
French (*Marzetti* California/Country) . . . . . . . . . . . . . . . . . .160
French (*Pfeiffer*) . . . . . . . . . . . . . . . . . . . . . . . . . . . . . . .150
French, creamy (*Henri's*) . . . . . . . . . . . . . . . . . . . . . . . . . .120

French, honey (*Marzetti*) . . . . . . . . . . . . . . . . . . . . . . . . . . . .170
French, savory (*Hellmann's/Best Foods*) . . . . . . . . . . . . . . .130
French, spicy (*Cardini's* Natural) . . . . . . . . . . . . . . . . . . . . . .130
French style (*Hellmann's/Best Foods* Fat Free) . . . . . . . . . . .45
French style, bacon tomato-flavored (*Henri's*) . . . . . . . . . . .140
garlic, roasted (*Cardini's*) . . . . . . . . . . . . . . . . . . . . . . . . . . .130
garlic, roasted (*Marzetti*) . . . . . . . . . . . . . . . . . . . . . . . . . . .150
garlic, roasted, vinaigrette (*Pfeiffer*) . . . . . . . . . . . . . . . . . .130
garlic cilantro lime (*Randall's*) . . . . . . . . . . . . . . . . . . . . . . . .80
grape vinaigrette (*El Torito* Serrano) . . . . . . . . . . . . . . . . . . .25
herb, garden (*Nasoya Vegi-Dressing*) . . . . . . . . . . . . . . . . . . .70
herb poppy seed (*Cardini's*) . . . . . . . . . . . . . . . . . . . . . . . . . .35
honey Dijon (*Hellmann's/Best Foods* Light) . . . . . . . . . . . . . .80
honey Dijon (*Marzetti*) . . . . . . . . . . . . . . . . . . . . . . . . . . . . . .140
honey Dijon peppercorn (*Girard's*) . . . . . . . . . . . . . . . . . . . .140
honey Dijon ranch (*Hellmann's*) . . . . . . . . . . . . . . . . . . . . . . .240
honey mustard (*Cardini's* Summer) . . . . . . . . . . . . . . . . . . . .150
honey mustard (*Marzetti's* Dip & Dressing) . . . . . . . . . . . . .130
honey mustard (*Ott's*) . . . . . . . . . . . . . . . . . . . . . . . . . . . . . .100
Italian (*Cardini's* Dressing/Marinade) . . . . . . . . . . . . . . . . . .120
Italian (*Girard's* Olde Venice) . . . . . . . . . . . . . . . . . . . . . . . .130
Italian (*Hellmann's/Best Foods*) . . . . . . . . . . . . . . . . . . . . . .110
Italian (*Marzetti*) . . . . . . . . . . . . . . . . . . . . . . . . . . . . . . . . .100
Italian (*Newman's Own* Family Recipe) . . . . . . . . . . . . . . . . .120
Italian, w/blue cheese crumbles (*Cardini's*) . . . . . . . . . . . . .130
Italian, creamy (*Marzetti*) . . . . . . . . . . . . . . . . . . . . . . . . . . .160
Italian, creamy (*Nasoya Vegi-Dressing*) . . . . . . . . . . . . . . . . .60
Italian, creamy (*Ott's*) . . . . . . . . . . . . . . . . . . . . . . . . . . . . . . .90
Italian, golden (*Hellmann's/Best Foods*) . . . . . . . . . . . . . . . . .90
Italian, Romano (*Cardini's* Natural) . . . . . . . . . . . . . . . . . . . .130
Italian, Romano or sweet (*Marzetti*) . . . . . . . . . . . . . . . . . . .150
Italian vinaigrette, blue cheese (*Marzetti*) . . . . . . . . . . . . . .100
Italian vinaigrette, roasted garlic (*Marzetti*) . . . . . . . . . . . .130
lemon herb or lime dill (*Cardini's* Dressing/Marinade) . . . . .130
mango lime vinaigrette (*Chi-Chi's*) . . . . . . . . . . . . . . . . . . . .120
mayonnaise type, see "Mayonnaise dressing"
mustard vinaigrette (*Henri's*) . . . . . . . . . . . . . . . . . . . . . . . . .90
oil and vinegar (*Newman's Own*) . . . . . . . . . . . . . . . . . . . . . .150
Oriental (*Girard's*) . . . . . . . . . . . . . . . . . . . . . . . . . . . . . . . .120
Parmesan basil (*Wish-Bone Just 2 Good!*) . . . . . . . . . . . . . . .40

**Salad dressing *(cont.)***
Parmesan, peppercorn (*Girard's*) .160
Parmesan, peppercorn (*Marzetti*) .160
Parmesan and roasted garlic (*Newman's Own*) .110
pepper, red, roasted (*Randall's* Italiana) .60
peppercorn, cracked (*Marzetti* Refrigerated) .150
pesto (*Cardini's* Pasta Dressing/Marinade) .140
poppy seed (*Marzetti* 16 fl. oz.) .160
poppy seed (*Marzetti* 15 fl. oz.) .140
poppy seed (*Marzetti* Fat Free) .60
poppy seed (*Ott's*) .90
potato salad (*Marzetti*) .150
ranch (*Chi-Chi's* Serrano) .140
ranch (*Hellmann's/Best Foods* Light) .80
ranch (*Henri's* Chef's Recipe) .150
ranch (*Hidden Valley* Original/Bacon) .140
ranch (*Marzetti*) .150
ranch (*Marzetti* Low Fat) .50
ranch (*Newman's Own*) .140
ranch (*Pfeiffer*) .150
ranch, buttermilk (*Marzetti*) .180
ranch, buttermilk and bacon (*Marzetti* Refrigerated) .160
ranch, buttermilk or garlic (*Hellmann's/Best Foods*) .140
ranch, garden (*Pfeiffer*) .160
ranch, Italian herb (*Hellmann's/Best Foods*) .130
ranch, Parmesan (*Cardini's* Aged/Natural) .150
ranch, peppercorn (*Marzetti*) .180
ranch, Southwest (*Henri's*) .100
ranch, spring onion (*Hellmann's/Best Foods*) .130
raspberry (*Girard's*) .120
raspberry vinaigrette (*Hellmann's/Best Foods* Fat Free) .35
raspberry vinaigrette (*Marzetti* House) .110
red pepper, roasted (*Cardini's* Natural) .110
red wine vinegar and oil (*Marzetti*) .90
red wine vinaigrette (*Girard's* Fat Free) .20
red wine vinaigrette (*Marzetti* Light) .30
red wine vinaigrette (*Pfeiffer*) .90
Russian (*Pfeiffer*) .140
Russian (*Wish-Bone*) .110
salsa vinaigrette (*Chi-Chi's*) .110

sesame garlic (*Nasoya Vegi-Dressing*) . . . . . . . . . . . . . . . . .60
sesame soy (*Sushi Chef*) . . . . . . . . . . . . . . . . . . . . . . . . .60
sesame soy (*Trader Vic's*) . . . . . . . . . . . . . . . . . . . . . . .110
slaw (*Henri's* Fat Free) . . . . . . . . . . . . . . . . . . . . . . . . .50
slaw (*Marzetti* Light) . . . . . . . . . . . . . . . . . . . . . . . . . .100
slaw (*Marzetti* Low Fat) . . . . . . . . . . . . . . . . . . . . . . . . .60
slaw (*Marzetti* Original/Refrigerated) . . . . . . . . . . . . . . . . .170
slaw (*Marzetti* Reduced Fat) . . . . . . . . . . . . . . . . . . . . . .100
slaw (*Marzetti* Southern Recipe) . . . . . . . . . . . . . . . . . . . .150
slaw (*Pfeiffer* Coleslaw) . . . . . . . . . . . . . . . . . . . . . . . .170
spinach salad (*Girard's*) . . . . . . . . . . . . . . . . . . . . . . . . .80
spinach salad (*Marzetti*) . . . . . . . . . . . . . . . . . . . . . . . . .80
sweet and saucy (*Marzetti*) . . . . . . . . . . . . . . . . . . . . . . .140
sweet and sour (*Henri's*) . . . . . . . . . . . . . . . . . . . . . . . .110
sweet and sour (*Marzetti*) . . . . . . . . . . . . . . . . . . . . . . . .160
sweet and sour (*Marzetti* Light) . . . . . . . . . . . . . . . . . . . .100
teriyaki ginger (*Henri's*) . . . . . . . . . . . . . . . . . . . . . . . . .80
Thousand Island (*Hellmann's/Best Foods*) . . . . . . . . . . . . . .130
Thousand Island (*Henri's*) . . . . . . . . . . . . . . . . . . . . . . . .100
Thousand Island (*Marzetti*) . . . . . . . . . . . . . . . . . . . . . . .140
Thousand Island (*Ott's*) . . . . . . . . . . . . . . . . . . . . . . . . .100
Thousand Island (*Nasoya Vegi-Dressing*) . . . . . . . . . . . . . . . .70
tomato, roasted, vinaigrette (*Henri's*) . . . . . . . . . . . . . . . . .90
tomato, sun-dried, vinaigrette (*Marzetti*) . . . . . . . . . . . . . .130
tomato, sun-dried, vinaigrette (*Wish-Bone*) . . . . . . . . . . . . . .50
**Salad toppers** (see also "Croutons"), crunchy or garden
vegetable (*McCormick Salad Toppins*), 1⅓ tbsp. . . . . . . .35
**Salami** (see also "Turkey salami"):
(*Boar's Head* Salame Panino), 1 oz. . . . . . . . . . . . . . . . . . .80
beef (*Boar's Head*), 2 oz. . . . . . . . . . . . . . . . . . . . . . . . .120
beef (*Hebrew National*), 3 slices, 2 oz. . . . . . . . . . . . . . . . .150
beef (*Hebrew National* Chub), 2 oz. . . . . . . . . . . . . . . . . . .170
beef (*Hebrew National* Lean), 4 slices, 2 oz. . . . . . . . . . . . . .90
beef (*Oscar Mayer* Machiach), 2 slices, 1.6 oz. . . . . . . . . . .120
cooked (*Boar's Head*), 2 oz. . . . . . . . . . . . . . . . . . . . . . . .130
cotto (*Oscar Mayer*), 2 slices, 1.6 oz. . . . . . . . . . . . . . . . .110
dry or hard (*Boar's Head*), 1 oz. . . . . . . . . . . . . . . . . . . . .110
dry or hard (*Homeland*), 1 oz. . . . . . . . . . . . . . . . . . . . . . .110
dry or hard (*Sara Lee*), 4 slices, 1.1 oz. . . . . . . . . . . . . . . .160
dry or hard (*Sara Lee* Deli), 4 slices, .9 oz. . . . . . . . . . . . .130

**Salami** ***(cont.)***
Genoa (*Boar's Head* Salame), 1 oz. . . . . . . . . . . . . . . . . . . . . .90
Genoa (*Citterio*), 3 slices, 1.1 oz. . . . . . . . . . . . . . . . . . . . .100
Genoa (*Di Lusso*), 2 oz. . . . . . . . . . . . . . . . . . . . . . . . . .210
Genoa (*Oscar Mayer*), 3 slices, 1 oz. . . . . . . . . . . . . . . . . . .100
Genoa (*San Remo Brand*), 1 oz. . . . . . . . . . . . . . . . . . . . . . .120
Milano (*Citterio*), 6 slices, 1.1 oz. . . . . . . . . . . . . . . . . . . .110
**"Salami," vegetarian,** frozen (*Yves* Deli Slices), 2.2 oz. . . .90
**Salisbury steak,** see "Beef dinner" and "Beef entree"
**Salmon,** fresh, meat only, 4 oz.:
Atlantic, farmed, raw . . . . . . . . . . . . . . . . . . . . . . . . . . .207
Atlantic, farmed, baked, broiled, or microwaved . . . . . . . . .234
Atlantic, wild, raw . . . . . . . . . . . . . . . . . . . . . . . . . . . . .161
Atlantic, wild, baked, broiled, or microwaved . . . . . . . . . . .206
Chinook, raw . . . . . . . . . . . . . . . . . . . . . . . . . . . . . . . .204
Chinook, baked, broiled, or microwaved . . . . . . . . . . . . . . .262
chum, raw . . . . . . . . . . . . . . . . . . . . . . . . . . . . . . . . . .136
chum, baked, broiled, or microwaved . . . . . . . . . . . . . . . . .175
coho, farmed, raw . . . . . . . . . . . . . . . . . . . . . . . . . . . . .182
coho, baked, broiled, or microwaved . . . . . . . . . . . . . . . . .202
coho, wild, raw . . . . . . . . . . . . . . . . . . . . . . . . . . . . . . .165
coho, wild, baked, broiled, or microwaved . . . . . . . . . . . . .158
coho, wild, boiled, poached, or steamed . . . . . . . . . . . . . . .209
pink, raw . . . . . . . . . . . . . . . . . . . . . . . . . . . . . . . . . . .132
pink, baked, broiled, or microwaved . . . . . . . . . . . . . . . . . .169
sockeye, raw . . . . . . . . . . . . . . . . . . . . . . . . . . . . . . . . .191
sockeye, baked, broiled, or microwaved . . . . . . . . . . . . . . .245
**Salmon, canned:**
pink (*Bumble Bee*), 2.2 oz. . . . . . . . . . . . . . . . . . . . . . . . .90
pink (*Chicken of the Sea* Traditional), 2 oz. . . . . . . . . . . . . .90
pink (*Crown Prince Natural*), ¼ cup . . . . . . . . . . . . . . . . . . .90
pink, skin/boneless (*Crown Prince*), ⅓ cup . . . . . . . . . . . . .90
red (*Chicken of the Sea*), 2 oz. . . . . . . . . . . . . . . . . . . . . .110
red (*Crown Prince*), ⅓ cup . . . . . . . . . . . . . . . . . . . . . . . .120
red, blueback (*Rubinstein's*), ¼ cup . . . . . . . . . . . . . . . . .110
red, sockeye (*Bumble Bee*), 2.2 oz. . . . . . . . . . . . . . . . . . .110
**Salmon, marinated** (*Spence & Co.* Gravlax), 2 oz. . . . . . . .120
**Salmon, smoked,** 2 oz., except as noted:
(*Ocean Beauty*) . . . . . . . . . . . . . . . . . . . . . . . . . . . . . . . .86
Atlantic (*Ducktrap River* Kendall Brook/Winter Harbor) . . . .130

Atlantic (*Ducktrap River Spruce Point*) . . . . . . . . . . . . . . . . .110
Atlantic, plain or cracked pepper/garlic (*Louis Kemp*) . . . . . .90
Chinook, lox . . . . . . . . . . . . . . . . . . . . . . . . . . . . . . . . . .67
lox or Nova (*Vita*) . . . . . . . . . . . . . . . . . . . . . . . . . . . . .50
pastrami style (*Ducktrap River Spruce Point*) . . . . . . . . . . .130
roasted (*Ducktrap River*) . . . . . . . . . . . . . . . . . . . . . . . .100
**Salmon, smoked, paté** (*Trois Petits Cochons*), 2 oz. . . . . . .90
**Salmon, smoked, spread** (*Sabra Salads* Lox), 1 oz. . . . . . .104
**Salmon burger,** frozen:
(*Ocean Beauty*), 3.2-oz. pc. . . . . . . . . . . . . . . . . . . . . . . .80
(*Omega Foods*), 3.2-oz. pc. . . . . . . . . . . . . . . . . . . . . . . .100
veggie (*Dr. Praeger's*), 2.8-oz. pc. . . . . . . . . . . . . . . . . . . .100
**Salmon seasoning** (*Old Bay* Classic), ⅕ pkg. . . . . . . . . . . . .40
**Salsa** (see also "Picante sauce"), 2 tbsp.:
(*Chi-Chi's* Garden) . . . . . . . . . . . . . . . . . . . . . . . . . . . . .15
(*Embasa* Mexican/Verde) . . . . . . . . . . . . . . . . . . . . . . . . . .5
(*Herdez* Casera/Verde) . . . . . . . . . . . . . . . . . . . . . . . . . .10
(*Herdez* Ranchera) . . . . . . . . . . . . . . . . . . . . . . . . . . . . .15
(*La Victoria* Ranchera/Verde/Victoria) . . . . . . . . . . . . . . . . .10
(*Ortega* Thick & Chunky) . . . . . . . . . . . . . . . . . . . . . . . . .10
(*Pace* Chunky/Chipotle/Cilantro/Garlic) . . . . . . . . . . . . . . . .10
all styles (*Old El Paso/Old El Paso* Thick n' Chunky) . . . . . . .10
black bean or chipotle corn (*Mrs. Renfro's*) . . . . . . . . . . . . .15
black bean and corn (*Muir Glen*) . . . . . . . . . . . . . . . . . . . .15
cheese, see "Cheese dip"
chipotle (*Embasa*) . . . . . . . . . . . . . . . . . . . . . . . . . . . . . .5
fire-roasted tomato (*Pace*) . . . . . . . . . . . . . . . . . . . . . . . .10
garlic, roasted (*Newman's Own*) . . . . . . . . . . . . . . . . . . . . .10
garlic, roasted (*Ortega*) . . . . . . . . . . . . . . . . . . . . . . . . . .10
habañero (*Shotgun Willie's* Hotter'n Hell) . . . . . . . . . . . . . .10
hot (*El Pato* Chili Fresco) . . . . . . . . . . . . . . . . . . . . . . . . .5
hot (*Newman's Own*) . . . . . . . . . . . . . . . . . . . . . . . . . . . .10
hot or medium (*Mrs. Renfro's*) . . . . . . . . . . . . . . . . . . . . .15
jalapeño (*El Paso*) . . . . . . . . . . . . . . . . . . . . . . . . . . . . .10
jalapeño, green or red (*La Victoria* Jalapeña) . . . . . . . . . . . .10
lime and garlic (*Pace*) . . . . . . . . . . . . . . . . . . . . . . . . . . .15
medium or mild (*Newman's Own*) . . . . . . . . . . . . . . . . . . . .10
mild (*Mrs. Renfro's*) . . . . . . . . . . . . . . . . . . . . . . . . . . . .10
mild (*Ortega* Mexican) . . . . . . . . . . . . . . . . . . . . . . . . . . .15
mild (*Snyder's*) . . . . . . . . . . . . . . . . . . . . . . . . . . . . . . .10

**Salsa *(cont.)***
peach (*Mrs. Renfro's*) . . . . . . . . . . . . . . . . . . . . . . . . .10
peach (*Newman's Own*) . . . . . . . . . . . . . . . . . . . . . . . . .25
picante, medium or mild (*La Victoria*) . . . . . . . . . . . . . . . . .10
pineapple (*Newman's Own*) . . . . . . . . . . . . . . . . . . . . . .15
red pepper, roasted, and garlic (*Pace*) . . . . . . . . . . . . . . . .10
roasted (*Mrs. Renfro's*) . . . . . . . . . . . . . . . . . . . . . . . .10
roasted tomato (*Chi-Chi's*) . . . . . . . . . . . . . . . . . . . . . .10
**Salsa seasoning** (*McCormick Produce Partners*), ½ tsp. . . . .5
**Salsify:**
raw, sliced, ½ cup . . . . . . . . . . . . . . . . . . . . . . . . . . .55
boiled, drained, sliced, ½ cup . . . . . . . . . . . . . . . . . . . . .46
**Salt,** table, 1 tbsp. . . . . . . . . . . . . . . . . . . . . . . . . . .0
**Salt, seasoned,** all varieties (*McCormick*), ¼ tsp. . . . . . . . .0
**Sandwich sauce,** ¼ cup, except as noted:
(*Durkee Famous*), 1 tbsp. . . . . . . . . . . . . . . . . . . . . . . .60
sloppy Joe (*Del Monte* Original) . . . . . . . . . . . . . . . . . . .50
sloppy Joe (*Heinz*), ½ cup . . . . . . . . . . . . . . . . . . . . . .70
sloppy Joe (*Hormel Not-So-Sloppy Joe*) . . . . . . . . . . . . . . .60
sloppy Joe (*Libby's*), ⅓ cup . . . . . . . . . . . . . . . . . . . . .50
sloppy Joe (*Manwich* Original) . . . . . . . . . . . . . . . . . . . .30
sloppy Joe, hickory flavor (*Del Monte*) . . . . . . . . . . . . . . .70
**Sandwich sauce seasoning mix,** see "Sloppy Joe seasoning mix"
**Sandwich spread** (see also specific listings):
(*Hellmann's/Best Foods*), 1 tbsp. . . . . . . . . . . . . . . . . . .50
(*Kraft*), 1 tbsp. . . . . . . . . . . . . . . . . . . . . . . . . . . . .50
(*Loma Linda*), ¼ cup . . . . . . . . . . . . . . . . . . . . . . . . .80
**Sapodilla,** 1 medium, 3" × 2½" . . . . . . . . . . . . . . . . . . .140
**Sapote** (*Frieda's*), 5 oz. . . . . . . . . . . . . . . . . . . . . . .190
**Sardine,** fresh, see "Herring"
**Sardine, canned:**
Atlantic, in oil, 2 medium, 3" long . . . . . . . . . . . . . . . . . .50
in hot sauce (*Chicken of the Sea* Brisling), 3.75-oz. can . . .220
in mustard (*Chicken of the Sea* Brisling), 3.75-oz. can . . . .260
in mustard (*Crown Prince*), ⅓ cup . . . . . . . . . . . . . . . . . .90
in mustard (*Underwood*), 1 can . . . . . . . . . . . . . . . . . . .180
in olive oil, drained:
(*Crown Prince*), 1 can . . . . . . . . . . . . . . . . . . . . . . . .210
(*Crown Prince Natural* Brisling 2-Layer), 1 can . . . . . . .290

skin/boneless (*Crown Prince*), 6 pcs. . . . . . . . . . . . . . . .230
skin/boneless (*Granadaisa*), ¼ cup . . . . . . . . . . . . . . . . .120
in soy oil, drained (*Crown Prince*), 1 can . . . . . . . . . . . . . . .210
in soy oil, drained (*Crown Prince* No Salt), 1 can . . . . . . . .230
in tomato sauce (*Chicken of the Sea* Oval), 5 oz. . . . . . . . . . .110
in tomato sauce (*Crown Prince* Brisling), 3.75-oz. can . . . .210
in tomato sauce (*Crown Prince* Oval), ⅓ cup . . . . . . . . . . . .80
in water (*Chicken of the Sea* Brisling), 2.9 oz. . . . . . . . . . . .150
**Sauce** (see also specific sauce listings), all purpose:
(*Aunt Nellie's* Old Style), 1 tbsp. . . . . . . . . . . . . . . . . . . . . .70
(*Silver Dollar City*), 2 tbsp. . . . . . . . . . . . . . . . . . . . . . . . .30
**Sauerkraut,** 2 tbsp.:
(*Bush's Best*) . . . . . . . . . . . . . . . . . . . . . . . . . . . . . . . . . .5
(*Cascadian Farm* Old World/Low Sodium) . . . . . . . . . . . . . .5
(*Del Monte*) . . . . . . . . . . . . . . . . . . . . . . . . . . . . . . . . . . . .0
(*Hebrew National*) . . . . . . . . . . . . . . . . . . . . . . . . . . . . . . .5
(*Libby's*) . . . . . . . . . . . . . . . . . . . . . . . . . . . . . . . . . . . . .5
(*Silver Floss*) . . . . . . . . . . . . . . . . . . . . . . . . . . . . . . . . . .5
Bavarian (*Bush's Best*) . . . . . . . . . . . . . . . . . . . . . . . . . . .15
Bavarian (*Del Monte*) . . . . . . . . . . . . . . . . . . . . . . . . . . . .15
**Sauerkraut juice** (*Bush's Best*), 8 fl. oz. . . . . . . . . . . . . . . .15
**Sausage** (see also specific listings), cooked, except
as noted:
beef, hot (*Johnsonville* Hot Links), 2.7 oz. . . . . . . . . . . . . .230
beef, smoked (*Healthy Choice*), 2 oz. . . . . . . . . . . . . . . . . . .80
beef, smoked (*Thorn Apple Valley*), 3.2-oz. link . . . . . . . . .290
brown and serve (*Little Sizzlers*), 3 links . . . . . . . . . . . . . .230
brown and serve (*Little Sizzlers*), 2 patties . . . . . . . . . . . .190
cheese, smoked:
(*Johnsonville Beddar with Cheddar*), 2.7-oz. link . . . . . .240
(*Oscar Mayer* Little Smokies), 6 links . . . . . . . . . . . . . .180
(*Oscar Mayer* Smokies), 1 link . . . . . . . . . . . . . . . . . . . .130
(*Thorn Apple Valley*), 3.2-oz. link . . . . . . . . . . . . . . . . . .290
chicken, 2-oz. link, except as noted:
Andouille, Cajun style (*Bilinski's*) . . . . . . . . . . . . . . . . . .80
apple, fresh, raw (*Aidell's*) . . . . . . . . . . . . . . . . . . . . . . .100
apple, smoked, cocktail (*Aidell's*), 6 links, 2 oz. . . . . . . .100
apple and Chardonnay (*Bilinski's*) . . . . . . . . . . . . . . . . . . .70
apple or lemon, smoked (*Aidell's*), 3.5-oz. link . . . . . . . .210
cilantro or jalapeño (*Bilinski's*) . . . . . . . . . . . . . . . . . . . .70

**Sausage, chicken *(cont.)***
pesto (*Bilinski's*) . . . . . . . . . . . . . . . . . . . . . . . . . . . . .90
spinach or sun-dried tomato (*Bilinski's*) . . . . . . . . . . . . . .70
teriyaki, fresh, raw (*Aidell's*), 3.5-oz. link . . . . . . . . . . . .210
chicken and turkey, 3.5-oz. link, except as noted:
artichoke, smoked (*Aidell's*) . . . . . . . . . . . . . . . . . . . . . .180
curry or pesto, smoked (*Aidell's*) . . . . . . . . . . . . . . . . . .220
habañero (*Aidell's*), 3.2-oz. link . . . . . . . . . . . . . . . . . . .160
smoked (*Aidell's* New Mexico) . . . . . . . . . . . . . . . . . . . .210
sun-dried tomato basil or Thai, fresh, raw (*Aidell's*) . . . .200
chorizo (*Fiorucci* Cantimpalo), 1 oz. . . . . . . . . . . . . . . . . . . .110
chorizo, beef, raw (*Aidell's*), 3.5-oz. link . . . . . . . . . . . . . . .400
chorizo, pork, spicy (*Battisoni*), 1 oz. . . . . . . . . . . . . . . . . . .80
dinner (*Jones Dairy Farm*), 1 link . . . . . . . . . . . . . . . . . . . .150
duck and turkey, smoked (*Aidell's*), 3.5-oz. link . . . . . . . . . .220
garlic (*Johnsonville* Irish O' Garlic), 3-oz. link . . . . . . . . . . .290
garlic (*Trois Petits Cochons* Saucisson à l'Ail), 2 oz. . . . . . . .80
Italian, chicken, mild or hot (*Bilinski's*), 2 oz. . . . . . . . . . . . .70
Italian, dry (*Boar's Head*), 1 oz. . . . . . . . . . . . . . . . . . . . . .100
Italian, pork, grilled, (*Johnsonville* Fresh), 1 link . . . . . . . . .290
Italian, pork, mild (*Johnsonville* Cooked), 1 link . . . . . . . . .240
Italian, pork, raw (*Aidell's*), 3.5-oz. link . . . . . . . . . . . . . . . .230
Italian, turkey, hot or sweet, cooked (*Perdue*), 1 link . . . . . .150
Italian style, ground, grilled (*Johnsonville*), 2.5 oz. . . . . . . .240
lamb and beef, w/rosemary, fresh, raw (*Aidell's*),
3.5-oz. link . . . . . . . . . . . . . . . . . . . . . . . . . . . . . . . . . .220
maple flavor (*Johnsonville* Vermont), 3 links . . . . . . . . . . .200
pickled, smoked or hot (*Hormel*), 6 links . . . . . . . . . . . . . .140
pork (*Little Sizzlers*), 3 links or 2 patties . . . . . . . . . . . . . .230
pork (*Oscar Mayer Little Friers*), 2 links . . . . . . . . . . . . . . .180
pork, brown sugar and honey (*Johnsonville*), 3 links . . . . .190
pork, ground, seasoned, raw (*Johnsonville*), 2.5 oz. . . . . . .210
pork, smoked, Andouille (*Aidell's* Cajun), 3.5-oz. link . . . . .220
pork, smoked, whiskey fennel (*Aidell's*), 3.5-oz. link . . . . . .220
pork and turkey (*Healthy Choice*), 2 links or 1 patty . . . . . . .50
pork and veal, smoked, (*Aidell's* Bier), 3.5-oz. link . . . . . . .240
smoked (*Boar's Head*), 4.6-oz. link . . . . . . . . . . . . . . . . . . .360
smoked (*Johnsonville*), 2.7-oz. link . . . . . . . . . . . . . . . . . .240
smoked (*Johnsonville* Little Smokies), 6 links, 2 oz. . . . . . .180
smoked (*Thorn Apple Valley*), 3.2-oz. link . . . . . . . . . . . . .280

smoked, hot (*Boar's Head* Skinless), 3.2 oz. . . . . . . . . . . . . .250
smoked, turkey (*Jennie-O*), 2 oz. . . . . . . . . . . . . . . . . . . . . . .70
turkey, raw, except as noted:
(*Jennie-O Breakfast Lover's*), 1 link . . . . . . . . . . . . . . . .130
(*Jennie-O Breakfast Lover's* Patties), 2 oz. . . . . . . . . . . . .130
(*Shady Brook Farms* Breakfast), 2 links . . . . . . . . . . . . . . .80
(*Shady Brook Farms* Dinner), 1 link . . . . . . . . . . . . . . . .190
(*Wampler* Breakfast), 4 oz. . . . . . . . . . . . . . . . . . . . . . .230
cranberry, smoked (*Aidell's*), 3.5-oz. link . . . . . . . . . . . .210
maple (*Shady Brook Farms* Breakfast), 1 link . . . . . . . . .100
w/scallions and herbs, fresh (*Aidell's*), 3.5-oz. link . . . . .200
turkey and chicken, see "chicken and turkey," above
**Sausage, canned:**
Polish (*Maxwell Street*), 2 oz. . . . . . . . . . . . . . . . . . . . . . .170
smoked (*Vienna*), 2 oz. . . . . . . . . . . . . . . . . . . . . . . . . . .150
Vienna (*Armour*), 3 links . . . . . . . . . . . . . . . . . . . . . . . . .150
Vienna, chicken (*Libby's*), 3 links . . . . . . . . . . . . . . . . . . .100
**Sausage, frozen,** Italian (*Rosina* Bites), 4 pcs., 2 oz. . . . . .180
**"Sausage," vegetarian,** frozen:
(*Boca* Breakfast), 2 links . . . . . . . . . . . . . . . . . . . . . . . .100
(*Boca* Breakfast), 1 patty . . . . . . . . . . . . . . . . . . . . . . . . .60
(*Morningstar Farms* Breakfast), 2 links . . . . . . . . . . . . . . .60
(*Morningstar Farms* Breakfast), 1 patty . . . . . . . . . . . . . . .80
(*Yves* Breakfast Links), 1.75 oz. . . . . . . . . . . . . . . . . . . . .60
(*Yves* Breakfast Patties), 2 oz. . . . . . . . . . . . . . . . . . . . . .70
bits (*Morningstar Farms* Crumbles), ⅔ cup . . . . . . . . . . . .90
Italian (*Boca*), 1 link . . . . . . . . . . . . . . . . . . . . . . . . . . .120
smoked (*Boca*), 1 link . . . . . . . . . . . . . . . . . . . . . . . . . .130
**Sausage hash,** canned (*Mary Kitchen*), 1 cup . . . . . . . . . .410
**Sausage stick:**
(*Johnsonville* Snack Stix), 1 oz. . . . . . . . . . . . . . . . . . . . .120
beef jerky, hickory-smoked, peppered, teriyaki, or sweet
mesquite (*Pemmican*), 1 oz. . . . . . . . . . . . . . . . . . . . . . . .70
beef jerky, sweet and hot (*Pemmican*), 1 oz. . . . . . . . . . . . .80
hot (*Rustler's Flamin' Hot*) . . . . . . . . . . . . . . . . . . . . . . . . .40
smoked (*Rustler's* Steak Strip), .8 oz. . . . . . . . . . . . . . . . . .60
spicy (*Rustler's*), .3 oz. . . . . . . . . . . . . . . . . . . . . . . . . . .50
spicy (*Rustler's*), .5 oz. . . . . . . . . . . . . . . . . . . . . . . . . . .70
turkey, peppered (*Pemmican*), 1 oz. . . . . . . . . . . . . . . . . . .60
turkey, sweet smoked (*Pemmican*), 1 oz. . . . . . . . . . . . . . . .70

**Sausage biscuit,** see "Breakfast sandwich"
**Savory,** ground, 1 tsp. . . . . . . . . . . . . . . . . . . . . . . . . . . . . .4
**Scallion,** see "Onion, green"
**Scallop,** meat only:
raw, 4 oz. . . . . . . . . . . . . . . . . . . . . . . . . . . . . . . . . . . .100
raw, 2 large or 5 small, 1.1 oz. . . . . . . . . . . . . . . . . . . . . . . .26
**Scallop, frozen** (*Contessa*), 4 oz., 1 cup . . . . . . . . . . . . . . . .80
**"Scallop," imitation,** frozen, bay style (*Louis Kemp Scallop Delights*), ½ cup, 3 oz. . . . . . . . . . . . . . . . . . . . . . .80
**Scallop, smoked** (*Ducktrap River*), ¼ cup . . . . . . . . . . . . . .60
**Scallop entree,** frozen:
fried (*Mrs. Paul's*), 13 pcs., 3.75 oz. . . . . . . . . . . . . . . . . . .220
stuffed w/seafood (*Oceans Cuisine*), 3.5 oz. . . . . . . . . . . . .200
**Scallop squash,** boiled, drained, sliced, ½ cup . . . . . . . . . .14
**Scampi sauce,** in jars (*Zatarain's*), 1 tbsp. . . . . . . . . . . . . . . .5
**Scone,** all fruit varieties (*Health Valley* Fat Free), 2.1-oz. pc. . . . . . . . . . . . . . . . . . . . . . . . . . . . . . . . . .180
**Scrapple** (*Dietz & Watson*), 2 oz. . . . . . . . . . . . . . . . . . . . .150
**Scrod,** fresh, see "Cod, Atlantic"
**Scup,** meat only:
raw, 4 oz. . . . . . . . . . . . . . . . . . . . . . . . . . . . . . . . . . . .119
baked, broiled, or microwaved, 4 oz. . . . . . . . . . . . . . . . . . .153
**Sea bass,** meat only:
raw, 4 oz. . . . . . . . . . . . . . . . . . . . . . . . . . . . . . . . . . . .110
baked, broiled, or microwaved, 4 oz. . . . . . . . . . . . . . . . . . .141
**Sea Breeze drink mixer** (*Mr & Mrs T*), 4 fl. oz. . . . . . . . . . .80
**Sea trout,** meat only:
raw, 4 oz. . . . . . . . . . . . . . . . . . . . . . . . . . . . . . . . . . . .118
baked, broiled, or microwaved, 4 oz. . . . . . . . . . . . . . . . . . .151
**Seafood,** see specific listings
**Seafood sauce** (see also specific listings), cocktail, ¼ cup:
(*Del Monte*) . . . . . . . . . . . . . . . . . . . . . . . . . . . . . . . . . .100
(*Golden Dipt*) . . . . . . . . . . . . . . . . . . . . . . . . . . . . . . . .100
(*Old Bay*) . . . . . . . . . . . . . . . . . . . . . . . . . . . . . . . . . . .110
(*Red Gold*) . . . . . . . . . . . . . . . . . . . . . . . . . . . . . . . . . . .70
hot, extra (*Golden Dipt*) . . . . . . . . . . . . . . . . . . . . . . . . . .100
**Seafood seasoning,** see "Fish seasoning and coating mix" and specific listings
**Seafood stuffing,** frozen (*Massachusetts Bay Clam Co.*), 1 oz. . . . . . . . . . . . . . . . . . . . . . . . . . . . . . . . . . . . . .80

**Seasoning,** see specific listings
**Seaweed:**
agar, flakes or bar (*Eden*), 1 tbsp. . . . . . . . . . . . . . . . . . . . . . .10
arame or hiziki (*Eden*), ½ cup . . . . . . . . . . . . . . . . . . . . . . .30
kombu (*Eden*), ½ of 7" pc. . . . . . . . . . . . . . . . . . . . . . . . . .10
nori (*Sushi Chef*), 1 sheet . . . . . . . . . . . . . . . . . . . . . . . .10
wakame (*Eden*), ½ cup . . . . . . . . . . . . . . . . . . . . . . . . . .25
**Semolina,** whole-grain, 1 cup . . . . . . . . . . . . . . . . . . . . .601
**Semolina flour,** mix (*Arrowhead Mills*), ½ cup . . . . . . . . . .240
**Sesame paste** (see also "Tahini"), whole seed,
1 tbsp. . . . . . . . . . . . . . . . . . . . . . . . . . . . . . . . . . . .95
**Sesame seasoning** (*Eden* Shake), ½ tsp. . . . . . . . . . . . . . . .10
**Sesame seeds:**
whole, brown (*Arrowhead Mills*), ¼ cup . . . . . . . . . . . . . . .200
whole, dried, 1 tbsp. . . . . . . . . . . . . . . . . . . . . . . . . . . . .52
kernels, decorticated (*Arrowhead Mills*), ¼ cup . . . . . . . . . .210
kernels, toasted, 1 oz. . . . . . . . . . . . . . . . . . . . . . . . . . .160
**Shad,** meat only:
raw, 4 oz. . . . . . . . . . . . . . . . . . . . . . . . . . . . . . . . . . .223
baked, broiled, or microwaved, 4 oz. . . . . . . . . . . . . . . . . .286
**Shallot,** fresh:
(*Frieda's*), 1 tbsp., 1 oz. . . . . . . . . . . . . . . . . . . . . . . . .20
chopped, 1 tbsp. . . . . . . . . . . . . . . . . . . . . . . . . . . . . . . .7
**Shallot, freeze-dried,** 1 tbsp. . . . . . . . . . . . . . . . . . . . . . .3
**Shark,** meat only, raw, 4 oz. . . . . . . . . . . . . . . . . . . . . . .148
**Sheepshead,** meat only:
raw, 4 oz. . . . . . . . . . . . . . . . . . . . . . . . . . . . . . . . . . .123
baked, broiled, or microwaved, 4 oz. . . . . . . . . . . . . . . . . .143
**Shells, pasta, mix:**
and cheddar, white (*Pasta Roni*), 1 cup* . . . . . . . . . . . . . . .310
w/cheese, creamy (*Land O Lakes*), 3.5 oz. . . . . . . . . . . . . .350
**Shells, pasta, entree,** frozen, 1 pkg., except as noted:
and American cheese (*Stouffer's*), ½ of 12-oz. pkg. . . . . . .280
and cheese w/jalapeños (*Michelina's*), 8 oz. . . . . . . . . . . .350
and cheese sauce (*Freezer Queen* Meal), 8.5 oz. . . . . . . . . .270
stuffed, broccoli (*Celentano*), 10 oz. . . . . . . . . . . . . . . . . .230
stuffed, cheese (*Celentano*), 10 oz. . . . . . . . . . . . . . . . . . .320
stuffed, cheese (*Celentano* Low Fat), 10 oz. . . . . . . . . . . . .250
stuffed, cheese, no sauce (*Celentano*), 4 pcs., ½ of
12.5-oz. pkg. . . . . . . . . . . . . . . . . . . . . . . . . . . . . . . . .320

**Sherbet** (see also "Sorbet"), ½ cup, except as noted:
all flavors, except cherry chip (*Darigold*) . . . . . . . . . . . . . . .120
all flavors, except pineapple (*Blue Bell*) . . . . . . . . . . . . . . . .130
cherry chip (*Darigold*) . . . . . . . . . . . . . . . . . . . . . . . . . . . . .130
lemon bar or Swiss orange (*Dreyer's/Edy's*) . . . . . . . . . . . .150
orange (*Turkey Hill* Grove) . . . . . . . . . . . . . . . . . . . . . . . . .120
orange and vanilla ice cream (*Breyers* Take Two) . . . . . . . .130
orange and vanilla ice cream swirl (*Dreyer's/Edy's*) . . . . . . .120
orange or rainbow (*Breyers*) . . . . . . . . . . . . . . . . . . . . . . . .130
pineapple (*Blue Bell*) . . . . . . . . . . . . . . . . . . . . . . . . . . . . .120
rainbow, fruit (*Turkey Hill*) . . . . . . . . . . . . . . . . . . . . . . . . .120
rainbow, tropical (*Dreyer's/Edy's*) . . . . . . . . . . . . . . . . . . . .130
strawberry (*Dreyer's/Edy's Starburst*) . . . . . . . . . . . . . . . . .160
**Sherbet bar** (see also "Iced confection bar"), 1 bar:
(*Popsicle* Cyclone) . . . . . . . . . . . . . . . . . . . . . . . . . . . . . . .50
all flavors (*Creamsicle* No Sugar) . . . . . . . . . . . . . . . . . . . . .25
orange (*Good Humor Pop-Ups*) . . . . . . . . . . . . . . . . . . . . . . .80
w/vanilla ice cream:
  orange (*Creamsicle* Single) . . . . . . . . . . . . . . . . . . . . . . .120
  orange raspberry (*Creamsicle*), 2.75 fl. oz. . . . . . . . . . . .110
  orange raspberry (*Creamsicle* Pop), 1.75 fl. oz. . . . . . . . . .80
rainbow (*Good Humor Pop-Ups*) . . . . . . . . . . . . . . . . . . . . . .90
**Shortening,** 1 tbsp. . . . . . . . . . . . . . . . . . . . . . . . . . . . . .110
**Shrimp,** meat only:
raw, 4 oz. . . . . . . . . . . . . . . . . . . . . . . . . . . . . . . . . . . . . .120
raw, 4 large, 1 oz. . . . . . . . . . . . . . . . . . . . . . . . . . . . . . . .30
boiled or steamed, 4 oz. . . . . . . . . . . . . . . . . . . . . . . . . . . .112
boiled or steamed, 4 large, .8 oz. . . . . . . . . . . . . . . . . . . . . .22
**Shrimp, canned:**
(*Crown Prince Natural*), ½ can, 2.1 oz. . . . . . . . . . . . . . . .120
medium (*Bumble Bee*), 2 oz. . . . . . . . . . . . . . . . . . . . . . . . .45
medium, small, or tiny (*Chicken of the Sea*), 2 oz. . . . . . . . .45
tiny (*3 Diamonds*), 2 oz. . . . . . . . . . . . . . . . . . . . . . . . . . . .55
tiny or broken (*Crown Prince*), ½ can, 2.1 oz. . . . . . . . . . . .60
drained, 1 cup . . . . . . . . . . . . . . . . . . . . . . . . . . . . . . . . . .154
**Shrimp, frozen:**
raw (*Contessa*), 4 oz. . . . . . . . . . . . . . . . . . . . . . . . . . . . . .70
cooked (*Contessa*), 4 oz. . . . . . . . . . . . . . . . . . . . . . . . . . .60
cooked, w/sauce (*Contessa Party Platter*), 3.75 oz. . . . . . . . .80
**"Shrimp," imitation,** from surimi, 4 oz. . . . . . . . . . . . . . . .115

**Shrimp, smoked** (*Ducktrap River*), ¼ cup . . . . . . . . . . . . . .60
**Shrimp dinner,** frozen, and vegetables (*Healthy Choice*), 11.8 oz. . . . . . . . . . . . . . . . . . . . . . . . . . . . . . . .270
**Shrimp entree, frozen:**
Alfredo, w/fettuccine (*Michelina's*), 8 oz. . . . . . . . . . . . . . . .310
w/angel-hair pasta (*Lean Cuisine Cafe Classics*), 10 oz. . . . . . . . . . . . . . . . . . . . . . . . . . . . . . . . . .280
Buffalo (*Mrs. Paul's/Van de Kamps*), 20 pcs., 4 oz. . . . . . . .320
butterfly (*Mrs. Paul's*), 7 pcs. . . . . . . . . . . . . . . . . . . . . .270
butterfly (*Van de Kamp's*), 7 pcs. . . . . . . . . . . . . . . . . . . .300
Cajun sauce (*Contessa Shrimp on the Bar-B*), ¼ of 24-oz. pkg. . . . . . . . . . . . . . . . . . . . . . . . . . . .140
fantail, breaded (*Mrs. Friday's*), 4 oz., about 7 pcs. . . . . . . .300
fried rice (*Yu Sing*), 8 oz. . . . . . . . . . . . . . . . . . . . . . . . . .350
herb sauce, Italian (*Contessa Shrimp on the Bar-B*), ¼ of 24-oz. pkg. . . . . . . . . . . . . . . . . . . . . . . . . . . .150
w/linguine (*Contessa* Mediterranean), 1⅓ cups . . . . . . . . .170
w/linguine (*Mrs. Paul's*), 1½ cups . . . . . . . . . . . . . . . . . . .180
lo mein (*Yu Sing*), 8 oz. . . . . . . . . . . . . . . . . . . . . . . . . . .210
popcorn (*Gorton's*), 3.6 oz., about 22 pcs. . . . . . . . . . . . . .250
popcorn (*Mrs. Paul's*), 20 pcs. . . . . . . . . . . . . . . . . . . . . .290
popcorn (*Van de Kamp's*), 20 pcs. . . . . . . . . . . . . . . . . . . .270
popcorn garlic and herb (*Gorton's*), 3.2 oz., 20 pcs. . . . . . .240
scampi (*Contessa*), ⅓ of 12-oz. pkg. . . . . . . . . . . . . . . . . .340
stir-fry (*Contessa*), 1¾ cups . . . . . . . . . . . . . . . . . . . . . .140
stir-fry (*Mrs. Paul's/Van de Kamp's*), 1⅔ cups . . . . . . . . . .260
stuffed (*Van de Kamp's*), 3 pcs., 4.5 oz. . . . . . . . . . . . . . . .290
sweet and sour (*Contessa*), 1½ cups . . . . . . . . . . . . . . . . .180
**Shrimp sauce** (*Crosse & Blackwell*), ¼ cup . . . . . . . . . . . .110
**Sloppy Joe sauce,** see "Sandwich sauce"
**Sloppy Joe seasoning mix:**
(*Lawry's*), 2 tsp. . . . . . . . . . . . . . . . . . . . . . . . . . . . . . . .20
(*Manwich*), ¼ oz. . . . . . . . . . . . . . . . . . . . . . . . . . . . . . .20
(*McCormick*), ⅛ pkg. . . . . . . . . . . . . . . . . . . . . . . . . . . .15
**Smelt,** rainbow, meat only:
raw, 4 oz. . . . . . . . . . . . . . . . . . . . . . . . . . . . . . . . . . . .110
baked, broiled, or microwaved, 4 oz. . . . . . . . . . . . . . . . .141
**Smoothie mix,** dry, all flavors (*McCormick Produce Partners*), ⅓ pkt. . . . . . . . . . . . . . . . . . . . . . . . . . . . .80
**Snack bar,** see "Cookie" and "Granola and Cereal bar"

**Snack chips and crisps** (see also specific listings), 1 oz.:
multigrain (*Garden of Eatin' Garden Grains*) . . . . . . . . . . . .150
multigrain, all flavors (*Sunchips*) . . . . . . . . . . . . . . . . . . . .140
onion flavor (*Funyuns*) . . . . . . . . . . . . . . . . . . . . . . . . . . .140
onion-flavor rings (*Utz*) . . . . . . . . . . . . . . . . . . . . . . . . .140
**Snack mix,** ½ cup, except as noted:
(*Cheez-It* Big Crunch/Double Cheese), ¾ cup . . . . . . . . . . .110
(*Cheez-It* Get Nutty) . . . . . . . . . . . . . . . . . . . . . . . . . . . .150
(*Cheez-It* Party Mix) . . . . . . . . . . . . . . . . . . . . . . . . . . . .140
(*Cheez-It/Cheez-It* Blitz Mix/Hoops Edition) . . . . . . . . . . . . .130
(*Chex* Bold Party Blend/Cheddar/Peanut Lover's) . . . . . . . .140
(*Chex* Traditional), ⅔ cup . . . . . . . . . . . . . . . . . . . . . . . .130
(*Doo Dads*) . . . . . . . . . . . . . . . . . . . . . . . . . . . . . . . . . .150
(*Gardetto's Snak•ens*) . . . . . . . . . . . . . . . . . . . . . . . . . . .160
(*Gardetto's Snak•ens* Reduced Fat) . . . . . . . . . . . . . . . . . .130
(*Ritz/Ritz* Cheddar) . . . . . . . . . . . . . . . . . . . . . . . . . . . . .150
(*Rold Gold*), ¾ cup . . . . . . . . . . . . . . . . . . . . . . . . . . . . .160
cheese, Italian blend (*Gardetto's*) . . . . . . . . . . . . . . . . . . .140
honey, toasted (*Wheatables*) . . . . . . . . . . . . . . . . . . . . . .130
honey nut (*Chex*) . . . . . . . . . . . . . . . . . . . . . . . . . . . . . . .130
hot and spicy (*Chex*), ⅔ cup . . . . . . . . . . . . . . . . . . . . . .130
Italian recipe (*Gardetto's*) . . . . . . . . . . . . . . . . . . . . . . . .150
nacho fiesta (*Chex*), ⅔ cup . . . . . . . . . . . . . . . . . . . . . . .120
peanut butter crunch (*Wheatables*) . . . . . . . . . . . . . . . . . .160
pretzel, mustard (*Gardetto's*) . . . . . . . . . . . . . . . . . . . . . .130
rice cracker (*Sushi Chef*) . . . . . . . . . . . . . . . . . . . . . . . . .140
**Snail, sea,** see "Whelk"
**Snap beans** (see also "Green beans"), all varieties
(*Frieda's*), ⅔ cup, 3 oz. . . . . . . . . . . . . . . . . . . . . . . . . . .25
**Snapper,** meat only:
raw, 4 oz. . . . . . . . . . . . . . . . . . . . . . . . . . . . . . . . . . . . .113
baked, broiled, or microwaved, 4 oz. . . . . . . . . . . . . . . . . .145
**Snow pea,** see "Peas, edible pod"
**Snow pea sprouts,** fresh (*Jonathan's*), 1 cup . . . . . . . . . . .40
**Soft drinks,** carbonated, 8 fl. oz., except as noted:
all flavors, except orange mango (*Koala*) . . . . . . . . . . . . . . .90
apple raspberry (*Fruitworks*), 12 fl. oz. . . . . . . . . . . . . . . .160
birch beer (*Pennsylvania Dutch*) . . . . . . . . . . . . . . . . . . . .110
blackberry (*Clearly Canadian*) . . . . . . . . . . . . . . . . . . . . . .100
cherry (*Clearly Canadian*) . . . . . . . . . . . . . . . . . . . . . . . . .80

cherry (*Sundrop*) . . . . . . . . . . . . . . . . . . . . . . . . . . . . .120
cherry, black (*IBC*) . . . . . . . . . . . . . . . . . . . . . . . . . . .120
cherry, cream (*Stewart's*), 12 fl. oz. . . . . . . . . . . . . . . . . . .190
cherry, lime (*Slice*), 12 fl. oz. . . . . . . . . . . . . . . . . . . . . .160
cherry spice (*Slice*), 12 fl. oz. . . . . . . . . . . . . . . . . . . . . .150
chocolate (*Hershey's*) . . . . . . . . . . . . . . . . . . . . . . . . . . .120
citrus (*Citra*) . . . . . . . . . . . . . . . . . . . . . . . . . . . . . . .90
club soda (*Canada Dry/Schweppes*) . . . . . . . . . . . . . . . . . . . .0
cola (*Coca-Cola* Classic/Caffeine Free/Cherry) . . . . . . . . . . .100
cola (*Coca-Cola* Classic/Caffeine Free), 12 fl. oz. . . . . . . . . .150
cola (*Pepsi/Pepsi* Caffeine Free), 12 fl. oz. . . . . . . . . . . . .150
cola (*Slice*), 12 fl. oz. . . . . . . . . . . . . . . . . . . . . . . . . .160
cola, cherry, wild (*Pepsi*), 12 fl. oz. . . . . . . . . . . . . . . . .160
Collins mixer (*Canada Dry/Schweppes*) . . . . . . . . . . . . . . . .100
cream (*Hires*) . . . . . . . . . . . . . . . . . . . . . . . . . . . . . . .120
cream (*Mug*), 12 fl. oz. . . . . . . . . . . . . . . . . . . . . . . . . .170
(*Dr Pepper*) . . . . . . . . . . . . . . . . . . . . . . . . . . . . . . . .100
(*Dr. Slice*), 12 fl. oz. . . . . . . . . . . . . . . . . . . . . . . . . .140
fruit punch (*Hawaiian Punch* Fruit Juicy Red) . . . . . . . . . . .130
fruit punch (*Slice*), 12 fl. oz. . . . . . . . . . . . . . . . . . . . . .190
fruit punch (*Tahitian Treat*) . . . . . . . . . . . . . . . . . . . . . .110
ginger ale (*Canada Dry*) . . . . . . . . . . . . . . . . . . . . . . . . . .90
ginger ale (*Schweppes*) . . . . . . . . . . . . . . . . . . . . . . . . . .80
ginger ale (*Vernors*), 12 fl. oz. . . . . . . . . . . . . . . . . . . . . .150
ginger ale, cranberry (*Canada Dry*) . . . . . . . . . . . . . . . . . . .90
ginger beer (*Stewart's*), 12 fl. oz. . . . . . . . . . . . . . . . . . . .200
grape (*Minute Maid*) . . . . . . . . . . . . . . . . . . . . . . . . . . . .130
grape (*Slice*), 12 fl. oz. . . . . . . . . . . . . . . . . . . . . . . . . .190
grape (*Welch's*) . . . . . . . . . . . . . . . . . . . . . . . . . . . . . .130
grape, white (*Clearly Canadian*) . . . . . . . . . . . . . . . . . . . . .90
grapefruit (*Wink*) . . . . . . . . . . . . . . . . . . . . . . . . . . . . .110
grapefruit kiwi lime (*Koala*) . . . . . . . . . . . . . . . . . . . . . . .90
guava berry (*Fruitworks*), 12 fl. oz. . . . . . . . . . . . . . . . . . .170
lemon, bitter (*Schweppes*) . . . . . . . . . . . . . . . . . . . . . . . .110
lemon ginger (*tré limone*) . . . . . . . . . . . . . . . . . . . . . . . . .90
lemonade (*Country Time*) . . . . . . . . . . . . . . . . . . . . . . . . . .90
lemonade, pink (*Fruitworks*), 12 fl. oz. . . . . . . . . . . . . . . . .170
(*Mountain Dew/Mountain Dew Code Red*), 12 fl. oz. . . . . . .170
orange (*Crush*) . . . . . . . . . . . . . . . . . . . . . . . . . . . . . . .120
orange (*Minute Maid*) . . . . . . . . . . . . . . . . . . . . . . . . . . .120

**Soft drinks** ***(cont.)***
orange (*Slice*), 12 fl. oz. . . . . . . . . . . . . . . . . . . . . . . . . .190
orange (*Sunkist*) . . . . . . . . . . . . . . . . . . . . . . . . . . . . . . .130
orange cream (*Stewart's*), 12 fl. oz. . . . . . . . . . . . . . . . . . .190
orange mango (*Koala*) . . . . . . . . . . . . . . . . . . . . . . . . . . . .80
orange passion fruit (*Fruitworks*), 12 fl. oz. . . . . . . . . . . . . .160
peach papaya (*Fruitworks*), 12 fl. oz. . . . . . . . . . . . . . . . . .170
pineapple (*Slice*), 12 fl. oz. . . . . . . . . . . . . . . . . . . . . . . .190
raspberry cream (*Clearly Canadian*) . . . . . . . . . . . . . . . . . . .75
root beer (*A&W*) . . . . . . . . . . . . . . . . . . . . . . . . . . . . . . .120
root beer (*Barq's/Barq's* Caffeine Free) . . . . . . . . . . . . . . .100
root beer (*Hires*) . . . . . . . . . . . . . . . . . . . . . . . . . . . . . . .120
root beer (*IBC*) . . . . . . . . . . . . . . . . . . . . . . . . . . . . . . . .110
root beer (*Mug*), 12 fl. oz. . . . . . . . . . . . . . . . . . . . . . . . .160
seltzer, plain or flavored (*Canada Dry/Schweppes*) . . . . . . . . .0
(*7Up/7Up* Cherry) . . . . . . . . . . . . . . . . . . . . . . . . . . . . . .100
(*Sierra Mist*), 12 fl. oz. . . . . . . . . . . . . . . . . . . . . . . . . . .150
(*Slice* Red), 12 fl. oz. . . . . . . . . . . . . . . . . . . . . . . . . . . .190
(*Sprite*) . . . . . . . . . . . . . . . . . . . . . . . . . . . . . . . . . . . . .100
(*Squirt*) . . . . . . . . . . . . . . . . . . . . . . . . . . . . . . . . . . . . .100
(*Squirt* Ruby Red) . . . . . . . . . . . . . . . . . . . . . . . . . . . . . .120
strawberry (*Slice*), 12 fl. oz. . . . . . . . . . . . . . . . . . . . . . . .170
strawberry melon (*Clearly Canadian*) . . . . . . . . . . . . . . . . . .80
strawberry melon (*Fruitworks*), 12 fl. oz. . . . . . . . . . . . . . .160
(*Sundrop*) . . . . . . . . . . . . . . . . . . . . . . . . . . . . . . . . . . .130
tangerine citrus (*Fruitworks*), 12 fl. oz. . . . . . . . . . . . . . . .150
tonic (*Canada Dry*) . . . . . . . . . . . . . . . . . . . . . . . . . . . . .100
tonic (*Schweppes*) . . . . . . . . . . . . . . . . . . . . . . . . . . . . . . .80
(*Vernors*) . . . . . . . . . . . . . . . . . . . . . . . . . . . . . . . . . . . .100
**Sole,** fresh, see "Flatfish"
**Sole entree,** frozen, 5-oz. pc., except as noted:
au gratin (*Oven Poppers*) . . . . . . . . . . . . . . . . . . . . . . . . . .220
w/shrimp and lobster, Newburg sauce (*Oven Poppers*) . . . .130
stuffed:
  broccoli/cheese or shrimp/lobster (*Oven Poppers*) . . . . .150
  crab or garlic/shrimp/almonds (*Oven Poppers*) . . . . . . .250
  w/crab, miniatures (*Oven Poppers*), 2-oz. pc. . . . . . . . .120
**Sopressata sausage:**
(*Boar's Head* Calabrese/Grande/Veneta), 1 oz. . . . . . . . . . .100

(*Citterio* Salame), 6 slices, 1.1 oz. . . . . . . . . . . . . . . . . . . . .110
(*Citterio Fresco*), 3 slices, 1.1 oz. . . . . . . . . . . . . . . . . . . . .110
**Sorbet** (see also "Sherbet"), ½ cup, except as noted:
berry, mixed (*Sharon's Sorbet*) . . . . . . . . . . . . . . . . . . . . .90
blackberry, raspberry, or strawberry (*Cascadian Farm*) . . . . .80
boysenberry (*Dreyer's/Edy's Whole Fruit*) . . . . . . . . . . . . . .150
chocolate (*Cascadian Farm*) . . . . . . . . . . . . . . . . . . . . . . .100
chocolate (*Häagen-Dazs*) . . . . . . . . . . . . . . . . . . . . . . . . .120
chocolate (*Sharon's Sorbet*) . . . . . . . . . . . . . . . . . . . . . . .130
coconut (*Sharon's Sorbet*) . . . . . . . . . . . . . . . . . . . . . . . .160
and ice cream, all flavors, except orange (*Cascadian Farm*) . . . . . . . . . . . . . . . . . . . . . . . . . . . . . . . . . .110
and ice cream, orange (*Cascadian Farm*) . . . . . . . . . . . . . .120
and ice cream orange swirl (*Dreyer's/Edy's* 50/50) . . . . . . .100
lemon (*Cascadian Farm Luscious Lemon*) . . . . . . . . . . . . . .90
lemon (*Dreyer's/Edy's Whole Fruit*) . . . . . . . . . . . . . . . . .140
lemon (*Häagen-Dazs* Zesty) . . . . . . . . . . . . . . . . . . . . . . .120
lemon (*Sharon's Sorbet*) . . . . . . . . . . . . . . . . . . . . . . . . . .75
mango (*Cascadian Farm Mango Magic*) . . . . . . . . . . . . . . . .90
mango (*Dreyer's Whole Fruit*) . . . . . . . . . . . . . . . . . . . . . .130
mango (*Sharon's Sorbet*) . . . . . . . . . . . . . . . . . . . . . . . . . .80
mango orange or peach (*Edy's Whole Fruit*) . . . . . . . . . . . .130
mango or orange (*Häagen-Dazs*) . . . . . . . . . . . . . . . . . . . .120
passion fruit or raspberry (*Sharon's Sorbet*) . . . . . . . . . . . .80
peach (*Cascadian Farm*) . . . . . . . . . . . . . . . . . . . . . . . . . . .90
peach (*Häagen-Dazs* Orchard) . . . . . . . . . . . . . . . . . . . . . .130
raspberry, strawberry, or tropical (*Häagen-Dazs*) . . . . . . . .120
raspberry or strawberry (*Dreyer's Whole Fruit*) . . . . . . . . . .130
strawberry (*Edy's Whole Fruit*) . . . . . . . . . . . . . . . . . . . . .120
**Sorbet bar** (see also "Fruit bar"), 1 bar:
orange/vanilla and cream (*Häagen-Dazs*) . . . . . . . . . . . . . .120
raspberry/vanilla and yogurt (*Häagen-Dazs*) . . . . . . . . . . . . .90
tangerine (*Dreyer's/Edy's Whole Fruit*) . . . . . . . . . . . . . . . .80
**Sorghum,** whole-grain, 1 cup . . . . . . . . . . . . . . . . . . . . . .650
**Sorghum syrup** (*Arrowhead Mills*), 1 tbsp. . . . . . . . . . . . . .60
**Sorrel,** see "Dock"
**Soup, can or jar, ready-to-serve,** 1 cup, except as noted:
bean, w/bacon (*Campbell's* Classic) . . . . . . . . . . . . . . . . . .170
bean, black (*Hain* Healthy) . . . . . . . . . . . . . . . . . . . . . . . . .90

**Soup, can or jar, ready-to-serve *(cont.)***

bean, black (*Health Valley* Organic) . . . . . . . . . . . . . . . . . . . .130
bean, black (*Progresso* Hearty) . . . . . . . . . . . . . . . . . . . . . . .170
bean, black, vegetable (*Amy's* Organic) . . . . . . . . . . . . . . . . .110
bean, black, vegetable (*Health Valley* Fat Free) . . . . . . . . . . .110
bean, 5, vegetable (*Health Valley* Fat Free) . . . . . . . . . . . . . .140
bean and ham (*Campbell's Chunky/Select*) . . . . . . . . . . . . . .180
bean and ham (*Healthy Choice*) . . . . . . . . . . . . . . . . . . . . . .160
bean, Italian, and pasta (*Healthy Choice*) . . . . . . . . . . . . . . .100
bean, navy (*Sylvia's*) . . . . . . . . . . . . . . . . . . . . . . . . . . . . . .170
bean, w/pasta (*Healthy Choice* Mediterranean) . . . . . . . . . . .120
beef barley (*Progresso*) . . . . . . . . . . . . . . . . . . . . . . . . . . . .130
beef broth (*College Inn* No Fat) . . . . . . . . . . . . . . . . . . . . . . .20
beef broth (*Swanson*) . . . . . . . . . . . . . . . . . . . . . . . . . . . . . . .10
beef broth w/onion (*Swanson*) . . . . . . . . . . . . . . . . . . . . . . . .20
beef mushroom (*Progresso*) . . . . . . . . . . . . . . . . . . . . . . . . .100
beef pasta (*Campbell's Chunky*) . . . . . . . . . . . . . . . . . . . . . .100
beef and potato (*Healthy Choice*) . . . . . . . . . . . . . . . . . . . . .110
beef vegetable (*Progresso*) . . . . . . . . . . . . . . . . . . . . . . . . . .120
beef vegetable (*Progresso* 99% Fat Free) . . . . . . . . . . . . . . .160
beef vegetable, country (*Campbell's Chunky*) . . . . . . . . . . . .180
beef w/white and wild rice (*Campbell's Chunky*) . . . . . . . . . .150
borscht (*Gold's*) . . . . . . . . . . . . . . . . . . . . . . . . . . . . . . . . . .70
broccoli (*Walnut Acres* Homestyle) . . . . . . . . . . . . . . . . . . . .110
broccoli carotene (*Health Valley* Fat Free) . . . . . . . . . . . . . . .70
chicken:
(*Healthy Choice* Fiesta) . . . . . . . . . . . . . . . . . . . . . . . . . . . .90
(*Progresso* Homestyle) . . . . . . . . . . . . . . . . . . . . . . . . . . . .90
grilled, w/sun-dried tomato (*Campbell's* Select) . . . . . . .100
grilled, and vegetables w/pasta (*Campbell's Chunky*) . . .110
roasted, w/vegetables (*Progresso* Garden) . . . . . . . . . . . .70
roasted, w/vegetables (*Progresso* 99% Fat Free) . . . . . . .90
roasted, w/white/wild rice (*Campbell's* Select) . . . . . . . .110
chicken barley (*Progresso*) . . . . . . . . . . . . . . . . . . . . . . . . . .110
chicken broccoli, creamy (*Progresso* 99% Fat Free) . . . . . . .90
chicken broccoli cheese potato (*Campbell's Chunky*) . . . . .190
chicken broth (*Boston Market*) . . . . . . . . . . . . . . . . . . . . . . . .15
chicken broth (*Butterball* Reduced Sodium) . . . . . . . . . . . . .10
chicken broth (*College Inn*) . . . . . . . . . . . . . . . . . . . . . . . . . .10
chicken broth (*Hain* Home Style) . . . . . . . . . . . . . . . . . . . . . .25

chicken broth (*Manischewitz*), ½ cup . . . . . . . . . . . . . . . . . . .15
chicken broth (*Swanson/Swanson Natural Goodness*) . . . . . .15
chicken broth, Italian herb or roasted garlic (*Swanson*) . . . . .20
chicken consommé (*Rokeach*) . . . . . . . . . . . . . . . . . . . . . . .50
chicken corn chowder (*Campbell's Chunky*) . . . . . . . . . . . .240
chicken, w/meatballs (*Progresso Chickarina*) . . . . . . . . . . .130
chicken mushroom chowder (*Campbell's Chunky*) . . . . . . .230
chicken noodle:
  (*Campbell's* Classic) . . . . . . . . . . . . . . . . . . . . . . . . . . . .80
  (*Campbell's Chunky* Classic) . . . . . . . . . . . . . . . . . . . . .130
  (*Campbell's Simply Home*) . . . . . . . . . . . . . . . . . . . . . . .90
  (*Campbell's Soup to Go*), 1 cont. . . . . . . . . . . . . . . . . . . .100
  (*Hain* Home Style) . . . . . . . . . . . . . . . . . . . . . . . . . . . . .150
  (*Hain* Home Style No Salt) . . . . . . . . . . . . . . . . . . . . . .110
  (*Health Valley* 99% Fat Free) . . . . . . . . . . . . . . . . . . . .130
  (*Healthy Choice* Old Fashioned) . . . . . . . . . . . . . . . . . . .120
  egg (*Campbell's* Select) . . . . . . . . . . . . . . . . . . . . . . . . . .90
  egg (*Wolfgang Puck's*) . . . . . . . . . . . . . . . . . . . . . . . . . .150
  vegetable (*Rokeach*) . . . . . . . . . . . . . . . . . . . . . . . . . . . .90
chicken pasta (*Campbell's Simply Home*) . . . . . . . . . . . . . . .90
chicken pasta and mushroom (*Campbell's Chunky*) . . . . . . .120
chicken pasta w/roasted garlic (*Campbell's* Select) . . . . . . .110
chicken rice (*Campbell's* Classic) . . . . . . . . . . . . . . . . . . . .80
chicken rice (*Campbell's Healthy Request* Hearty) . . . . . . . .100
chicken rice (*Campbell's* Select) . . . . . . . . . . . . . . . . . . . .100
chicken rice (*Campbell's Soup to Go*), 1 cont. . . . . . . . . . . .140
chicken rice (*Health Valley* 99% Fat Free) . . . . . . . . . . . . .130
chicken rice, savory, white/wild (*Campbell's Chunky*) . . . . .140
chicken rice w/vegetables (*Progresso*) . . . . . . . . . . . . . . . .90
chicken rice w/vegetables (*Progresso* 99% Fat Free) . . . . . .110
chicken rice, white/wild (*Campbell's Simply Home*) . . . . . . .100
chicken and rotini (*Progresso* Hearty) . . . . . . . . . . . . . . . . .90
chicken and rotini, roasted (*Progresso*) . . . . . . . . . . . . . . . .80
chicken vegetable (*Campbell's Chunky* Hearty) . . . . . . . . . . .90
chicken vegetable (*Campbell's Healthy Request*) . . . . . . . . .110
chicken vegetable (*Campbell's* Select) . . . . . . . . . . . . . . . . .100
chicken vegetable, Italian style (*Campbell's* Select) . . . . . . .130
chicken vegetable, w/pasta (*Wolfgang Puck's*) . . . . . . . . . .140
chicken vegetable, spicy (*Campbell's Chunky*) . . . . . . . . . . .110
chicken vegetable, white meat (*Progresso*) . . . . . . . . . . . . . .90

**Soup, can or jar, ready-to-serve *(cont.)***
chili beef (*Healthy Choice*) . . . . . . . . . . . . . . . . . . . . . . . . .190
chili beef, w/beans (*Campbell's Chunky*), 10 ¾-oz. can . . . .300
chili pepper (*A Taste of Thai*) . . . . . . . . . . . . . . . . . . . . . . . .45
clam chowder, Manhattan (*Campbell's Chunky*) . . . . . . . . .140
clam chowder, New England:
(*Campbell's Chunky*) . . . . . . . . . . . . . . . . . . . . . . . . . . .240
(*Campbell's Healthy Request*) . . . . . . . . . . . . . . . . . . .110
(*Campbell's* Select) . . . . . . . . . . . . . . . . . . . . . . . . . . .190
(*Campbell's* Select 98% Fat Free) . . . . . . . . . . . . . . . .110
(*Healthy Choice*) . . . . . . . . . . . . . . . . . . . . . . . . . . . . .120
(*Progresso*) . . . . . . . . . . . . . . . . . . . . . . . . . . . . . . . .190
(*Progresso* 99% Fat Free) . . . . . . . . . . . . . . . . . . . . . .110
coconut ginger (*A Taste of Thai*) . . . . . . . . . . . . . . . . . . . .100
corn chowder (*Greene's Farm*), ½ of 15-oz. can . . . . . . . . .120
corn chowder (*Walnut Acres* Country) . . . . . . . . . . . . . . . .150
corn vegetable (*Health Valley* Fat Free) . . . . . . . . . . . . . . . .70
escarole, in chicken broth (*Progresso*) . . . . . . . . . . . . . . . .25
garlic, roasted, and lentil (*Progresso*) . . . . . . . . . . . . . . . .120
gazpacho (*Dominique's*) . . . . . . . . . . . . . . . . . . . . . . . . . . .60
ginger carrot (*Walnut Acres*) . . . . . . . . . . . . . . . . . . . . . . .100
gumbo (*Healthy Choice* Zesty) . . . . . . . . . . . . . . . . . . . . . .100
hot and sour (*Rice Road*) . . . . . . . . . . . . . . . . . . . . . . . . . .90
lemon grass (*A Taste of Thai*) . . . . . . . . . . . . . . . . . . . . . . .35
lentil (*Coco Pazzo*) . . . . . . . . . . . . . . . . . . . . . . . . . . . . . .220
lentil (*Health Valley* Organic) . . . . . . . . . . . . . . . . . . . . . . .80
lentil (*Health Valley* Organic No Salt) . . . . . . . . . . . . . . . .100
lentil (*Progresso*) . . . . . . . . . . . . . . . . . . . . . . . . . . . . . . .140
lentil, savory (*Campbell's* Select) . . . . . . . . . . . . . . . . . . .130
lentil, vegetarian (*Hain* Healthy) . . . . . . . . . . . . . . . . . . . .170
lentil and carrot (*Health Valley* Fat Free) . . . . . . . . . . . . . .100
lobster bisque (*Baxter's*) . . . . . . . . . . . . . . . . . . . . . . . . . .120
macaroni and bean (*Progresso*) . . . . . . . . . . . . . . . . . . . . .160
matzo ball (*Manischewitz*) . . . . . . . . . . . . . . . . . . . . . . . . .110
menudo (*Juanita's* Menudito/Hot & Spicy) . . . . . . . . . . . . .170
menudo (*Pico Pica*) . . . . . . . . . . . . . . . . . . . . . . . . . . . . . .200
minestrone (*Campbell's* Classic) . . . . . . . . . . . . . . . . . . . . .90
minestrone (*Campbell's* Plus! Hearty) . . . . . . . . . . . . . . . . .130
minestrone (*Campbell's* Select Old World) . . . . . . . . . . . . .120
minestrone (*Campbell's Simply Home*) . . . . . . . . . . . . . . . .140

minestrone (*Campbell's Soup to Go*), 1 cont. . . . . . . . . . . .140
minestrone (*Hain* Home Style) . . . . . . . . . . . . . . . . . . . . . . .110
minestrone (*Health Valley* Fat Free) . . . . . . . . . . . . . . . . . . . .90
minestrone (*Progresso*) . . . . . . . . . . . . . . . . . . . . . . . . . .120
minestrone (*Rokeach*) . . . . . . . . . . . . . . . . . . . . . . . . . . .170
minestrone, herb and shells (*Progresso*) . . . . . . . . . . . . . .120
minestrone, Tuscany style (*Campbell's* Select) . . . . . . . . . .160
mulligatawny, hot (*Patak's* Sabzi) . . . . . . . . . . . . . . . . . . . .100
mushroom, cream of (*Campbell's* Select 98% Fat Free) . . . .80
mushroom, cream of (*Hain* Home Style) . . . . . . . . . . . . . . .150
mushroom, cream of (*Rokeach*) . . . . . . . . . . . . . . . . . . . . .120
mushroom barley (*Hain* Healthy) . . . . . . . . . . . . . . . . . . . . .130
mushroom barley (*Health Valley* Organic) . . . . . . . . . . . . . . .70
mushroom broth (*Health Valley* Fat Free) . . . . . . . . . . . . . . .10
mushroom rice, country (*Campbell's* Select) . . . . . . . . . . . . .80
noodle, Oriental, w/vegetables (*Campbell's* Select) . . . . . . .100
onion, French (*Progresso*) . . . . . . . . . . . . . . . . . . . . . . . . .50
onion, French (*Rokeach*) . . . . . . . . . . . . . . . . . . . . . . . . . .80
pasta and vegetables (*Campbell's* Plus! Hearty) . . . . . . . . .110
pea, split (*Health Valley* Organic) . . . . . . . . . . . . . . . . . . . .110
pea, split (*Progresso* 99% Fat Free) . . . . . . . . . . . . . . . . . .170
pea, split, and carrot (*Health Valley* Fat Free) . . . . . . . . . . .110
pea, split, w/ham (*Campbell's Chunky*) . . . . . . . . . . . . . . . .180
pea, split, w/ham (*Campbell's Healthy Request*/Select) . . . .170
pea, split, w/ham (*Healthy Choice*) . . . . . . . . . . . . . . . . . . .170
pea, split, vegetarian (*Hain* Healthy) . . . . . . . . . . . . . . . . .110
penne in chicken broth (*Progresso* Hearty) . . . . . . . . . . . . . .80
pepper steak (*Campbell's Chunky*) . . . . . . . . . . . . . . . . . . .140
potato (*Rokeach*) . . . . . . . . . . . . . . . . . . . . . . . . . . . . . . .115
potato, baked:
  w/bacon, chives (*Healthy Choice*) . . . . . . . . . . . . . . . . .140
  w/bacon bits and chives (*Campbell's Chunky*) . . . . . . . .150
  w/cheddar and bacon bits (*Campbell's Chunky*) . . . . . . .180
  w/steak and cheese (*Campbell's Chunky*) . . . . . . . . . . .200
potato, w/broccoli and cheese (*Progresso*) . . . . . . . . . . . . .160
potato, creamy, and ham (*Healthy Choice*) . . . . . . . . . . . . .140
potato, creamy, w/roasted garlic (*Campbell's Healthy Request*) . . . . . . . . . . . . . . . . . . . . . . . . . . . . . . . .110
potato, creamy, w/roasted garlic (*Campbell's* Select) . . . . . .180
potato, white cheddar (*Progresso* 99% Fat Free) . . . . . . . . .100

**Soup, can or jar, ready-to-serve *(cont.)***
potato ham chowder (*Campbell's Chunky*) .............210
potato leek (*Health Valley* Organic) ....................70
pozole (*Juanita's*) ....................................170
pumpkin (*Walnut Acres* Autumn Harvest) ..............100
ravioli, tomato, w/vegetables (*Campbell's Chunky/Healthy Request*) ......................................150
rotini, vegetable (*Health Valley* Fat Free) ...............100
sirloin burger (*Campbell's Chunky*) ...................180
sirloin steak, grilled, w/vegetables (*Campbell's Chunky*) ...120
steak and potato (*Campbell's Chunky*) ................160
tomato (*Campbell's/Campbell's* Classic) ................120
tomato (*Health Valley* Organic) ........................80
tomato, creamy (*Campbell's*) ..........................140
tomato, creamy (*Campbell's* Classic) ...................140
tomato, basil (*Progresso*) .............................160
tomato, chunky (*Hain* Home Style) ......................120
tomato, garden (*Campbell's* Select) ....................100
tomato lentil, mild Indian (*Patak's*) ...................120
tomato w/roasted garlic, herbs (*Campbell's*) ............150
tomato rotini (*Progresso*) .............................140
tomato vegetable (*Health Valley* Fat Free) ...............80
tomato vegetable (*Wolfgang Puck's* Country) ............150
tomato vegetable, garden (*Progresso* 99% Fat Free) ......100
tortellini and herb (*Progresso*) .........................140
turkey noodle (*Progresso*) ..............................90
turkey rice, white and wild (*Healthy Choice*) ............100
vegetable (*Campbell's Chunky*) .........................130
vegetable (*Campbell's* Select) ..........................110
vegetable (*Campbell's* Select Fiesta) ...................120
vegetable (*Health Valley* Organic) .......................80
vegetable (*Progresso*) ..................................90
vegetable (*Progresso* 99% Fat Free) ......................70
vegetable (*Progresso* Vegetarian) .......................100
vegetable (*Rokeach*) ...................................110
vegetable, country (*Campbell's Healthy Request*) ........110
vegetable, country or garden (*Campbell's Simply Home*) ...110
vegetable, garden (*Campbell's Soup to Go*), 1 cont. ......130
vegetable, garden (*Healthy Choice*) .....................120
vegetable, garden, 14 (*Health Valley* Fat Free) ............80

vegetable barley (*Health Valley* Fat Free) . . . . . . . . . . . . . . . . .90
vegetable beef (*Campbell's Chunky* Old Fashioned) . . . . . . . .160
vegetable beef (*Campbell's Healthy Request* Hearty) . . . . . .130
vegetable beef (*Campbell's* Select) . . . . . . . . . . . . . . . . . . . . .100
vegetable beef pasta (*Campbell's Soup to Go*), 1 cont. . . . .130
vegetable w/beef stock (*Campbell's* Classic) . . . . . . . . . . . . . .80
vegetable broth (*Hain* Healthy) . . . . . . . . . . . . . . . . . . . . . . . . .30
vegetable broth (*Health Valley* Fat Free) . . . . . . . . . . . . . . . . .20
vegetable clam (*Healthy Choice*) . . . . . . . . . . . . . . . . . . . . . . . .80
vegetable w/pasta (*Campbell's Chunky* Hearty) . . . . . . . . . . .140
wild rice (*Hain* Healthy) . . . . . . . . . . . . . . . . . . . . . . . . . . . . . .80

**Soup, canned, condensed,** undiluted, ½ cup:

asparagus, cream of (*Campbell's*) . . . . . . . . . . . . . . . . . . . . . .110
barley and bean (*Rokeach*) . . . . . . . . . . . . . . . . . . . . . . . . . . .120
bean, black (*Campbell's*) . . . . . . . . . . . . . . . . . . . . . . . . . . . . .110
bean, w/bacon (*Campbell's*) . . . . . . . . . . . . . . . . . . . . . . . . . .170
bean, navy (*Walnut Acres*) . . . . . . . . . . . . . . . . . . . . . . . . . . . .110
beef w/vegetables and barley (*Campbell's*) . . . . . . . . . . . . . . .80
broccoli, cream of (*Campbell's*) . . . . . . . . . . . . . . . . . . . . . . . .90
broccoli, cream of (*Campbell's* 98% Fat Free) . . . . . . . . . . . . .70
broccoli, cream of (*Campbell's Healthy Request*) . . . . . . . . . .60
broccoli cheese (*Campbell's*) . . . . . . . . . . . . . . . . . . . . . . . . .110
broccoli cheese (*Campbell's* 98% Fat Free) . . . . . . . . . . . . . . .60
celery, cream of (*Campbell's*) . . . . . . . . . . . . . . . . . . . . . . . . .100
celery, cream of (*Campbell's* 98% Fat Free) . . . . . . . . . . . . . .60
celery, cream of (*Campbell's Healthy Request*) . . . . . . . . . . . .70
cheese, cheddar (*Campbell's*) . . . . . . . . . . . . . . . . . . . . . . . . .130
cheese, nacho (*Campbell's* Fiesta) . . . . . . . . . . . . . . . . . . . . .130
chicken:
  clear (*Rokeach*) . . . . . . . . . . . . . . . . . . . . . . . . . . . . . . . . .20
  cream of (*Campbell's*) . . . . . . . . . . . . . . . . . . . . . . . . . . . .120
  cream of (*Campbell's* 98% Fat Free) . . . . . . . . . . . . . . . . . .80
  cream of (*Campbell's Healthy Request*) . . . . . . . . . . . . . . . .70
  cream of, and broccoli (*Campbell's*) . . . . . . . . . . . . . . . . .120
  cream of, and broccoli (*Campbell's Healthy Request*) . . .80
  cream of, Dijon (*Campbell's*) . . . . . . . . . . . . . . . . . . . . . .130
  cream of, w/herbs (*Campbell's*) . . . . . . . . . . . . . . . . . . . . .80
  cream of, mushroom (*Campbell's*) . . . . . . . . . . . . . . . . . .120
  and dumplings (*Campbell's*) . . . . . . . . . . . . . . . . . . . . . . . .80
  gumbo (*Campbell's*) . . . . . . . . . . . . . . . . . . . . . . . . . . . . . . .60

**Soup, canned, condensed, chicken *(cont.)***

noodle (*Campbell's* Homestyle) . . . . . . . . . . . . . . . . . . . . . .70
noodle (*Campbell's/Campbell's Healthy Request*) . . . . . . .60
noodle (*Campbell's* Noodle O's) . . . . . . . . . . . . . . . . . . . . . .80
noodle, creamy (*Campbell's*) . . . . . . . . . . . . . . . . . . . . . .130
noodle, curly (*Campbell's*) . . . . . . . . . . . . . . . . . . . . . . . . .80
rice (*Campbell's*) . . . . . . . . . . . . . . . . . . . . . . . . . . . . . . . . .70
rice (*Campbell's Healthy Request*) . . . . . . . . . . . . . . . . . . .60
rice, wild and white (*Campbell's*) . . . . . . . . . . . . . . . . . . .60
and stars (*Campbell's*) . . . . . . . . . . . . . . . . . . . . . . . . . . . .70
vegetable (*Campbell's*) . . . . . . . . . . . . . . . . . . . . . . . . . . . .80
vegetable (*Campbell's Healthy Request*) . . . . . . . . . . . . . .80
vegetable, Southwestern (*Campbell's*) . . . . . . . . . . . . . . .110

chili beef w/beans (*Campbell's* Fiesta) . . . . . . . . . . . . . . . . .170
clam bisque (*Chincoteague* Premium) . . . . . . . . . . . . . . . . .100
clam chowder, Manhattan (*Campbell's*) . . . . . . . . . . . . . . . . .70
clam chowder, New England (*Campbell's*) . . . . . . . . . . . . . . .90
clam chowder, New England (*Campbell's* 98% Fat Free) . . . .80
corn chowder (*Chincoteague* Premium) . . . . . . . . . . . . . . . .100
corn chowder (*Walnut Acres*) . . . . . . . . . . . . . . . . . . . . . . . . .80
crab, cream of (*Chincoteague* Chesapeake Bay) . . . . . . . . .200
crab, red, vegetable (*Chincoteague*) . . . . . . . . . . . . . . . . . . .90
crab and cheddar (*Chincoteague* Chesapeake Bay) . . . . . . . .90
lobster bisque (*Chincoteague* Premium) . . . . . . . . . . . . . . . .90
minestrone (*Campbell's*) . . . . . . . . . . . . . . . . . . . . . . . . . . . .90
minestrone (*Campbell's Healthy Request*) . . . . . . . . . . . . . .80
minestrone (*Walnut Acres*) . . . . . . . . . . . . . . . . . . . . . . . . .120
mushroom (*Rokeach*) . . . . . . . . . . . . . . . . . . . . . . . . . . . . . .80
mushroom, beefy (*Campbell's*) . . . . . . . . . . . . . . . . . . . . . . .70
mushroom, cream of (*Campbell's*) . . . . . . . . . . . . . . . . . . . .100
mushroom, cream of (*Campbell's Healthy Request*) . . . . . . .70
mushroom, cream of, w/roasted garlic (*Campbell's*) . . . . . . .70
mushroom, golden (*Campbell's*) . . . . . . . . . . . . . . . . . . . . . .80
noodle, double, in chicken broth (*Campbell's*) . . . . . . . . . . .100
noodle, mega, in chicken broth (*Campbell's*) . . . . . . . . . . . . .60
noodle and ground beef (*Campbell's*) . . . . . . . . . . . . . . . . .100
onion, cream of (*Campbell's*) . . . . . . . . . . . . . . . . . . . . . . .110
onion, French (*Campbell's*) . . . . . . . . . . . . . . . . . . . . . . . . .45
oyster chowder (*Olde Cape Cod*) . . . . . . . . . . . . . . . . . . . . . .70
oyster stew (*Campbell's*) . . . . . . . . . . . . . . . . . . . . . . . . . . .80

pasta w/chicken (*Campbell's* Fun Shapes) . . . . . . . . . . . . . . . .60
pea, green (*Campbell's*) . . . . . . . . . . . . . . . . . . . . . . . . .180
pea, split, and egg barley (*Rokeach*) . . . . . . . . . . . . . . . . .150
pea, split, and barley (*Walnut Acres*) . . . . . . . . . . . . . . . .150
pea, split, w/ham (*Campbell's*) . . . . . . . . . . . . . . . . . . . .180
pepperpot (*Campbell's*) . . . . . . . . . . . . . . . . . . . . . . . . . .90
potato, cream of (*Campbell's*) . . . . . . . . . . . . . . . . . . . . .90
Scotch broth (*Campbell's*) . . . . . . . . . . . . . . . . . . . . . . .70
shrimp, cream of (*Campbell's*) . . . . . . . . . . . . . . . . . . . .90
tomato (*Campbell's*) . . . . . . . . . . . . . . . . . . . . . . . . . . . .80
tomato (*Campbell's Healthy Request*) . . . . . . . . . . . . . . . . .90
tomato (*Rokeach*) . . . . . . . . . . . . . . . . . . . . . . . . . . . . .60
tomato (*Walnut Acres*) . . . . . . . . . . . . . . . . . . . . . . . . . .70
tomato bisque (*Campbell's*) . . . . . . . . . . . . . . . . . . . . . .130
tomato, Italian, w/basil and oregano (*Campbell's*) . . . . . . . .100
tomato noodle (*Campbell's*) . . . . . . . . . . . . . . . . . . . . . .120
tomato rice (*Campbell's* Old Fashioned) . . . . . . . . . . . . . . .110
tomato rice (*Rokeach*) . . . . . . . . . . . . . . . . . . . . . . . . .110
tomato w/roasted garlic and herb (*Campbell's*) . . . . . . . . . .100
turkey, noodle or vegetable (*Campbell's*) . . . . . . . . . . . . . . .70
vegetable (*Campbell's*) . . . . . . . . . . . . . . . . . . . . . . . . . .80
vegetable (*Campbell's* Old Fashioned) . . . . . . . . . . . . . . . . .70
vegetable (*Campbell's Healthy Request*) . . . . . . . . . . . . . . . .90
vegetable (*Rokeach*) . . . . . . . . . . . . . . . . . . . . . . . . . . . .80
vegetable, California style (*Campbell's*) . . . . . . . . . . . . . . .60
vegetable, vegetarian (*Campbell's*) . . . . . . . . . . . . . . . . . .80
vegetable beef (*Campbell's*) . . . . . . . . . . . . . . . . . . . . . . .70
vegetable beef (*Campbell's Healthy Request*) . . . . . . . . . . . .75
vegetable pasta (*Campbell's* Hearty) . . . . . . . . . . . . . . . . . .80
vegetable pasta (*Campbell's Healthy Request* Hearty) . . . . . .90
**Soup, frozen,** 7.5 oz., except as noted:
barley mushroom (*Tabatchnick*) . . . . . . . . . . . . . . . . . . . . .70
bean, Yankee (*Tabatchnick*) . . . . . . . . . . . . . . . . . . . . . .160
beef noodle (*Reames*), 3.3 oz. . . . . . . . . . . . . . . . . . . . .140
broccoli, cream of (*Tabatchnick*) . . . . . . . . . . . . . . . . . . . .90
cabbage (*Tabatchnick*) . . . . . . . . . . . . . . . . . . . . . . . . . .60
chicken (*Tabatchnick* New York) . . . . . . . . . . . . . . . . . . . .35
chicken, w/dumplings (*Tabatchnick*) . . . . . . . . . . . . . . . . . .70
chicken noodle (*Reames* Hearty Homestyle), 3 oz. . . . . . . .130
corn chowder (*Tabatchnick*) . . . . . . . . . . . . . . . . . . . . . .150

**Soup, frozen *(cont.)***
lentil (*Tabatchnick*) . . . . . . . . . . . . . . . . . . . . . . . . . . . .140
minestrone (*Tabatchnick*) . . . . . . . . . . . . . . . . . . . . . . . . .150
mushroom (*Tabatchnick* No Salt) . . . . . . . . . . . . . . . . . . . . .70
mushroom, cream of (*Tabatchnick*) . . . . . . . . . . . . . . . . . .110
onion (*Tabatchnick*) . . . . . . . . . . . . . . . . . . . . . . . . . . . . .50
pea (*Tabatchnick*) . . . . . . . . . . . . . . . . . . . . . . . . . . . . .180
potato, New England (*Tabatchnick*) . . . . . . . . . . . . . . . . .150
potato, old fashioned (*Tabatchnick*) . . . . . . . . . . . . . . . . . .70
spinach, cream of (*Tabatchnick*) . . . . . . . . . . . . . . . . . . . .90
tomato rice (*Tabatchnick*) . . . . . . . . . . . . . . . . . . . . . . . . .60
vegetable (*Tabatchnick*) . . . . . . . . . . . . . . . . . . . . . . . . .110
wild rice (*Tabatchnick*) . . . . . . . . . . . . . . . . . . . . . . . . . .120
**Soup, mix** (see also "Soup base"), dry, 1 pkg. or cont., except as noted:
bean, black (*Knorr* TasteBreaks Cup) . . . . . . . . . . . . . . . .190
bean, black (*Near East*) . . . . . . . . . . . . . . . . . . . . . . . . . .190
bean, black (*Nile Spice*) . . . . . . . . . . . . . . . . . . . . . . . . . .170
bean, black, spicy, w/couscous (*Health Valley*), ⅓ cup . . . .130
bean, black, zesty, w/rice (*Health Valley*), ⅓ cup . . . . . . . . .100
bean, navy (*Knorr TasteBreaks*) . . . . . . . . . . . . . . . . . . . .130
bean, navy (*Nile Spice* Home Style) . . . . . . . . . . . . . . . . .200
bean, rice and, see "rice and beans," below
beef noodle (*House of Tsang*) . . . . . . . . . . . . . . . . . . . . . .120
beef noodle vegetable (*Herb-Ox*) . . . . . . . . . . . . . . . . . . .130
beef vegetable (*Hormel* Micro Cup) . . . . . . . . . . . . . . . . . . .90
broccoli, cream of (*Knorr Recipe Classics*), 3 tbsp. . . . . . . . .70
broccoli cheese w/ham (*Hormel* Micro Cup) . . . . . . . . . . . .170
cheddar broccoli (*Nile Spice* Home Style) . . . . . . . . . . . . .110
chicken, roasted, w/rotini (*Near East*) . . . . . . . . . . . . . . .100
chicken noodle (*Herb-Ox*) . . . . . . . . . . . . . . . . . . . . . . . .110
chicken noodle (*House of Tsang*) . . . . . . . . . . . . . . . . . . .130
chicken noodle (*Nile Spice* Home Style) . . . . . . . . . . . . . . . .90
chicken noodle or rice (*Hormel* Micro Cup) . . . . . . . . . . . . .110
chicken rice (*Mrs. Grass*), ¼ pkg. . . . . . . . . . . . . . . . . . . . .80
chicken rice, creamy (*Knorr* Savory), 3 tbsp. . . . . . . . . . . . .90
chicken vegetable (*Nile Spice* Home Style) . . . . . . . . . . . . .110
clam chowder, New England (*Hormel* Micro Cup) . . . . . . . .130
coconut ginger (*A Taste of Thai*), 2 tsp. . . . . . . . . . . . . . . . .15
corn (*House of Tsang* Velvet) . . . . . . . . . . . . . . . . . . . . . .170

corn, sweet (*Nile Spice* Home Style) . . . . . . . . . . . . . . . . . . .110
corn chowder, roasted (*Near East*) . . . . . . . . . . . . . . . . . . .140
corn chowder, w/tomatoes (*Health Valley*), ¼ cup . . . . . . .100
garlic, roasted, herb (*Knorr Recipe Classics*), 3 tbsp. . . . . . .80
gazpacho (*Nile Spice*) . . . . . . . . . . . . . . . . . . . . . . . . . . .100
herb w/garlic or red pepper (*Lipton Recipe Secrets*),
  1 cup* . . . . . . . . . . . . . . . . . . . . . . . . . . . . . . . . . . . . .30
hot and sour (*Knorr Recipe Classics*), 2 tbsp. . . . . . . . . . . . .45
leek (*Knorr Recipe Classics*), 2 tbsp. . . . . . . . . . . . . . . . . . .70
lentil (*Herb-Ox*) . . . . . . . . . . . . . . . . . . . . . . . . . . . . . . .140
lentil (*Nile Spice* Home Style) . . . . . . . . . . . . . . . . . . . . . .170
lentil w/couscous (*Health Valley*), ⅓ cup . . . . . . . . . . . . . .130
minestrone (*Near East*) . . . . . . . . . . . . . . . . . . . . . . . . . .140
minestrone (*Nile Spice* Home Style) . . . . . . . . . . . . . . . . . .140
mushroom, beefy (*Lipton Recipe Secrets*), 1 cup* . . . . . . . .35
mushroom, country (*Nile Spice* Home Style) . . . . . . . . . . .140
mushroom and noodle (*House of Tsang*) . . . . . . . . . . . . . .120
noodle:
  all varieties (*Nissin Cup Noodles*) . . . . . . . . . . . . . . . . . .300
  buckwheat or brown rice (*Westbrae Natural* Ramen),
    ½ pkg. . . . . . . . . . . . . . . . . . . . . . . . . . . . . . . . . . . .140
  beef (*Nissin Cup Noodles*) . . . . . . . . . . . . . . . . . . . . . . .300
  beef (*Nissin Cup Noodles* Twin), ½ pkg. . . . . . . . . . . . . . .150
  beef (*Nissin Top Ramen*), ½ pkg. . . . . . . . . . . . . . . . . . .190
  beef, hot sauce (*Nissin Cup Noodles*) . . . . . . . . . . . . . . .290
  beef, picante (*Nissin Top Ramen*), ½ pkg. . . . . . . . . . . . .180
  chicken (*Mrs. Grass* Homestyle), ¼ pkg. . . . . . . . . . . . . . .70
  chicken (*Nissin Cup Noodles* Twin), ½ pkg. . . . . . . . . . . .150
  chicken (*Nissin Top Ramen*), ½ pkg. . . . . . . . . . . . . . . . .180
  chicken, Cajun (*Nissin Top Ramen*), ½ pkg. . . . . . . . . . . .180
  chicken, creamy (*Nissin Top Ramen*), ½ pkg. . . . . . . . . . .190
  chicken, w/real broth (*Mrs. Grass*), ¼ pkg. . . . . . . . . . . .60
  chicken mushroom (*Nissin Top Ramen*), ½ pkg. . . . . . . .190
  chicken sesame (*Nissin Top Ramen*), ½ pkg. . . . . . . . . . .190
  chicken teriyaki (*Nissin Top Ramen*), ½ pkg. . . . . . . . . . .190
  chicken vegetable (*Nissin Cup Noodles* Twin),
    ½ pkg. . . . . . . . . . . . . . . . . . . . . . . . . . . . . . . . . . . .160
  chicken vegetable (*Nissin Top Ramen*), ½ pkg. . . . . . . . .190
  chicken w/vegetables (*Health Valley*), ⅓ cup . . . . . . . . .110
  chili (*Nissin Top Ramen*), ½ pkg. . . . . . . . . . . . . . . . . . .190

**Soup, mix, noodle *(cont.)***

mushroom (*Westbrae Natural* Ramen), ½ pkg. . . . . . . .140
Oriental (*Nissin Top Ramen*), ½ pkg. . . . . . . . . . . . . . . . .190
pork (*Nissin Top Ramen*), ½ pkg. . . . . . . . . . . . . . . . . .180
seaweed (*Westbrae Natural* Ramen), ½ pkg. . . . . . . . . .140
shrimp (*Nissin Cup Noodles* Twin), ½ pkg. . . . . . . . . . .150
shrimp (*Nissin Top Ramen*), ½ pkg. . . . . . . . . . . . . . . .190
onion (*Lipton Recipe Secrets*), 1 cup* . . . . . . . . . . . . . . . . .20
onion (*Mrs. Grass* Soup/Dip), ¼ pkg. . . . . . . . . . . . . . . . . . .30
onion, beefy (*Lipton Recipe Secrets*), 1 cup* . . . . . . . . . . . .25
onion, French (*Knorr Recipe Classics*), 2 tbsp. . . . . . . . . . . .35
onion, golden (*Lipton Recipe Secrets*), 1 cup* . . . . . . . . . . .50
onion mushroom (*Lipton Recipe Secrets*), 1 cup* . . . . . . . .30
onion mushroom (*Mrs. Grass* Soup/Dip), ¼ pkg. . . . . . . . . .50
pasta Italiano (*Health Valley*), ½ cup . . . . . . . . . . . . . . . . .140
pasta marinara, Mediterranean or Parmesan
(*Health Valley*), ½ cup . . . . . . . . . . . . . . . . . . . . . . . . .100
pea, split (*Knorr TasteBreaks*) . . . . . . . . . . . . . . . . . . . . . . .150
pea, split (*Near East/Nile Spice*) . . . . . . . . . . . . . . . . . . . .200
pea, split, garden, w/carrots (*Health Valley*), ½ cup . . . . . .110
potato, creamy w/broccoli (*Health Valley*), ⅓ cup . . . . . . . . .80
potato cheese, w/ham (*Hormel* Micro Cup) . . . . . . . . . . . . .190
potato leek (*Herb-Ox*) . . . . . . . . . . . . . . . . . . . . . . . . . . . .140
potato leek (*Knorr TasteBreaks*) . . . . . . . . . . . . . . . . . . . .130
potato leek (*Nile Spice* Home Style) . . . . . . . . . . . . . . . . . .110
rice and beans, black (*Uncle Ben's* Hearty), 1.5 oz. . . . . . . .150
rice and beans, red (*Near East*) . . . . . . . . . . . . . . . . . . . . .190
spinach, cream of (*Knorr Recipe Classics*), 2 tbsp. . . . . . . . .70
tomato basil (*Knorr Recipe Classics*), 3 tbsp. . . . . . . . . . . . .80
tomato herb (*Nile Spice* Home Style) . . . . . . . . . . . . . . . . . .90
vegetable (*Knorr Recipe Classics*), 2 tbsp. . . . . . . . . . . . . . .60
vegetable (*Lipton Recipe Secrets*), 1 cup* . . . . . . . . . . . . . .30
vegetable (*Mrs. Grass* Homestyle Soup/Dip), ¼ pkt. . . . . . . .35
vegetable, chicken flavor (*Knorr TasteBreaks*) . . . . . . . . . . .120
vegetable, cream of (*Knorr* Savory), 3 tbsp. . . . . . . . . . . . .100
vegetable, spring (*Knorr Recipe Classics*), 2 tbsp. . . . . . . . .25
vegetable, vegetarian (*Knorr TasteBreaks*) . . . . . . . . . . . . . .160
vegetable herb (*Arrowhead Mills*), ⅓ cup . . . . . . . . . . . . . .150
vichyssoise (*Nile Spice*) . . . . . . . . . . . . . . . . . . . . . . . . . . .100

wild rice (*Herb-Ox*) . . . . . . . . . . . . . . . . . . . . . . . . . . .230
wild rice and herb (*Arrowhead Mills*), ⅓ cup . . . . . . . . . . .140
**Soup base mix:**
beef (*Watkins* Soup/Gravy), 2 tsp. . . . . . . . . . . . . . . . . . . . .15
beef vegetable (*Wyler's Soup Starter*), ⅛ pkg. . . . . . . . . . .100
broccoli, cream of (*McCormick Produce Partners*),
⅓ pkt. . . . . . . . . . . . . . . . . . . . . . . . . . . . . . . . . . . .35
cheddar broccoli (*McCormick Produce Partners*), ⅓ pkt. . . .70
cheese (*Watkins* Soup/Gravy), 2½ tbsp. . . . . . . . . . . . . . . . .80
chicken (*Watkins* Soup/Gravy), 2 tsp. . . . . . . . . . . . . . . . . . .15
chicken noodle (*Watkins* Soup/Gravy), 1 tbsp. . . . . . . . . . . .30
chicken noodle (*Wyler's Soup Starter*), ⅛ pkg. . . . . . . . . . . .80
chicken vegetable, hearty (*Wyler's Soup Starter*), ⅐ pkg. . . .70
chicken, w/white and wild rice (*Wyler's Soup Starter*),
⅛ pkg. . . . . . . . . . . . . . . . . . . . . . . . . . . . . . . . . . . .70
chili, 3-bean (*Wyler's Soup Starter*), ⅙ pkg. . . . . . . . . . . . .150
cream (*Watkins* Soup/Gravy), 2½ tbsp. . . . . . . . . . . . . . . . .90
mushroom (*Watkins* Soup/Gravy), 2 tbsp. . . . . . . . . . . . . . .60
onion (*Watkins* Soup/Gravy), 2 tsp. . . . . . . . . . . . . . . . . . . .20
onion, French (*McCormick Produce Partners*), ⅓ pkt. . . . . . .40
potato, cream of (*McCormick Produce Partners*), ¼ pkt. . . . .25
potato, garlic and chives (*Wyler's Soup Starter*),
⅙ pkg. . . . . . . . . . . . . . . . . . . . . . . . . . . . . . . . . . . .130
vegetable, garden (*McCormick Produce Partners*), ⅓ pkt. . . .40
**Sour cream,** see "Cream, sour"
**Soy bean,** see "Soybean"
**Soy beverage,** 8 fl. oz.:
(*Edensoy/Edensoy* Extra) . . . . . . . . . . . . . . . . . . . . . . . . .130
(*Silk*) . . . . . . . . . . . . . . . . . . . . . . . . . . . . . . . . . . . . . .100
(*Soy Dream* Original) . . . . . . . . . . . . . . . . . . . . . . . . . . . .130
(*Vitasoy* Creamy Original) . . . . . . . . . . . . . . . . . . . . . . . .110
carob or chocolate (*Soy Dream*) . . . . . . . . . . . . . . . . . . . .210
chai or mocha (*Silk*) . . . . . . . . . . . . . . . . . . . . . . . . . . . .130
chocolate (*Silk*) . . . . . . . . . . . . . . . . . . . . . . . . . . . . . . .140
vanilla (*Soy Dream*) . . . . . . . . . . . . . . . . . . . . . . . . . . . .150
**Soy butter,** mix, roasted (*Natural Touch*), 2 tbsp. . . . . . . . .170
**Soy flour** (*Arrowhead Mills*), ½ cup . . . . . . . . . . . . . . . . . .200
**Soy meal,** defatted, raw, 1 cup . . . . . . . . . . . . . . . . . . . . .414
**Soy milk,** see "Soy beverage"

**Soy nuts:**
(*Skee's Soy Nutz* Salted), 1 oz. . . . . . . . . . . . . . . . . . . . . . . . .150
honey-roasted (*Skee's Soy Nutz*), 1 oz. . . . . . . . . . . . . . . . .140
onion–garlic (*Skee's Soy Nutz*), 1 oz. . . . . . . . . . . . . . . . . . .150
roasted, barbecue, honey, spicy, or wasabi (*Frieda's*), ¼ cup . . . . . . . . . . . . . . . . . . . . . . . . . . . . . . . . . . . .140
**Soy sauce,** 1 tbsp.:
(*House of Tsang* Dark) . . . . . . . . . . . . . . . . . . . . . . . . . . .10
(*House of Tsang* Light/Low Sodium) . . . . . . . . . . . . . . . . . .5
(*Kikkoman/Kikkoman* Lite) . . . . . . . . . . . . . . . . . . . . . . . .10
(*La Choy*) . . . . . . . . . . . . . . . . . . . . . . . . . . . . . . . . . . . .10
garlic, spicy (*Watkins*) . . . . . . . . . . . . . . . . . . . . . . . . . . .10
ginger flavor (*House of Tsang*) . . . . . . . . . . . . . . . . . . . . .20
shoyu (*Eden* Imported) . . . . . . . . . . . . . . . . . . . . . . . . . . .15
tamari (*San-J*) . . . . . . . . . . . . . . . . . . . . . . . . . . . . . . . . .15
tamari (*San-J* Reduced Sodium) . . . . . . . . . . . . . . . . . . . . .20
**Soy spread** (*Soy Wonder*), 2 tbsp. . . . . . . . . . . . . . . . . . . .170
**Soybean** (see also "Edamame"), green, shelled, boiled, drained, ½ cup . . . . . . . . . . . . . . . . . . . . . . . . . . . . . . .127
**Soybean, canned** (*Westbrae Natural*), ½ cup . . . . . . . . . . .150
**Soybean cake or curd,** see "Tofu"
**Soybean kernels,** roasted, toasted, 1 oz., 95 kernels . . . . .129
**Soybean spread/dip,** 2 tbsp.:
all flavors, except horseradish and red pepper (*Maxbean*) . . .45
horseradish or roasted red pepper (*Maxbean*) . . . . . . . . . . . .40
**Soybean sprouts,** fresh (*Jonathan's*), 1 cup . . . . . . . . . . . .100
**Spaghetti,** see "Pasta"
**Spaghetti dish, mix,** w/tomato sauce (*Classico It's Pasta Anytime*), 15.25-oz. cont. . . . . . . . . . . . . . . . . . . . . . . . .490
**Spaghetti entree, can or pkg.,** 1 cup, except as noted:
(*Franco-American SpaghettiOs* w/Calcium) . . . . . . . . . . . . .190
w/franks (*Franco-American SpaghettiOs*) . . . . . . . . . . . . . .240
w/franks, rings (*Kid's Kitchen*) . . . . . . . . . . . . . . . . . . . . .240
marinara, w/roasted vegetables (*Cascadian Farm*), 10 oz. . . . . . . . . . . . . . . . . . . . . . . . . . . . . . . . . . . . . .230
w/meatballs:
(*Chef Boyardee*) . . . . . . . . . . . . . . . . . . . . . . . . . . . . . . .250
(*Chef Boyardee* Micro Cup), 7.5-oz. cont. . . . . . . . . . . .210
(*Dinty Moore American Classics*), 1 bowl . . . . . . . . . . .290
(*Kid's Kitchen*) . . . . . . . . . . . . . . . . . . . . . . . . . . . . . . .220

(*Franco-American SpaghettiOs*) . . . . . . . . . . . . . . . . . .240
rings (*Kid's Kitchen*) . . . . . . . . . . . . . . . . . . . . . . . . . .230
tomato cheese sauce (*Franco-American SpaghettiOs*) . . . . .180
**Spaghetti entree, frozen,** 1 pkg., except as noted:
Bolognese (*Michelina's*), 8.5 oz. . . . . . . . . . . . . . . . . . . . .280
cheesy, bake (*Stouffer's*), 12 oz. . . . . . . . . . . . . . . . . . . .460
cheesy bake (*Stouffer's Family Favorites*), ¼ of
40-oz. pkg. . . . . . . . . . . . . . . . . . . . . . . . . . . . . . . . . .370
marinara (*Budget Gourmet*), 8 oz. . . . . . . . . . . . . . . . . . .270
marinara (*Michelina's*), 8 oz. . . . . . . . . . . . . . . . . . . . . .260
w/meat sauce (*Healthy Choice* Solo), 10 oz. . . . . . . . . . . .290
w/meat sauce (*Lean Cuisine Everyday Favorites*),
11.5 oz. . . . . . . . . . . . . . . . . . . . . . . . . . . . . . . . . . . . .300
w/meat sauce (*Stouffer's*), 12 oz. . . . . . . . . . . . . . . . . . . .440
w/meat sauce, garlic bread (*Marie Callender's*), 17 oz. . . . .670
and meatballs (*Master Choice*), 1 cup . . . . . . . . . . . . . . . .350
and meatballs, w/sauce (*Michelina's*), 9 oz. . . . . . . . . . . . .300
w/meatballs (*Lean Cuisine Everyday Favorites*), 9.5 oz. . . . .270
w/meatballs (*Stouffer's*), 12⅝ oz. . . . . . . . . . . . . . . . . . .390
w/tomato and basil sauce (*Michelina's*), 8 oz. . . . . . . . . . .260
**Spaghetti sauce,** see "Pasta sauce"
**Spaghetti squash:**
raw (*Frieda's*), ¾ cup, 3 oz. . . . . . . . . . . . . . . . . . . . . . . .30
baked or boiled, drained, ½ cup . . . . . . . . . . . . . . . . . . . . .23
**Spanakopita,** see "Spinach–feta appetizer"
**Spareribs,** see "Pork" and "pork, refrigerated"
**Spelt chips** (*VitaSpelt* Snackin' Flatchips), 1 oz. . . . . . . . . . .70
**Spelt flakes,** see "Cereal, ready-to-eat"
**Spelt flour** (*Hodgson Mill* Organic), ¼ cup . . . . . . . . . . . .115
**Spelt kernels** (*Purity Foods* Berries), ¼ cup . . . . . . . . . . .130
**Spice,** see specific listings
**Spinach,** fresh:
raw (*Mann's* Salad Spinach), 3 oz. . . . . . . . . . . . . . . . . . . .40
raw, baby (*Dole* Organic Blend), 3 oz. . . . . . . . . . . . . . . . . .35
raw, baby (*Fresh Express*), 1½ cups, 3 oz. . . . . . . . . . . . . . .20
raw, baby (*Ready Pac*), 4 cups, 3 oz. . . . . . . . . . . . . . . . . . .40
raw, chopped, ½ cup . . . . . . . . . . . . . . . . . . . . . . . . . . . . . .6
raw, shredded (*Dole*), 1½ cups, 3 oz. . . . . . . . . . . . . . . . . .40
boiled, drained, ½ cup . . . . . . . . . . . . . . . . . . . . . . . . . . . .21
cooked (*Ready Pac* Microwave), ½ cup, 3 oz. . . . . . . . . . . . .20

**Spinach, canned,** ½ cup:
whole leaf or chopped (*Bush's Best*) .................... 30
whole leaf or chopped (*Popeye/Sunshine*) ................ 30
**Spinach, frozen** (see also "Spinach dish"):
(*Tree of Life* Organic), 1 cup .......................... 20
leaf, blocks (*Bonduelle*), 3-oz. block .................. 25
leaf, cut (*Birds Eye*), 1 cup ........................... 20
leaf, cut (*Green Giant*), ¾ cup ......................... 15
leaf or chopped (*Seabrook Farms*), ⅓ cup ................ 20
chopped (*Birds Eye*), ⅓ cup ............................. 20
**Spinach, New Zealand,** chopped:
raw, 1 oz. or ½ cup ...................................... 4
boiled, drained, ½ cup ................................... 11
**Spinach, water** (*Frieda's* Ong Choy), 2 cups, 3 oz. ........ 20
**Spinach dip** (*Marie's*), 2 tbsp. ........................... 140
**Spinach dip mix** (*McCormick*), 2 tbsp.* ..................... 40
**Spinach dish,** frozen:
creamed (*Seabrook*), ½ cup .............................. 120
creamed (*Stouffer's* Side Dish), ½ of 9-oz. pkg. ........ 230
creamed (*Tabatchnick*), 7.5 oz. ......................... 60
pancake (*Dr. Praeger's*), 1.3-oz. cake .................. 70
soufflé (*Stouffer's* Side Dish), ⅓ of 12-oz. pkg. ....... 140
**Spinach entree, packaged,** w/rice, 1 pkg.:
w/cheese (*Tamarind Tree* Palak Paneer) .................. 380
w/garbanzos (*Tamarind Tree* Saag Chole) ................. 370
**Spinach–feta appetizer,** frozen (*Apollo/Athens*),
5 pcs., 5 oz. ............................................ 390
**Spinach–feta snack** (*Amy's*), 5–6 pcs., ½ pkg. ............ 170
**Spiny lobster,** meat only:
raw, 4 oz. ............................................... 127
boiled or steamed, 2-lb. lobster w/shell ................. 233
boiled or steamed, 4 oz. ................................. 138
**Spiral pasta entree,** frozen, spicy tomato sauce
(*Michelina's*), 8 oz. ................................... 210
**Split peas:**
dry, green or yellow (*Jack Rabbit*), ¼ cup .............. 110
boiled, ½ cup ............................................ 116
**Sports drink,** 8 fl. oz.:
all flavors (*Gatorade*) ................................. 50
lemon-lime (*AriZona*) ................................... 60

**Spot,** meat only:
raw, 4 oz. . . . . . . . . . . . . . . . . . . . . . . . . . . . . .140
baked, broiled, or microwaved, 4 oz. . . . . . . . . . . . . . . . . .179
**Sprouts,** see "Bean sprouts" and specific listings
**Sprouts, mixed,** fresh, 1 cup:
(*Jonathan's*) . . . . . . . . . . . . . . . . . . . . . . . . . . . .100
(*Jonathan's* Gourmet) . . . . . . . . . . . . . . . . . . . . . . .20
hot and spicy (*Jonathan's*) . . . . . . . . . . . . . . . . . . . .25
salad (*Jonathan's*) . . . . . . . . . . . . . . . . . . . . . . . . .80
**Squab,** fresh, raw:
meat w/skin, 4 oz. . . . . . . . . . . . . . . . . . . . . . . . . . .333
breast meat only, 4 oz. . . . . . . . . . . . . . . . . . . . . . . .161
**Squash** (see also specific squash listings), frozen, cooked (*Birds Eye*), ½ cup . . . . . . . . . . . . . . . . . . . . . . . . .50
**Squid,** fresh, meat only, raw, 4 oz. . . . . . . . . . . . . . . . . .104
**Squid, frozen,** tubes, tentacles (*Soundings*), 4 oz. . . . . . . .110
**Starfruit,** see "Carambola"
**Steak,** see "Beef"
**Steak marinade,** see "Marinade"
**Steak sauce,** 1 tbsp., except as noted:
(*A.1.*) . . . . . . . . . . . . . . . . . . . . . . . . . . . . . . . . .15
(*A.1.* Bold/Spicy) . . . . . . . . . . . . . . . . . . . . . . . . . .20
(*A.1.* Sweet/Tangy) . . . . . . . . . . . . . . . . . . . . . . . . .30
(*A.1.* Thick/Hearty) . . . . . . . . . . . . . . . . . . . . . . . . .25
(*HP*) . . . . . . . . . . . . . . . . . . . . . . . . . . . . . . . . .15
(*Lea & Perrins* Sweet & Spicy/Traditional) . . . . . . . . . . . .25
(*Newman's Own*) . . . . . . . . . . . . . . . . . . . . . . . . . . .20
(*Peter Luger* Steak House) . . . . . . . . . . . . . . . . . . . . .30
(*Texas Best*) . . . . . . . . . . . . . . . . . . . . . . . . . . . . .15
peppercorn (*Lawry's* Weekday Gourmet), 2 tbsp. . . . . . . . . .40
**Steak seasoning,** all varieties (*McCormick*), ¼ tsp. . . . . . . . .0
**Stir-fry sauce** (see also "Marinade,"), 1 tbsp.:
(*House of Tsang* Classic) . . . . . . . . . . . . . . . . . . . . . .25
(*House of Tsang Bangkok Padang/Saigon Sizzle*) . . . . . . . . .45
(*Kikkoman*) . . . . . . . . . . . . . . . . . . . . . . . . . . . . . .20
garlic and ginger (*Rice Road*) . . . . . . . . . . . . . . . . . . .25
herb and roasted garlic (*Lawry's* Seasoning) . . . . . . . . . . . .5
lemon (*Rice Road*) . . . . . . . . . . . . . . . . . . . . . . . . . .15
lemon basil (*Lawry's* Seasoning) . . . . . . . . . . . . . . . . . .10
sesame ginger (*Lawry's* Seasoning) . . . . . . . . . . . . . . . .15

**Stir-fry sauce *(cont.)***
spicy, Szechuan (*House of Tsang*) . . . . . . . . . . . . . . . . . . . .20
sweet and sour (*House of Tsang*) . . . . . . . . . . . . . . . . . . . .35
sweet and spicy (*Lawry's* Seasoning) . . . . . . . . . . . . . . . . .20
teriyaki (*House of Tsang Korean*) . . . . . . . . . . . . . . . . . . . .30
**Stir-fry seasoning mix** (*McCormick Produce Partners*), ⅕ pkg. . . . . . . . . . . . . . . . . . . . . . . . . . . . . . . . .20
**Strawberry,** fresh:
(*Dole*), 8 medium, 5.2 oz. . . . . . . . . . . . . . . . . . . . . . . .45
halves, ½ cup . . . . . . . . . . . . . . . . . . . . . . . . . . . . . . .23
**Strawberry, dried** (*Frieda's*), ½ cup, 1.4 oz. . . . . . . . . . . . .150
**Strawberry, frozen:**
(*Big Valley*), ⅔ cup . . . . . . . . . . . . . . . . . . . . . . . . . . .50
(*Cascadian Farm*), 1 cup . . . . . . . . . . . . . . . . . . . . . . . .90
(*Tree of Life* Organic), ¾ cup . . . . . . . . . . . . . . . . . . . . .50
whole (*Birds Eye*), ½ cup . . . . . . . . . . . . . . . . . . . . . . .100
whole (*Sun-Vale* No Sugar), 1 cup . . . . . . . . . . . . . . . . . . .40
sliced, in sugar (*Big Valley* Tub), ⅔ cup . . . . . . . . . . . . . . .150
sliced, sweetened (*Sun-Vale*), ⅔ cup . . . . . . . . . . . . . . . . .150
in light syrup (*Birds Eye* Lite), 10 oz. . . . . . . . . . . . . . . . .120
in syrup (*Birds Eye*), 4.75 oz. . . . . . . . . . . . . . . . . . . . . .120
**Strawberry drink** (*Hawaiian Punch* Surfin'), 8 fl. oz. . . . . . .120
**Strawberry drink blends:**
banana (*AriZona*), 8 fl. oz. . . . . . . . . . . . . . . . . . . . . . .140
banana (*Libby's* Nectar), 11.5-fl.-oz. can . . . . . . . . . . . . . .220
banana (*WhipperSnapple*), 10 fl. oz. . . . . . . . . . . . . . . . . .160
kiwi (*Dole*), 8 fl. oz. . . . . . . . . . . . . . . . . . . . . . . . . . .130
kiwi (*Dole*), 11.5 fl. oz. . . . . . . . . . . . . . . . . . . . . . . . .180
kiwi (*Libby's* Nectar), 11.5-fl.-oz. can . . . . . . . . . . . . . . . .200
kiwi (*Tropicana Twister*) . . . . . . . . . . . . . . . . . . . . . . . .130
**Strawberry pie glaze** (*Smucker's*), 2 oz. . . . . . . . . . . . . . . .80
**Strawberry juice blend** (*Ceres*), 5.25 fl. oz. . . . . . . . . . . . .87
**Strawberry milk,** see "Milk, flavored"
**Strawberry milk drink mix** (*Nesquik*), 2 tbsp. . . . . . . . . . . .90
**Strawberry syrup,** ¼ cup, except as noted:
(*Maple Grove Farms*) . . . . . . . . . . . . . . . . . . . . . . . . . .210
(*Nesquik*), 2 tbsp. . . . . . . . . . . . . . . . . . . . . . . . . . . . .110
(*Smucker's*) . . . . . . . . . . . . . . . . . . . . . . . . . . . . . . . .210
(*Smucker's* Sundae Syrup), 2 tbsp. . . . . . . . . . . . . . . . . . .100

**Strawberry topping,** 2 tbsp.:
(*Mrs. Richardson's*) . . . . . . . . . . . . . . . . . . . . . . . . . . . .70
(*Smucker's*) . . . . . . . . . . . . . . . . . . . . . . . . . . . . . . . . . .100
**String bean,** see "Green bean"
**Stroganoff mix,** vegetarian (*Natural Touch*), 4 tbsp. . . . . . . .90
**Stroganoff sauce,** beef (*Lawry's*), 1 tbsp. . . . . . . . . . . . . . .20
**Strudel,** see "Apple pastry"
**Stuffing** (see also "Stuffing mix"):
corn bread (*Pepperidge Farm*), ¾ cup . . . . . . . . . . . . . . . .170
herb-seasoned (*Chatham Village* Traditional), ¾ cup . . . . . .150
herb-seasoned (*Pepperidge Farm*), ¾ cup . . . . . . . . . . . . .170
**Stuffing mix:**
(*Bell's*), ½ cup . . . . . . . . . . . . . . . . . . . . . . . . . . . . . . .130
(*Kellogg's Croutettes*), 1 cup . . . . . . . . . . . . . . . . . . . . .120
beef (*Stove Top*), ½ cup* . . . . . . . . . . . . . . . . . . . . . . . . .180
chicken flavor (*Pepperidge Farm* One Step), ½ cup . . . . . . .140
chicken flavor (*Stove Top*), ½ cup* . . . . . . . . . . . . . . . . . .170
corn bread (*Stove Top*), ½ cup* . . . . . . . . . . . . . . . . . . . . .170
corn bread, Southwest (*Pepperidge Farm* One Step),
½ cup . . . . . . . . . . . . . . . . . . . . . . . . . . . . . . . . . . .150
cranberry and herb (*Chatham Village*), 1 cup . . . . . . . . . . .130
herb (*Chatham Village* Traditional), 1 cup . . . . . . . . . . . . . .150
herbs, savory (*Stove Top*), 1 cup* . . . . . . . . . . . . . . . . . . .170
long grain/wild rice (*Stove Top*), ½ cup* . . . . . . . . . . . . . .180
for pork or turkey (*Stove Top*), ½ cup* . . . . . . . . . . . . . . . .170
**Sturgeon,** meat only:
raw, 4 oz. . . . . . . . . . . . . . . . . . . . . . . . . . . . . . . . . . . . .120
baked, broiled, or microwaved, 4 oz. . . . . . . . . . . . . . . . . .153
smoked, 4 oz. . . . . . . . . . . . . . . . . . . . . . . . . . . . . . . . . .196
***Subway,*** 1 serving:
breakfast sandwich:
bacon and egg . . . . . . . . . . . . . . . . . . . . . . . . . . . . . .305
cheese and egg . . . . . . . . . . . . . . . . . . . . . . . . . . . . . .302
ham and egg . . . . . . . . . . . . . . . . . . . . . . . . . . . . . . . .291
western egg . . . . . . . . . . . . . . . . . . . . . . . . . . . . . . . .285
6" Classic sub:
*Cold Cut Trio* . . . . . . . . . . . . . . . . . . . . . . . . . . . . . . .415
*Italian BMT* . . . . . . . . . . . . . . . . . . . . . . . . . . . . . . . . .453
meatball . . . . . . . . . . . . . . . . . . . . . . . . . . . . . . . . . . .501

***Subway*, 6" classic sub, *(cont.)***

*Seafood & Crab*, w/light mayo . . . . . . . . . . . . . . . . . . . .378
steak and cheese . . . . . . . . . . . . . . . . . . . . . . . . . .362
*Subway Melt* . . . . . . . . . . . . . . . . . . . . . . . . . . . .380
tuna, w/light mayo . . . . . . . . . . . . . . . . . . . . . . . .419

6" Select sub:
asiago Caesar chicken . . . . . . . . . . . . . . . . . . . . . .391
honey mustard melt . . . . . . . . . . . . . . . . . . . . . . . .373
roast beef, horseradish . . . . . . . . . . . . . . . . . . . . .401
steak and cheese, Southwest . . . . . . . . . . . . . . . . . .412

deli-style sandwich:
ham . . . . . . . . . . . . . . . . . . . . . . . . . . . . . . . . . .194
roast beef . . . . . . . . . . . . . . . . . . . . . . . . . . . . . .206
turkey breast . . . . . . . . . . . . . . . . . . . . . . . . . . . .200
tuna w/light mayo . . . . . . . . . . . . . . . . . . . . . . . . .309

*7 Under 6* sub:
ham . . . . . . . . . . . . . . . . . . . . . . . . . . . . . . . . . .261
roast beef . . . . . . . . . . . . . . . . . . . . . . . . . . . . . .264
roast chicken breast . . . . . . . . . . . . . . . . . . . . . . . .311
*Subway Club* . . . . . . . . . . . . . . . . . . . . . . . . . . . .294
turkey breast . . . . . . . . . . . . . . . . . . . . . . . . . . . .254
turkey breast and ham . . . . . . . . . . . . . . . . . . . . . .267
*Veggie Delite* . . . . . . . . . . . . . . . . . . . . . . . . . . . .200

wraps:
asiago Caesar chicken . . . . . . . . . . . . . . . . . . . . . .413
steak and cheese . . . . . . . . . . . . . . . . . . . . . . . . . .353
turkey breast and bacon . . . . . . . . . . . . . . . . . . . . .321

condiments/extras:
bacon, 2 slices . . . . . . . . . . . . . . . . . . . . . . . . . . .45
cheese, 2 triangles . . . . . . . . . . . . . . . . . . . . . . . . .41
mayo, 1 tbsp. . . . . . . . . . . . . . . . . . . . . . . . . . . . .111
mayo, light, 1 tbsp. . . . . . . . . . . . . . . . . . . . . . . . .46
mustard, 2 tsp. . . . . . . . . . . . . . . . . . . . . . . . . . . . .8
oil blend, 1 tsp. . . . . . . . . . . . . . . . . . . . . . . . . . .45
vinegar, 1 tsp. . . . . . . . . . . . . . . . . . . . . . . . . . . . .1

Classic salad, w/out dressing:
*Cold Cut Trio* . . . . . . . . . . . . . . . . . . . . . . . . . . .234
*Italian BMT* . . . . . . . . . . . . . . . . . . . . . . . . . . . . .273
meatball . . . . . . . . . . . . . . . . . . . . . . . . . . . . . . .320
steak and cheese . . . . . . . . . . . . . . . . . . . . . . . . . .182

*Seafood and Crab,* w/light mayo . . . . . . . . . . . . . . . . . . .198
*Subway Melt* . . . . . . . . . . . . . . . . . . . . . . . . . . .203
tuna, w/light mayo . . . . . . . . . . . . . . . . . . . . . . .238
*7 Under 6* salad, w/out dressing:
ham . . . . . . . . . . . . . . . . . . . . . . . . . . . . . . . .112
roast beef . . . . . . . . . . . . . . . . . . . . . . . . . . . .114
roast chicken breast . . . . . . . . . . . . . . . . . . . . .137
*Subway Club* . . . . . . . . . . . . . . . . . . . . . . . . . . .145
turkey breast . . . . . . . . . . . . . . . . . . . . . . . . . .105
turkey breast and ham . . . . . . . . . . . . . . . . . . . .117
*Veggie Delite* . . . . . . . . . . . . . . . . . . . . . . . . . . .50
dressing, 2 oz.:
French, fat free . . . . . . . . . . . . . . . . . . . . . . . . .70
Italian, fat free . . . . . . . . . . . . . . . . . . . . . . . . .20
ranch, fat free . . . . . . . . . . . . . . . . . . . . . . . . . .60
cookie:
chocolate chip . . . . . . . . . . . . . . . . . . . . . . . . .209
chocolate chunk or *M&Ms* . . . . . . . . . . . . . . . . . .210
macadamia nut . . . . . . . . . . . . . . . . . . . . . . . . .221
oatmeal raisin . . . . . . . . . . . . . . . . . . . . . . . . .197
peanut butter . . . . . . . . . . . . . . . . . . . . . . . . . .220
sugar . . . . . . . . . . . . . . . . . . . . . . . . . . . . . . . .222
**Succotash, canned,** ½ cup:
kernel (*Libby's*) . . . . . . . . . . . . . . . . . . . . . . . . .90
cream-style . . . . . . . . . . . . . . . . . . . . . . . . . . . .103
cream-style (*Blue Boy*) . . . . . . . . . . . . . . . . . . . . .90
**Succotash, frozen:**
(*John Cope's*), ⅔ cup . . . . . . . . . . . . . . . . . . . . .80
boiled, drained, ½ cup . . . . . . . . . . . . . . . . . . . . .79
**Sucker,** white, meat only:
raw, 4 oz. . . . . . . . . . . . . . . . . . . . . . . . . . . . . .105
baked, broiled, or microwaved, 4 oz. . . . . . . . . . . . . .135
**Sugar,** beet or cane:
brown, 1 cup, not packed . . . . . . . . . . . . . . . . . . .546
granulated, 1 cup . . . . . . . . . . . . . . . . . . . . . . . .773
granulated, 1 tbsp. . . . . . . . . . . . . . . . . . . . . . . . .46
granulated, 1 tsp. . . . . . . . . . . . . . . . . . . . . . . . . .15
powdered or confectioner's, 1 cup, sifted . . . . . . . . . . . .389
powdered or confectioner's, 1 tbsp., unsifted . . . . . . . . . . .31
**Sugar, maple,** 1 oz. . . . . . . . . . . . . . . . . . . . . . . .99

**Sugar, substitute.**
(*Equal*), 1 pkt. . . . . . . . . . . . . . . . . . . . . . . . . . . . . . . .4
(*NutraSweet*), 1 tsp. . . . . . . . . . . . . . . . . . . . . . . . . . . . .2
(*Sweet'n Low*), 1 pkt. . . . . . . . . . . . . . . . . . . . . . . . . . . .4
(*Weight Watchers*) . . . . . . . . . . . . . . . . . . . . . . . . . . . . . .5
**Sugar, turbinado** (*Hain*), 1 tsp. . . . . . . . . . . . . . . . . . . . . . .15
**Sugar apple,** 1 medium, 9.9 oz. . . . . . . . . . . . . . . . . . . . . . .146
**Sugar snap peas,** see "Peas, edible pod"
**Summer sausage:**
(*Johnsonville* Chub Original/Beef/Garlic), 2 oz. . . . . . . . . . . .180
(*Oscar Mayer*), 2 slices, 1.6 oz. . . . . . . . . . . . . . . . . . . . . .140
smoked (*Old Smokehouse*), 2 oz. . . . . . . . . . . . . . . . . . . . . .200
**Sunburst squash,** baby, fresh (*Frieda's*), ⅔ cup, 3 oz. . . . . .15
**Sunfish,** pumpkinseed, meat only:
raw, 4 oz. . . . . . . . . . . . . . . . . . . . . . . . . . . . . . . . . . . .101
baked, broiled, or microwaved, 4 oz. . . . . . . . . . . . . . . . . . .129
**Sunflower butter** (*Kettle Roaster Fresh*), 1 oz. . . . . . . . . . .168
**Sunflower seed,** 1 oz. kernels, except as noted:
(*Frito-Lay*) . . . . . . . . . . . . . . . . . . . . . . . . . . . . . . . . . .180
(*Planters*), ¼ cup . . . . . . . . . . . . . . . . . . . . . . . . . . . . . .200
(*Planters*), 3-oz. pkg. . . . . . . . . . . . . . . . . . . . . . . . . . . .280
raw (*Blue Diamond*), ¼ cup . . . . . . . . . . . . . . . . . . . . . . . .190
roasted, in shell (*Planters*), ¾ cup . . . . . . . . . . . . . . . . . . .180
oil-roasted (*Blue Diamond*), ¼ cup . . . . . . . . . . . . . . . . . . .210
barbecue (*Frito-Lay*) . . . . . . . . . . . . . . . . . . . . . . . . . . . . .200
hot (*Frito-Lay* Flamin') . . . . . . . . . . . . . . . . . . . . . . . . . . .180
**Swamp cabbage,** raw, .6-oz. shoot . . . . . . . . . . . . . . . . . . . .2
**Sweet peas,** see "Peas, green"
**Sweet potato:**
raw, 5" long, 4.7 oz. . . . . . . . . . . . . . . . . . . . . . . . . . . . . .137
baked in skin, 5" long . . . . . . . . . . . . . . . . . . . . . . . . . . . .118
baked in skin, mashed, ½ cup . . . . . . . . . . . . . . . . . . . . . . .103
boiled w/out skin, mashed, ½ cup . . . . . . . . . . . . . . . . . . . .172
**Sweet potato, canned,** ½ cup, except as noted:
whole (*Royal Prince/Trappey's*), 3 pcs., 6.1 oz. . . . . . . . . . . .200
cut (*Allens/Princella/Sugary Sam*), ⅔ cup . . . . . . . . . . . . . .160
cut (*Glory Foods*) . . . . . . . . . . . . . . . . . . . . . . . . . . . . . . .120
mashed (*Princella/Sugary Sam*), ⅔ cup . . . . . . . . . . . . . . . .120
candied (*Royal Prince*) . . . . . . . . . . . . . . . . . . . . . . . . . . .210

orange–pineapple (*Royal Prince*) . . . . . . . . . . . . . . . . . . . . .210
in syrup (*Sylvia's* Yams) . . . . . . . . . . . . . . . . . . . . . . . . .120
**Sweet potato, frozen:**
baked, cubed, ½ cup . . . . . . . . . . . . . . . . . . . . . . . . . . . .88
candied (*Green Giant*), ¾ cup . . . . . . . . . . . . . . . . . . . . . .240
candied (*Mrs. Paul's*), 5 oz. . . . . . . . . . . . . . . . . . . . . . . .300
candied, w/apple (*Mrs. Paul's*), 1¼ cups . . . . . . . . . . . . . . .270
**Sweet potato chips,** all varieties (*Terra*), 1 oz. . . . . . . . . . . .140
**Sweet and sour drink mixer** (*Mr & Mrs T*), 4 fl. oz. . . . . . .150
**Sweet and sour sauce,** 2 tbsp.:
(*Contadina*) . . . . . . . . . . . . . . . . . . . . . . . . . . . . . . . . .40
(*Kikkoman*) . . . . . . . . . . . . . . . . . . . . . . . . . . . . . . . . .35
duck sauce (*Ka•Me*) . . . . . . . . . . . . . . . . . . . . . . . . . . . .60
duck sauce (*Ty Ling*) . . . . . . . . . . . . . . . . . . . . . . . . . . .70
w/ginger (*Ka•Me*) . . . . . . . . . . . . . . . . . . . . . . . . . . . . . .50
Hawaiian style (*World Harbors*) . . . . . . . . . . . . . . . . . . . . .60
**Swiss chard,** fresh:
raw (*Frieda's*), 1 cup, 3 oz. . . . . . . . . . . . . . . . . . . . . . . . .15
boiled, drained, chopped, ½ cup . . . . . . . . . . . . . . . . . . . . .18
**Swisswurst** (*Johnsonville*), 2.7-oz. link . . . . . . . . . . . . . . .240
**Swordfish,** fresh, meat only:
raw, 4 oz. . . . . . . . . . . . . . . . . . . . . . . . . . . . . . . . . . .137
baked, broiled, or microwaved, 4 oz. . . . . . . . . . . . . . . . . .176
**Syrup,** see "Pancake syrup" and specific syrup listings
**Szechuan sauce** (*Ka•Me*), 1 tbsp. . . . . . . . . . . . . . . . . . . .25

# T

**FOOD AND MEASURE** | **CALORIES**

**Tabouli** (*Frieda's*), ½ cup . . . . . . . . . . . . . . . . . . . . . . . . .160
**Tabouli salad mix:**
(*Cedar's*), 2 tbsp. . . . . . . . . . . . . . . . . . . . . . . . . . . . . .30
(*Near East*), ⅔ cup* . . . . . . . . . . . . . . . . . . . . . . . .110
(*Yorgo*), 2 tbsp. . . . . . . . . . . . . . . . . . . . . . . . . . . . . .25
**Taco,** frozen, 1 pc.:
beef/cheese, soft (*El Monterey Family Classics*), 5.5 oz. . . . .440
beef/cheese, spicy (*El Monterey Family Classics*), 5 oz. . . . .380
beef/cheese, spicy (*El Monterey Family Classics*), 5.5 oz. . . .420
beef/pork, soft (*El Monterey Family Classics*), 4 oz. . . . . . .230
***Taco Bell,*** 1 serving:
burrito, bean . . . . . . . . . . . . . . . . . . . . . . . . . . . . . .370
burrito, chili cheese . . . . . . . . . . . . . . . . . . . . . . . . . .330
burrito, fiesta, beef . . . . . . . . . . . . . . . . . . . . . . . . . .380
burrito, fiesta, chicken or steak . . . . . . . . . . . . . . . . . .370
burrito, grilled stuft, beef . . . . . . . . . . . . . . . . . . . . . .730
burrito, grilled stuft, chicken or steak . . . . . . . . . . . . . .690
burrito, 7-layer . . . . . . . . . . . . . . . . . . . . . . . . . . . . .520
*Burrito Supreme,* beef . . . . . . . . . . . . . . . . . . . . . . . .430
*Burrito Supreme,* chicken . . . . . . . . . . . . . . . . . . . . . .410
*Burrito Supreme,* steak . . . . . . . . . . . . . . . . . . . . . . .420
*Burrito Supreme,* double, beef . . . . . . . . . . . . . . . . . .510
*Burrito Supreme,* double, chicken . . . . . . . . . . . . . . . .460
*Burrito Supreme,* double, steak . . . . . . . . . . . . . . . . . .470
*Chalupa Baja,* beef . . . . . . . . . . . . . . . . . . . . . . . . . .420
*Chalupa Baja,* chicken or steak . . . . . . . . . . . . . . . . . .400
chalupa nacho cheese, beef . . . . . . . . . . . . . . . . . . . . .370
chalupa nacho, chicken or steak . . . . . . . . . . . . . . . . . .350
*Chalupa Supreme,* beef . . . . . . . . . . . . . . . . . . . . . . .380
*Chalupa Supreme,* chicken or steak . . . . . . . . . . . . . . .360
cheesy gordita crunch . . . . . . . . . . . . . . . . . . . . . . . . .560
cheesy gordita crunch *Supreme* . . . . . . . . . . . . . . . . . .610
*Gordita Baja,* beef . . . . . . . . . . . . . . . . . . . . . . . . . .360
*Gordita Baja,* chicken or steak . . . . . . . . . . . . . . . . . .340

gordita nacho cheese, beef . . . . . . . . . . . . . . . . . . . . . . . . . . .310
gordita nacho, chicken or steak . . . . . . . . . . . . . . . . . . . . . . . .290
*Gordita Supreme,* beef, chicken, or steak . . . . . . . . . . . . . .300
taco, *Double Decker* . . . . . . . . . . . . . . . . . . . . . . . . . . . . . .380
taco, regular . . . . . . . . . . . . . . . . . . . . . . . . . . . . . . . . . . . .210
taco, soft, beef . . . . . . . . . . . . . . . . . . . . . . . . . . . . . . . . . .210
taco, soft, chicken or steak . . . . . . . . . . . . . . . . . . . . . . . . .190
*Taco Supreme, Double Decker* . . . . . . . . . . . . . . . . . . . . . . .380
*Taco Supreme,* regular . . . . . . . . . . . . . . . . . . . . . . . . . . . .210
*Taco Supreme,* soft, beef . . . . . . . . . . . . . . . . . . . . . . . . . .210
*Taco Supreme,* soft, chicken . . . . . . . . . . . . . . . . . . . . . . . .190
*Tace Supreme,* soft, steak . . . . . . . . . . . . . . . . . . . . . . . . . .280
specialties:
*Enchirito,* beef . . . . . . . . . . . . . . . . . . . . . . . . . . . . . . . . .370
*Enchirito,* chicken or steak . . . . . . . . . . . . . . . . . . . . . . . .350
Mexican pizza . . . . . . . . . . . . . . . . . . . . . . . . . . . . . . . . . .390
*MexiMelt* . . . . . . . . . . . . . . . . . . . . . . . . . . . . . . . . . . . . .290
taco salad, w/salsa . . . . . . . . . . . . . . . . . . . . . . . . . . . . . .850
taco salad, w/salsa, w/out shell . . . . . . . . . . . . . . . . . . . . .400
tostada . . . . . . . . . . . . . . . . . . . . . . . . . . . . . . . . . . . . . . .250
quesadilla, cheese . . . . . . . . . . . . . . . . . . . . . . . . . . . . . . .490
quesadilla, chicken . . . . . . . . . . . . . . . . . . . . . . . . . . . . . .540
zesty chicken border bowl w/dressing . . . . . . . . . . . . . . .720
zesty chicken border bowl w/out dressing . . . . . . . . . . . .470
nachos and sides:
Mexican rice . . . . . . . . . . . . . . . . . . . . . . . . . . . . . . . . . . .190
nachos . . . . . . . . . . . . . . . . . . . . . . . . . . . . . . . . . . . . . . . .320
*Nachos BellGrande* . . . . . . . . . . . . . . . . . . . . . . . . . . . . . .760
nachos, mucho grande . . . . . . . . . . . . . . . . . . . . . . . . . . .1,320
*Nachos Supreme* . . . . . . . . . . . . . . . . . . . . . . . . . . . . . . . .440
Pintos 'n Cheese . . . . . . . . . . . . . . . . . . . . . . . . . . . . . . . .180
twists, cinnamon . . . . . . . . . . . . . . . . . . . . . . . . . . . . . . . .150
**Taco entree,** frozen, 1 pkg.:
beef, mini (*Swanson Fun Feast*), 7.2 oz. . . . . . . . . . . . . . . .400
beef, w/salsa and rice (*Michelina's*), 8 oz. . . . . . . . . . . . . .380
**Taco filling,** beef, frozen (*Ortega*), ⅓ cup . . . . . . . . . . . . .100
**Taco sauce,** 1 tbsp., except as noted:
(*Chi-Chi's*) . . . . . . . . . . . . . . . . . . . . . . . . . . . . . . . . . . . . . .10
hot, medium, or mild (*Ortega*) . . . . . . . . . . . . . . . . . . . . . . .10
hot, medium, or mild (*Old El Paso*) . . . . . . . . . . . . . . . . . . . .5

**Taco sauce *(cont.)***
hot or mild (*Mrs. Renfro's*), 2 tbsp. . . . . . . . . . . . . . . . . . . . .10
red, medium or mild (*La Victoria*) . . . . . . . . . . . . . . . . . . . . . .5
**Taco seasoning mix:**
(*Bearitos*), 2¼ tsp. . . . . . . . . . . . . . . . . . . . . . . . . . . . . .20
(*El Torito*), ⅕ pkt. . . . . . . . . . . . . . . . . . . . . . . . . . . . . .25
(*Hain*), 2 tsp. . . . . . . . . . . . . . . . . . . . . . . . . . . . . . . . .20
(*McCormick* Original/Less Sodium), ⅙ pkg. . . . . . . . . . . . .20
(*Old El Paso*), 2 tsp. . . . . . . . . . . . . . . . . . . . . . . . . . . .15
chicken (*McCormick*), ¼ pkg. . . . . . . . . . . . . . . . . . . . . . .25
hot or mild (*McCormick*), ⅙ pkg. . . . . . . . . . . . . . . . . . . .20
**Taco shell** (see also "Tortilla"):
(*Old El Paso*), 3 pcs. . . . . . . . . . . . . . . . . . . . . . . . . . .150
tostada (*Los Pericos*), 1 pc. . . . . . . . . . . . . . . . . . . . . . .90
tostada (*Old El Paso*), 3 pcs. . . . . . . . . . . . . . . . . . . . .150
white/yellow corn (*Chi-Chi's*), 2 pcs. . . . . . . . . . . . . . . . .170
**Tahini:**
(*Joyva*), 2 tbsp. . . . . . . . . . . . . . . . . . . . . . . . . . . . . .200
(*Telma* Tehina), ½ cup . . . . . . . . . . . . . . . . . . . . . . . . .230
**Tahini spread/dip** (*Sabra Salads*), 1 oz. . . . . . . . . . . . . . .80
**Tamale, frozen,** 1 pc.:
(*Goya*) . . . . . . . . . . . . . . . . . . . . . . . . . . . . . . . . . . . .240
beef (*El Monterey*) . . . . . . . . . . . . . . . . . . . . . . . . . . . .300
beef (*El Monterey Family Classics*) . . . . . . . . . . . . . . . . . .230
chicken (*El Monterey/El Monterey Family Classics*) . . . . . . .250
**Tamale dinner,** frozen, 1 pkg.:
beef (*Patio*), 12 oz. . . . . . . . . . . . . . . . . . . . . . . . . . . .440
beef, and enchilada (*Patio*), 12.25 oz. . . . . . . . . . . . . . . .480
**Tamale pot pie,** frozen, Mexican (*Amy's*), 8 oz. . . . . . . . . .220
**Tamari,** see "Soy sauce"
**Tamarillo,** fresh (*Frieda's*), 2 pcs., 4.2 oz. . . . . . . . . . . . . .40
**Tamarind,** pulp, ½ cup . . . . . . . . . . . . . . . . . . . . . . . . .144
**Tangerine,** fresh:
(*Dole*), 1 medium, 3.8 oz. . . . . . . . . . . . . . . . . . . . . . . . . .50
(*Frieda's* Delite/Pixie/Page Mandarin/Satsuma), 5 oz. . . . . .60
1 large, 2½" diam. . . . . . . . . . . . . . . . . . . . . . . . . . . . . . .37
sections w/out membrane, ½ cup . . . . . . . . . . . . . . . . . . . .43
**Tangerine, canned:**
in juice, ½ cup . . . . . . . . . . . . . . . . . . . . . . . . . . . . . . . .46
in light syrup (*Del Monte*), ½ cup . . . . . . . . . . . . . . . . . . .80

in light syrup (*Del Monte* Snack Cup), ½ cup . . . . . . . . . . . .70
in light syrup (*Dole*), ½ cup . . . . . . . . . . . . . . . . . . . . . . . .80
in light syrup (*Garden Treat* Mandarin), ⅔ cup . . . . . . . . . .100
**Tangerine drink,** ruby red:
(*Tropicana Twister*), 8 fl. oz. . . . . . . . . . . . . . . . . . . . . . . .130
(*Tropicana Twister*), 11.5 fl. oz. . . . . . . . . . . . . . . . . . . . .190
**Tangerine juice:**
fresh, 8 fl. oz. . . . . . . . . . . . . . . . . . . . . . . . . . . . . . . . .106
frozen*, 8 fl. oz. . . . . . . . . . . . . . . . . . . . . . . . . . . . . . . .111
**Taquito,** frozen, 4.5-oz. pc.:
beef/cheese (*El Monterey Family Classics*) . . . . . . . . . . . . .330
chicken/cheese (*El Monterey Family Classics*) . . . . . . . . . . .310
**Taquito, breakfast,** frozen, egg, bacon, cheese, salsa
(*El Monterey Family Classics*), 4.5 oz. . . . . . . . . . . . . . . .290
**Tapioca pudding,** see "Pudding" and "Pudding and pie
filling mix"
**Taro,** fresh:
raw, sliced, ½ cup . . . . . . . . . . . . . . . . . . . . . . . . . . . . . .56
cooked, sliced, ½ cup . . . . . . . . . . . . . . . . . . . . . . . . . . .94
**Taro, Tahitian:**
raw, sliced, ½ cup . . . . . . . . . . . . . . . . . . . . . . . . . . . . . .25
cooked, sliced, ½ cup . . . . . . . . . . . . . . . . . . . . . . . . . . .30
**Taro chips:**
(*Terra*), 1 oz. . . . . . . . . . . . . . . . . . . . . . . . . . . . . . . . .140
spiced (*Terra*), 1 oz. . . . . . . . . . . . . . . . . . . . . . . . . . . .130
**Taro root,** raw (*Frieda's*), ⅔ cup, 3 oz. . . . . . . . . . . . . . . . .90
**Tarragon,** ground, 1 tsp. . . . . . . . . . . . . . . . . . . . . . . . . . . .5
**Tartar sauce,** 2 tbsp.:
(*Golden Dipt*) . . . . . . . . . . . . . . . . . . . . . . . . . . . . . . . .160
(*Golden Dipt* Fat Free) . . . . . . . . . . . . . . . . . . . . . . . . . . .35
(*Hellmann's/Best Foods*) . . . . . . . . . . . . . . . . . . . . . . . . . .80
(*Hellmann's/Best Foods* Low Fat) . . . . . . . . . . . . . . . . . . . .40
(*Maille* Dipping) . . . . . . . . . . . . . . . . . . . . . . . . . . . . . . .140
(*Marzetti* Sauce Shoppe) . . . . . . . . . . . . . . . . . . . . . . . . .120
(*Old Bay*) . . . . . . . . . . . . . . . . . . . . . . . . . . . . . . . . . . .130
***TCBY,*** all flavors, ½ cup:
ice cream, hand-dipped, lowfat . . . . . . . . . . . . . . . . . . . . .120
ice cream, hand-dipped, lowfat, no sugar . . . . . . . . . . . . . .100
sorbet, soft serve . . . . . . . . . . . . . . . . . . . . . . . . . . . . . . .100
yogurt, soft serve, 96% fat free . . . . . . . . . . . . . . . . . . . . .130

***TCBY (cont.)***
yogurt, soft serve, nonfat . . . . . . . . . . . . . . . . . . . . . . . . .110
yogurt, soft serve, nonfat, no sugar . . . . . . . . . . . . . . . . . . . .80
**Tea** (see also "Tea, iced"), plain, 1 bag or tsp. . . . . . . . . . . . .0
**Tea, iced,** 8 fl. oz.:
(*AriZona*) . . . . . . . . . . . . . . . . . . . . . . . . . . . . . . . . . .90
(*AriZona Rx Health/Stress*) . . . . . . . . . . . . . . . . . . . . . . . .70
(*AriZona Rx Energy*) . . . . . . . . . . . . . . . . . . . . . . . . . . .120
(*AriZona Rx Memory*) . . . . . . . . . . . . . . . . . . . . . . . . . . .80
(*Turkey Hill*) . . . . . . . . . . . . . . . . . . . . . . . . . . . . . . . .90
(*Turkey Hill* Decaf) . . . . . . . . . . . . . . . . . . . . . . . . . . . .80
ginseng (*AriZona* Extract) . . . . . . . . . . . . . . . . . . . . . . . .60
green tea, all varieties (*AriZona*) . . . . . . . . . . . . . . . . . . .70
green tea, w/ginseng and honey (*Turkey Hill*) . . . . . . . . . . . .70
lemon (*Turkey Hill* Cooler) . . . . . . . . . . . . . . . . . . . . . . .100
lemon, peach, or raspberry (*AriZona*) . . . . . . . . . . . . . . . . .90
lemon, peach, or raspberry (*Snapple*) . . . . . . . . . . . . . . . .100
lemonade or mint (*Snapple*) . . . . . . . . . . . . . . . . . . . . . . .110
mint, w/chamomile (*Turkey Hill* Cooler) . . . . . . . . . . . . . . . .90
oolong, blueberry or w/ginkgo, ginseng (*Turkey Hill*) . . . . .100
orange (*Turkey Hill* Cooler) . . . . . . . . . . . . . . . . . . . . . . .100
peach or raspberry (*Turkey Hill* Cooler) . . . . . . . . . . . . . . .110
sweet (*Snapple*) . . . . . . . . . . . . . . . . . . . . . . . . . . . . . .120
**Tea, iced, mix:**
(*Nestea* 100%/Sun Tea), 2 tsp. . . . . . . . . . . . . . . . . . . . . . .0
(*Nestea* Sugar Free), 2 tsp. . . . . . . . . . . . . . . . . . . . . . . . .5
herb, lemon or orange spice (*Nestea*), 1 tbsp. . . . . . . . . . . .15
lemon (*Nestea*), 2 tsp. . . . . . . . . . . . . . . . . . . . . . . . . . . .5
lemon and sugar or lemonade (*Nestea*), 2 tbsp. . . . . . . . . . .80
peach, raspberry, or tangerine (*Watkins*), 4 tsp. . . . . . . . . .80
**Teff seed or flour** (*Arrowhead Mills*), 2 oz. . . . . . . . . . . . .200
**Tempeh,** ½ cup . . . . . . . . . . . . . . . . . . . . . . . . . . . . . .160
**Tempura batter mix** (*Golden Dipt* Fry Easy), ¼ cup . . . . . .100
**Teriyaki entree,** frozen (*Lean Cuisine Everyday Favorites*),
10-oz. pkg. . . . . . . . . . . . . . . . . . . . . . . . . . . . . . . . . .290
**Teriyaki sauce** (see also "Marinade"):
(*Kikkoman* Baste & Glaze), 2 tbsp. . . . . . . . . . . . . . . . . . . .50
(*San-J*), 1 tbsp. . . . . . . . . . . . . . . . . . . . . . . . . . . . . . . .10
(*Sun Luck* Honey Mirin), 1 tbsp. . . . . . . . . . . . . . . . . . . . . .30
(*Sushi Chef*), 1 tbsp. . . . . . . . . . . . . . . . . . . . . . . . . . . . .35

(*Watkins* Tangy), 1 tbsp. . . . . . . . . . . . . . . . . . . . . . . . . . .15
chicken (*Lawry's* Weekday Gourmet), 2 tbsp. . . . . . . . . . . . .40
Hawaiian style, and marinade (*World Harbors*), 2 tbsp. . . . . .70
w/honey, pineapple (*Kikkoman* Baste & Glaze), 2 tbsp. . . . . .80
hot, tropical (*World Harbors Maui Mountain*), 2 tbsp. . . . . . .70
Polynesian (*Trader Vic's*), 1 tbsp. . . . . . . . . . . . . . . . . . . . .15
sesame garlic (*Rice Road*), 1 tbsp. . . . . . . . . . . . . . . . . . . .15
**Texas toast,** see "Bread, frozen"
**Thai sauce** (see also "Peanut sauce" and specific listings):
chili, garlic pepper or sweet green/red (*A Taste of Thai*),
1 tsp. . . . . . . . . . . . . . . . . . . . . . . . . . . . . . . . . . . . .10
chili, pepper paste (*A Taste of Thai*), 1 tsp. . . . . . . . . . . . . . .20
curry, green (*Ka•Me*), 1 tbsp. . . . . . . . . . . . . . . . . . . . . . . .10
curry, red (*Ka•Me*), 1 tbsp. . . . . . . . . . . . . . . . . . . . . . . . . .15
curry base, see "Curry sauce base"
and marinade, East Asian (*World Harbors*), 2 tbsp. . . . . . . . .40
pad Thai (*A Taste of Thai*), 2 tbsp. . . . . . . . . . . . . . . . . . . . .90
seasoning (*A Taste of Thai*), 1 tbsp. . . . . . . . . . . . . . . . . . . .15
**Thuringer cervelat,** see "Summer sausage"
**Thyme,** ground, 1 tsp. . . . . . . . . . . . . . . . . . . . . . . . . . . . . .4
**Thymus,** 4 oz.:
beef, braised . . . . . . . . . . . . . . . . . . . . . . . . . . . . . . . . . .362
veal, braised . . . . . . . . . . . . . . . . . . . . . . . . . . . . . . . . . .197
**Tikka sauce,** see "Curry sauce, cooking"
**Tilefish,** meat only:
raw, 4 oz. . . . . . . . . . . . . . . . . . . . . . . . . . . . . . . . . . . . .109
baked, broiled, or microwaved, 4 oz. . . . . . . . . . . . . . . . . . .167
**Toaster bagel, muffin, and pastry,** 1 pc.:
all fruit varieties (*Weight Watchers*) . . . . . . . . . . . . . . . . .190
all varieties, except cream cheese (*Toaster Strudel*) . . . . . .190
apple cinnamon (*Pop-Tarts*) . . . . . . . . . . . . . . . . . . . . . . . .210
apple cinnamon (*Pop-Tarts Pastry Swirls*) . . . . . . . . . . . . .260
bagel, cream cheese, all varieties (*Toaster Bagel Shoppe*) . . .130
berry, frosted (*Pop-Tarts Snack-Stix*) . . . . . . . . . . . . . . . . .190
berry, wild (*Pop-Tarts*) . . . . . . . . . . . . . . . . . . . . . . . . . . . .210
blueberry (*Eggo* Toaster Muffin) . . . . . . . . . . . . . . . . . . . . .120
blueberry (*Pop-Tarts*) . . . . . . . . . . . . . . . . . . . . . . . . . . . . .200
blueberry (*Thomas' Toast-r-Cakes*) . . . . . . . . . . . . . . . . . . . .90
blueberry, frosted (*Pop-Tarts*) . . . . . . . . . . . . . . . . . . . . . . .200
brown sugar cinnamon, plain or frosted (*Pop-Tarts*) . . . . . .210

**Toaster bagel, muffin, and pastry *(cont.)***

cheese (*Pop-Tarts Pastry Swirls*) . . . . . . . . . . . . . . . . . . . . .260
cherry, plain or frosted (*Pop-Tarts*) . . . . . . . . . . . . . . . . . . .200
chocolate fudge, frosted (*Pop-Tarts*) . . . . . . . . . . . . . . . . . .200
chocolate fudge, frosted (*Pop-Tarts* Low Fat) . . . . . . . . . . .190
chocolate–vanilla creme, frosted (*Pop-Tarts*) . . . . . . . . . . .200
cinnamon (*Eggo* Toaster Muffin) . . . . . . . . . . . . . . . . . . . . .130
corn (*Thomas' Toast-r-Cakes*) . . . . . . . . . . . . . . . . . . . . . . .100
cream cheese, all varieties (*Toaster Strudel*) . . . . . . . . . . . .200
eggs, w/cheese:
  all varieties, except Western (*Toaster Scrambles*) . . . . . .180
  Western style (*Toaster Scrambles*) . . . . . . . . . . . . . . . . .170
grape, frosted (*Pop-Tarts*) . . . . . . . . . . . . . . . . . . . . . . . . .200
pizza, see "Pizza, stuffed/pocket"
raisin bran (*Thomas' Toast-r-Cake*) . . . . . . . . . . . . . . . . . . . .90
raspberry, frosted (*Pop-Tarts*) . . . . . . . . . . . . . . . . . . . . . .210
S'mores (*Pop-Tarts*) . . . . . . . . . . . . . . . . . . . . . . . . . . . . . .200
strawberry (*Eggo* Toaster Muffin) . . . . . . . . . . . . . . . . . . . .130
strawberry (*Pop-Tarts*) . . . . . . . . . . . . . . . . . . . . . . . . . . . .200
strawberry (*Pop-Tarts* Low Fat) . . . . . . . . . . . . . . . . . . . . .190
strawberry (*Pop Tarts Pastry Swirls*) . . . . . . . . . . . . . . . . . .260
strawberry, frosted (*Pop-Tarts*) . . . . . . . . . . . . . . . . . . . . .200
strawberry, frosted (*Pop-Tarts* Low Fat) . . . . . . . . . . . . . . .190
strawberry, frosted (*Pop-Tarts Snack-Stix*) . . . . . . . . . . . . .190
tropical, frosted (*Pop-Tarts Wild Tropical Blast*) . . . . . . . . .210
watermelon, wild, frosted (*Pop-Tarts*) . . . . . . . . . . . . . . . .210

**Tofu:**

fresh, unflavored:
  extra firm (*Azumaya* Lite), 2.8 oz. . . . . . . . . . . . . . . . . . . .60
  extra firm (*Nasoya*), 3 oz. . . . . . . . . . . . . . . . . . . . . . . . . .90
  extra firm or firm (*Azumaya*), 2.8 oz. . . . . . . . . . . . . . . . .70
  firm (*Nasoya*), 3 oz. . . . . . . . . . . . . . . . . . . . . . . . . . . . . .70
  firm (*Tree of Life* Organic/Vacuum Pack), ⅕ block . . . . .100
  silken (*Azumaya*), 3.2 oz. . . . . . . . . . . . . . . . . . . . . . . . . .50
  silken (*Azumaya* Lite), 3.2 oz. . . . . . . . . . . . . . . . . . . . . .40
  silken (*Nasoya*), 3.2 oz. . . . . . . . . . . . . . . . . . . . . . . . . . .45
  silken, enriched (*Nasoya*), ⅕ of 1-lb. block . . . . . . . . . . .40
  soft (*Nasoya*), 3 oz. . . . . . . . . . . . . . . . . . . . . . . . . . . . . .60
fresh, 5-spice or garlic–onion flavor (*Nasoya*), 3 oz. . . . . . . .70

baked:
(*Tree of Life* Organic), ⅓ block . . . . . . . . . . . . . . . . . . .150
chili picante (*Azumaya*), 2 pcs. . . . . . . . . . . . . . . . . . . . .200
mesquite (*Azumaya*), 2 pcs. . . . . . . . . . . . . . . . . . . . . . .190
mesquite smoke (*Nasoya*), 2 pcs. . . . . . . . . . . . . . . . . . . .220
Oriental (*Tree of Life* Organic), ⅓ block . . . . . . . . . . . . .130
savory or island spice (*Tree of Life* Organic),
⅓ block . . . . . . . . . . . . . . . . . . . . . . . . . . . . . . . . .140
teriyaki (*Azumaya*), 2 pcs. . . . . . . . . . . . . . . . . . . . . . .200
teriyaki or Tex-Mex (*Nasoya*), 2 pcs. . . . . . . . . . . . . . . .230
Thai peanut (*Nasoya*), 2 pcs. . . . . . . . . . . . . . . . . . . . . .240
Thai peanut, spicy (*Azumaya*), 2 pcs. . . . . . . . . . . . . . . .190
salted and fermented (fuyu), 1 oz. . . . . . . . . . . . . . . . . . . . .33
smoked (*Tree of Life* Original), ½ block . . . . . . . . . . . . . . .120
**Tofu, ground** (*Tree of Life Ready Ground*), 3 oz. . . . . . . . . . .60
**Tofu pudding,** see "Pudding, nondairy"
**Tofu sauce** (*Westbrae Natural*), 1 tsp. . . . . . . . . . . . . . . . . . .5
**Tofu seasoning mix,** ¼ pkg.:
breakfast scramble or eggless salad (*TofuMate*) . . . . . . . . . .15
mandarin stir-fry (*TofuMate*) . . . . . . . . . . . . . . . . . . . . . . . .30
Mediterranean herb or Texas taco (*TofuMate*) . . . . . . . . . . . .15
Szechuan stir-fry (*TofuMate*) . . . . . . . . . . . . . . . . . . . . . . . .25
**Tomatillo,** fresh:
1 medium, 1⅝" diam. . . . . . . . . . . . . . . . . . . . . . . . . . . . . .11
chopped, ½ cup . . . . . . . . . . . . . . . . . . . . . . . . . . . . . . . . .21
**Tomatillo, can or jar:**
whole (*Embasa*), 3 pcs., 2.1 oz. . . . . . . . . . . . . . . . . . . . . .15
whole (*La Costeña*), 4 pcs., 4.3 oz. . . . . . . . . . . . . . . . . . . .40
whole (*La Victoria* Entero), 5 pcs., 4.5 oz. . . . . . . . . . . . . .40
crushed (*Embasa*), ¼ cup . . . . . . . . . . . . . . . . . . . . . . . . . .10
**Tomato:**
raw (*Frieda's* Baby Roma/Teardrop), ⅔ cup, 3 oz. . . . . . . . .20
raw, 2⅗" tomato . . . . . . . . . . . . . . . . . . . . . . . . . . . . . . . . .26
raw, chopped or diced, ½ cup . . . . . . . . . . . . . . . . . . . . . . . .19
boiled, ½ cup . . . . . . . . . . . . . . . . . . . . . . . . . . . . . . . . . . .32
dried, see "Tomato, dried"
**Tomato, can or jar,** ½ cup, except as noted:
(*S&W Italian Recipe*) . . . . . . . . . . . . . . . . . . . . . . . . . . . . .35
whole, peeled (*Hunt's*) . . . . . . . . . . . . . . . . . . . . . . . . . . . .20

**Tomato, can or jar *(cont.)***
whole, peeled (*Progresso*) .25
whole, peeled (*Progresso* Italian) .20
whole, peeled, plain or basil (*Muir Glen*) .30
crushed (*Del Monte* Original or Italian Recipe) .45
crushed (*Hunt's*) .30
crushed garlic or Italian herb (*Contadina*), ¼ cup .20
crushed, fire-roasted (*Muir Glen*), ¼ cup .20
crushed, w/garlic (*Del Monte*) .50
diced (*Red Gold*) .25
diced (*Red Gold* Chili Ready) .35
diced (*S&W Ready Cut*) .25
diced, basil, garlic, oregano (*Hunt's*) .25
diced, fire-roasted (*Muir Glen*), ¼ cup .30
diced, garlic or green pepper and onion (*Del Monte*) .40
diced, green chili or jalapeño (*Del Monte*) .30
diced, Italian (*Red Gold*) .50
diced, onions, sauteed (*Contadina*) .40
paste or puree, see "Tomato paste and Tomato puree"
stewed (*Hunt's*) .30
stewed (*Muir Glen*) .30
stewed, all styles, except Italian (*Del Monte*) .35
stewed, Italian (*Del Monte*) .30
**Tomato, dried:**
1 pc., 32 pcs. per cup .5
½ cup .70
bits (*Sonoma*), 2–3 tsp. .15
halves (*Sonoma*), 2–3 pcs. .15
halves or chopped (*Frieda's*), ⅓ cup, 1.1 oz. .100
marinated:
(*Frieda's* Julienne), 1 tbsp. .35
(*Hogue Farms*), 3 pcs. .40
(*Sonoma*), 2–3 halves .35
in oil (*Roland* Sun-dried), 2 pcs. .45
yellow, halves or chopped (*Frieda's*), ½ cup, 3 oz. .220
**Tomato, pickled:**
(*Ba-Tampte*), ½ pc., 1.5 oz. .5
(*Claussen*), 1 oz. .5
(*Hebrew National/Shorr's*), 1 oz. .4
**Tomato, sun-dried,** see "Tomato, dried"

**Tomato blend,** dried (*Frieda's* Tomato Toss), ½ cup, 1.1 oz. . . . . . . . . . . . . . . . . . . . . . . . . . . . .100
**Tomato dip mix,** bacon or horseradish (*Watkins*), 1 tsp. . . . .10
**Tomato juice,** 8 fl. oz., except as noted:
(*Campbell's/Campbell's Healthy Request*) . . . . . . . . . . . . . . .50
(*Eden* Organic) . . . . . . . . . . . . . . . . . . . . . . . . . . . . . . . . .35
(*Muir Glen*) . . . . . . . . . . . . . . . . . . . . . . . . . . . . . . . . . . .40
(*Red Gold*) . . . . . . . . . . . . . . . . . . . . . . . . . . . . . . . . . . .45
(*Sacramento*) . . . . . . . . . . . . . . . . . . . . . . . . . . . . . . . . . .40
(*Sacramento*), 6 fl. oz. . . . . . . . . . . . . . . . . . . . . . . . . . . .35
(*Welch's*) . . . . . . . . . . . . . . . . . . . . . . . . . . . . . . . . . . . .50
**Tomato paste,** 2 tbsp., except as noted:
(*Hunt's*) . . . . . . . . . . . . . . . . . . . . . . . . . . . . . . . . . . . .25
(*Progresso*) . . . . . . . . . . . . . . . . . . . . . . . . . . . . . . . . . .30
(*Red Gold*) . . . . . . . . . . . . . . . . . . . . . . . . . . . . . . . . . . .30
double concentrate (*Amore*), 1½ tbsp. . . . . . . . . . . . . . . . . . .35
Italian, roasted garlic, or pesto (*Contadina*) . . . . . . . . . . . . . .35
**Tomato pesto,** see "Pesto sauce"
**Tomato puree,** ¼ cup:
(*Contadina*) . . . . . . . . . . . . . . . . . . . . . . . . . . . . . . . . . . .20
(*Progresso*) . . . . . . . . . . . . . . . . . . . . . . . . . . . . . . . . . .25
(*Red Gold*) . . . . . . . . . . . . . . . . . . . . . . . . . . . . . . . . . . .25
thick (*Progresso*) . . . . . . . . . . . . . . . . . . . . . . . . . . . . . . .20
**Tomato relish,** 1 tbsp.:
(*Heinz* Piccalilli) . . . . . . . . . . . . . . . . . . . . . . . . . . . . . . .15
(*Pickle Eater's* Piccalilli) . . . . . . . . . . . . . . . . . . . . . . . . .10
hot or mild (*Mrs. Renfro's*) . . . . . . . . . . . . . . . . . . . . . . . .10
medium, Indian (*Patak's*) . . . . . . . . . . . . . . . . . . . . . . . . . .10
**Tomato sauce,** canned (see also "Pasta sauce"), ¼ cup:
(*Del Monte*) . . . . . . . . . . . . . . . . . . . . . . . . . . . . . . . . . . .20
(*Hunt's*) . . . . . . . . . . . . . . . . . . . . . . . . . . . . . . . . . . . .15
(*Hunt's* for Chili) . . . . . . . . . . . . . . . . . . . . . . . . . . . . . . .25
(*Hunt's* for Lasagna) . . . . . . . . . . . . . . . . . . . . . . . . . . . . .40
(*Hunt's* for Meat Loaf) . . . . . . . . . . . . . . . . . . . . . . . . . . . .30
(*Hunt's* for Pasta) . . . . . . . . . . . . . . . . . . . . . . . . . . . . . . .50
(*Hunt's* for Tacos) . . . . . . . . . . . . . . . . . . . . . . . . . . . . . . .15
(*Muir Glen/Muir Glen* Chunky) . . . . . . . . . . . . . . . . . . . . . . .20
(*Progresso*) . . . . . . . . . . . . . . . . . . . . . . . . . . . . . . . . . .20
(*Red Gold*) . . . . . . . . . . . . . . . . . . . . . . . . . . . . . . . . . . .20
**Tomato–beef drink** (*Beefamato*), 8 fl. oz. . . . . . . . . . . . . . .50

**Tomato–chile cocktail** (*Snap-E-Tom*), 6 fl. oz. . . . . . . . . . . .40
**Tomato–clam drink,** 8 fl. oz.:
(*Clamato* Bloody Caesar) . . . . . . . . . . . . . . . . . . . . . . . . . .50
plain or picante (*Clamato*) . . . . . . . . . . . . . . . . . . . . . . . . .60
**Tomato–olive relish** (*Sonoma* Muffaletta), 2 tbsp. . . . . . . . . .70
**Tongue,** braised or simmered:
beef, 4 oz. . . . . . . . . . . . . . . . . . . . . . . . . . . . . . . . . . . .321
veal (calf), 4 oz. . . . . . . . . . . . . . . . . . . . . . . . . . . . . . . .229
**Tongue lunch meat,** beef, 2 oz.:
and bloodwurst (*Boar's Head*) . . . . . . . . . . . . . . . . . . . . . .170
corned (*Hebrew National*) . . . . . . . . . . . . . . . . . . . . . . . . .120
**Tortellini** (see also "Tortelloni"), refrigerated:
cheese (*Celentano*), 1 cup . . . . . . . . . . . . . . . . . . . . . . . .420
cheese, 3 (*Buitoni*), 1 cup . . . . . . . . . . . . . . . . . . . . . . . .290
chicken and herb or spinach cheese (*Buitoni*), ¾ cup . . . . .260
meat (*Celentano*), 1 cup . . . . . . . . . . . . . . . . . . . . . . . . . .340
**Tortellini entree, canned,** meat (*Chef Boyardee*),
½ of 15-oz. can . . . . . . . . . . . . . . . . . . . . . . . . . . . . . . .260
**Tortellini entree, frozen,** 1 pkg.:
cheese (*Healthy Choice* Bowl), 10.35 oz. . . . . . . . . . . . . . . .320
cheese (*Wolfgang Puck's*), 12 oz. . . . . . . . . . . . . . . . . . . . .360
chicken, spicy (*Wolfgang Puck's*), 12 oz. . . . . . . . . . . . . . .490
mushroom (*Wolfgang Puck's*), 12 oz. . . . . . . . . . . . . . . . . .430
**Tortelloni** (see also "Tortellini"), refrigerated, 1 cup:
cheese and roasted garlic (*Buitoni*) . . . . . . . . . . . . . . . . .270
chicken and prosciutto (*Buitoni*) . . . . . . . . . . . . . . . . . . . .360
mozzarella and cheese (*Buitoni*) . . . . . . . . . . . . . . . . . . . .320
**Tortilla:**
corn (*Azteca*), 2 pcs., 1.2 oz. . . . . . . . . . . . . . . . . . . . . . . .90
flour (*Azteca*), 2 pcs., 1.7 oz. . . . . . . . . . . . . . . . . . . . . .150
flour (*Azteca*), 1.4-oz. pc. . . . . . . . . . . . . . . . . . . . . . . . .130
flour (*Azteca* Burrito Size), 1.75-oz. pc. . . . . . . . . . . . . . . .160
flour (*Azteca* Fat Free), 1.4-oz. pc. . . . . . . . . . . . . . . . . . .110
flour or soft taco (*Old El Paso*), 2 pcs. . . . . . . . . . . . . . . .160
**Tortilla chips,** see "Corn chips and similar snacks"
**Tortilla entree,** frozen (*Michelina's* Sunset), 8-oz. pkg. . . . .310
**Trail mix,** 3 tbsp.:
apple cranberry crunch (*Planters*) . . . . . . . . . . . . . . . . . . .140
Cajun crunch (*Planters*), ⅓ cup . . . . . . . . . . . . . . . . . . . .130

caramel nut crunch (*Planters*) ........................140
Caribbean crunch (*Planters*) ........................140
fruit and nuts (*Planters* 6 oz.) ........................130
fruit and nuts (*Planters* 10 oz.) ........................120
nuts and chocolate (*Planters*) ........................170
nuts and raisins (*Planters*) ........................160
**Tree fern,** cooked, chopped, ½ cup ....................28
**Trout** (see also "Sea trout"), meat only:
mixed species, raw, 4 oz. ........................168
mixed species, baked, broiled, or microwaved, 4 oz. ......215
rainbow, farmed, raw, 4 oz. ........................156
rainbow, farmed, baked, broiled, or microwaved, 4 oz. ....192
rainbow, wild, raw, 4 oz. ........................135
rainbow, wild, baked, broiled, or microwaved, 4 oz. ......170
**Trout, smoked,** fillet, 2 oz.:
(*Ducktrap River*) ........................110
peppered, rainbow (*Spence & Co.*) ....................100
**Trout, smoked, paté,** ¼ cup:
(*Ducktrap River*) ........................130
(*Ducktrap River* Lowfat) ........................70
**Tuna,** meat only:
bluefin, raw, 4 oz. ........................163
bluefin, baked, broiled, or microwaved, 4 oz. ...........208
skipjack, raw, 4 oz. ........................117
skipjack, baked, broiled, or microwaved, 4 oz. ..........150
yellowfin, raw, 4 oz. ........................123
yellowfin, baked, broiled, or microwaved, 4 oz. ..........158
**Tuna, canned,** drained, 2 oz. or ¼ cup, except as noted:
light, in oil (*Bumble Bee*) ........................110
light, in oil (*Chicken of the Sea*) ....................110
light, in oil (*Star-Kist* Pouch) ........................110
light, in water (*Bumble Bee*) ........................60
light, in water (*Chicken of the Sea*) ....................60
white, chunk, in water (*Chicken of the Sea*) ............60
white, solid, in oil (*Bumble Bee*) ........................90
white, solid, in oil (*Chicken of the Sea*) ................90
white, solid, in olive oil (*Chicken of the Sea* Genova) .....130
white, solid, in olive oil (*Progresso*) ..................160
white, solid, in water (*Bumble Bee*) ..................70

**Tuna, canned *(cont.)***
white, solid, in water (*Chicken of the Sea*) . . . . . . . . . . . . . .70
white, solid, in water (*Crown Prince Natural* Albacore) . . . . .65
**"Tuna," vegetarian:**
canned, drained (*Worthington Tuno*), ⅓ cup . . . . . . . . . . . . .80
frozen (*Worthington Tuno*), ½ cup . . . . . . . . . . . . . . . . . . . .80
frozen (*Veggie Master* Vege Fillet), ¼ pkg. . . . . . . . . . . . . .104
**Tuna burger,** frozen (*Omega Foods*), 3.2-oz. pc. . . . . . . . . . .90
**Tuna entree, frozen,** 1 pkg.:
(*Healthy Choice* Solo Casserole), 9 oz. . . . . . . . . . . . . . . . .240
and noodles (*Stouffer's* Casserole), 10 oz. . . . . . . . . . . . . .360
and noodles, homestyle (*Marie Callender's*), 10 oz. . . . . . . .430
**Tuna entree mix,** 1 cup*:
au gratin (*Tuna Helper*) . . . . . . . . . . . . . . . . . . . . . . . . . . .310
broccoli, cheesy (*Tuna Helper*) . . . . . . . . . . . . . . . . . . . . . .270
broccoli, creamy, or garden cheddar (*Tuna Helper*) . . . . . . .290
fettuccine Alfredo (*Tuna Helper*) . . . . . . . . . . . . . . . . . . . .310
pasta, cheesy (*Tuna Helper*) . . . . . . . . . . . . . . . . . . . . . . . .270
pasta, creamy (*Tuna Helper*) . . . . . . . . . . . . . . . . . . . . . . .290
tetrazzini or tuna melt (*Tuna Helper*) . . . . . . . . . . . . . . . . .300
**Tuna salad,** refrigerated:
(*Sabra Salads*), 1 oz. . . . . . . . . . . . . . . . . . . . . . . . . . . . . .85
(*Wampler*), ⅓ cup . . . . . . . . . . . . . . . . . . . . . . . . . . . . . .180
chunky (*Wampler*), ⅓ cup . . . . . . . . . . . . . . . . . . . . . . . . . .180
**Tuna seasoning** (*Old Bay Classic*), ⅕ pkg. . . . . . . . . . . . . . .30
**Turbot,** European, meat only:
raw, 4 oz. . . . . . . . . . . . . . . . . . . . . . . . . . . . . . . . . . . . . . .108
baked, broiled, or microwaved, 4 oz. . . . . . . . . . . . . . . . . . .138
**Turkey** (see also "Turkey, frozen and refrigerated"), fresh, all classes, roasted:
meat w/skin, 4 oz. . . . . . . . . . . . . . . . . . . . . . . . . . . . . . . .236
meat only, 4 oz. . . . . . . . . . . . . . . . . . . . . . . . . . . . . . . . . .193
meat only, diced, 1 cup . . . . . . . . . . . . . . . . . . . . . . . . . . . .238
skin only, 1 oz. . . . . . . . . . . . . . . . . . . . . . . . . . . . . . . . . . .125
dark meat, w/skin, 4 oz. . . . . . . . . . . . . . . . . . . . . . . . . . . .251
dark meat only, 4 oz. . . . . . . . . . . . . . . . . . . . . . . . . . . . . . .212
dark meat only, diced, 1 cup . . . . . . . . . . . . . . . . . . . . . . . .262
light meat, w/skin, 4 oz. . . . . . . . . . . . . . . . . . . . . . . . . . . .223
light meat only, 4 oz. . . . . . . . . . . . . . . . . . . . . . . . . . . . . .178
light meat only, diced, 1 cup . . . . . . . . . . . . . . . . . . . . . . . .219

breast, meat w/skin, ½ breast, 1.9 lb. (4.2 lbs. raw w/bone) . . . . . . . . . . . . . . . . . . . . . . . . . . . . . . .1,637
breast, meat w/skin, 4 oz. . . . . . . . . . . . . . . . . . . . . . . . . .214
ground, see "Turkey, ground"
leg, meat w/skin, 1.2 lb. (1.5 lbs. raw w/bone) . . . . . . . . .1,133
leg, meat w/skin, 4 oz. . . . . . . . . . . . . . . . . . . . . . . . . . . .236
wing, meat w/skin, 6.6 oz. (9.9 oz. raw w/bone) . . . . . . . . .426
wing, meat w/skin, 4 oz. . . . . . . . . . . . . . . . . . . . . . . . . . .260
**Turkey, canned,** 2 oz., ¼ cup:
(*Hormel* Chunk) . . . . . . . . . . . . . . . . . . . . . . . . . . . . . .70
white meat (*Hormel* Chunk) . . . . . . . . . . . . . . . . . . . . . . .60
**Turkey, cured,** dark meat (*Wampler*), 2 oz. . . . . . . . . . . . .80
**Turkey, frozen or refrigerated, raw,** 4 oz., except as noted:
whole (*Jennie-O*) . . . . . . . . . . . . . . . . . . . . . . . . . . . . .170
whole (*Norbest* Gold Label Hen) . . . . . . . . . . . . . . . . . . .195
whole, young (*Shady Brook Farms* Prime) . . . . . . . . . . . . .180
whole, young, basted (*Jennie-O* Young Frozen) . . . . . . . . . .160
boneless (*Jennie-O* Frozen) . . . . . . . . . . . . . . . . . . . . . .140
boneless (*Jennie-O* Young) . . . . . . . . . . . . . . . . . . . . . . .170
boneless, roast (*Norbest/Norbest* Breast) . . . . . . . . . . . . .135
breast (*Jennie-O*) . . . . . . . . . . . . . . . . . . . . . . . . . . . . .170
breast (*Norbest* Tender-Times) . . . . . . . . . . . . . . . . . . . .170
breast (*Shady Brook Farms*) . . . . . . . . . . . . . . . . . . . . . .180
breast, basted (*Jennie-O*) . . . . . . . . . . . . . . . . . . . . . . .170
breast, split, rotisserie (*Shady Brook Farms*) . . . . . . . . . . .180
breast, boneless fillet (*Perdue*) . . . . . . . . . . . . . . . . . . . .120
breast, boneless, slices (*Jennie-O*) . . . . . . . . . . . . . . . . . .90
breast half, marinated rotisserie (*Perdue*) . . . . . . . . . . . . .170
ground, see "Turkey, ground"
pan roast (*Jennie-O* Extra Lean), 5 oz. . . . . . . . . . . . . . . .120
pan roast, combo or white meat (*Jennie-O*), 5 oz. . . . . . . .150
tenderloin (*Perdue Fit 'n Easy*) . . . . . . . . . . . . . . . . . . . .120
tenderloin, butter garlic or cracked pepper (*Perdue*) . . . . . .110
thigh (*Shady Brook Farms*) . . . . . . . . . . . . . . . . . . . . . . .145
wing (*Shady Brook Farms*) . . . . . . . . . . . . . . . . . . . . . . . .220
**Turkey, frozen or refrigerated, cooked,** 3 oz., except as noted:
(*Boar's Head Deli Dinners Ovengold*) . . . . . . . . . . . . . . . . .90
whole, oven-roasted (*Shady Brook Farm*) . . . . . . . . . . . . . .130
whole, smoked (*Norbest*) . . . . . . . . . . . . . . . . . . . . . . . . .145
breast (*Perdue* Whole/Half) . . . . . . . . . . . . . . . . . . . . . . .150

**Turkey, frozen or refrigerated, cooked *(cont.)***
breast, cutlet, thin-sliced (*Perdue Fit 'n Easy*), 2.4 oz. . . . . . .90
breast, fillet or London broil cut (*Perdue Fit 'n Easy*) . . . . .110
breast, tenderloin (*Perdue Fit 'n Easy*) . . . . . . . . . . . . . . . .110
breast, honey roast (*Shady Brook Farms*) . . . . . . . . . . . . . . .70
breast, smoked, hickory (*Shady Brook Farms*) . . . . . . . . . . .60
breast half, marinated rotisserie (*Perdue*) . . . . . . . . . . . . . .130
drumstick, smoked (*Shady Brook Farms*) . . . . . . . . . . . . . .180
nuggets (*Louis Rich*), 4 pcs., 3.25 oz. . . . . . . . . . . . . . . . .260
tenderloin, cracked pepper (*Perdue*) . . . . . . . . . . . . . . . . . . .90
tenderloin, butter garlic (*Perdue*) . . . . . . . . . . . . . . . . . . . .100
thigh, smoked (*Shady Brook Farms*) . . . . . . . . . . . . . . . . . .160
wing, smoked (*Shady Brook Farms*) . . . . . . . . . . . . . . . . . .200
wing drumettes (*Perdue*), 3.3-oz. pc. . . . . . . . . . . . . . . . . .180
**Turkey, ground,** 4 oz., except as noted:
raw (*Perdue Fit 'n Easy*) . . . . . . . . . . . . . . . . . . . . . . . . . .170
raw (*Wampler*) . . . . . . . . . . . . . . . . . . . . . . . . . . . . . . . .210
raw, breast (*Jennie-O* Frozen) . . . . . . . . . . . . . . . . . . . . . .140
raw, breast (*Perdue Fit 'n Easy*) . . . . . . . . . . . . . . . . . . . .120
raw, burger (*Jennie-O*) . . . . . . . . . . . . . . . . . . . . . . . . . . .160
raw, burger (*Shady Brook Farms*) . . . . . . . . . . . . . . . . . . . .170
raw, burger, barbecue (*Wampler*) . . . . . . . . . . . . . . . . . . . .220
raw, burger, specially seasoned (*Wampler*) . . . . . . . . . . . . .180
cooked (*Perdue Fit 'n Easy*), 3 oz. . . . . . . . . . . . . . . . . . . .160
**"Turkey," vegetarian,** frozen:
(*Yves* Deli Slices), 2.2 oz. . . . . . . . . . . . . . . . . . . . . . . . . .85
smoked, sliced (*Worthington* Meatless), 3 slices . . . . . . . . . .140
**Turkey bacon** (*Jennie-O* Extra Lean/Fat Free), 1 slice . . . . . .20
**Turkey bologna,** 2 oz.:
(*Norbest*) . . . . . . . . . . . . . . . . . . . . . . . . . . . . . . . . . . . .130
(*Wampler*) . . . . . . . . . . . . . . . . . . . . . . . . . . . . . . . . . . .100
**Turkey burger,** see "Turkey, ground"
**Turkey dinner,** frozen, 1 pkg.:
breast (*Healthy Choice* Traditional), 10.5 oz. . . . . . . . . . . . .320
breast (*Swanson Traditional Favorites*), 11.75 oz. . . . . . . . .330
breast, grilled (*Healthy Choice*), 10 oz. . . . . . . . . . . . . . . .260
breast, roast (*Stouffer's* HomeStyle), 16 oz. . . . . . . . . . . . .460
and gravy w/dressing (*Banquet Extra Helping*), 17 oz. . . . . .620
stuffing, baked (*Swanson Traditional Favorites*), 13.5 oz. . . .450
white meat, mostly (*Swanson Hungry-Man*), 16.75 oz. . . . .500

**Turkey entree, can or pkg.** (see also "Chili"):
and dressing (*Dinty Moore American Classics*), 1 bowl . . . .290
stew (*Dinty Moore* Can), 1 cup . . . . . . . . . . . . . . . . . . . . . . .140
stew (*Dinty Moore* Microwave Cup), 1 cup . . . . . . . . . . . . .130
**Turkey entree, frozen,** 1 pkg., except as noted:
breast medallions, grilled (*Marie Callender's*), 9.5 oz. . . . . .290
breast medallions and stuffing (*Marie Callender's* Bowl), 11 oz. . . . . . . . . . . . . . . . . . . . . . . . . . . . . . . . . .320
croquettes, gravy and (*Freezer Queen* Family), 1 patty w/gravy, ⅙ pkg. . . . . . . . . . . . . . . . . . . . . . . . . . . . .140
divan (*Healthy Choice* Bowl), 11 oz. . . . . . . . . . . . . . . . . . .270
glazed, tenderloins (*Lean Cuisine Café Classics*), 9 oz. . . . .260
and gravy, w/dressing (*Freezer Queen* Meal), 9.25 oz. . . . . .230
and gravy, rolls (*Freezer Queen* Deluxe Family), 1 pc. . . . . .170
and gravy, w/whipped potato (*Freezer Queen* Homestyle), 9 oz. . . . . . . . . . . . . . . . . . . . . . . . . . . . . . . . . . .210
w/gravy and stuffing (*Marie Callender's*), 14 oz. . . . . . . . . .420
gravy and, w/dressing (*Morton*), 9 oz. . . . . . . . . . . . . . . . .240
home style (*Lean Cuisine Everyday Favorites*), 9⅜ oz. . . . . . . . . . . . . . . . . . . . . . . . . . . . . . . . . .250
pie (*Marie Callender's*), 9.5 oz. . . . . . . . . . . . . . . . . . . . . . .660
pie (*Marie Callender's* 16.5 oz.), 1 cup . . . . . . . . . . . . . . .540
pie (*Stouffer's*), 10 oz. . . . . . . . . . . . . . . . . . . . . . . . . . . .750
pie (*Stouffer's*), ½ of 16-oz. pkg. . . . . . . . . . . . . . . . . . . .590
pie (*Swanson Potato-Topped*), 12 oz. . . . . . . . . . . . . . . . . .350
pie, white, deep dish (*Swanson Hungry-Man*), 1 cup . . . . .520
roast (*Lean Cuisine Skillet Sensations*), ½ of 24-oz. pkg. . . . . . . . . . . . . . . . . . . . . . . . . . . .220
roast, breast (*Healthy Choice* Medley), 8.5 oz. . . . . . . . . . .220
roast, breast (*Lean Cuisine Café Classics*), 9.75 oz. . . . . . . .270
roast, breast (*Lean Cuisine Hearty Portions*), 14 oz. . . . . . .320
roast, breast (*Stouffer's* HomeStyle), 9⅝ oz. . . . . . . . . . . .310
roast, white meat (*Banquet*), 9 oz. . . . . . . . . . . . . . . . . . . .230
roasted, slow, breast, and mashed potato (*Healthy Choice* Duo), 8.5 oz. . . . . . . . . . . . . . . . . . . . . . . .200
sliced, gravy and (*Banquet* Family), 2 slices w/gravy . . . . . .140
sliced, gravy and (*Freezer Queen* Family), ⅙ pkg. . . . . . . . . .60
tetrazzini (*Stouffer's*), 10 oz. . . . . . . . . . . . . . . . . . . . . . . .400
**Turkey fat,** 1 tbsp. . . . . . . . . . . . . . . . . . . . . . . . . . . . . . .115
**Turkey frankfurter,** see "Frankfurter"

**Turkey gravy,** can or jar, ¼ cup:
(*Franco-American/Franco-American Slow Roast*) . . . . . . . . . .25
(*Heinz* Home Style) . . . . . . . . . . . . . . . . . . . . . . . . . . . . .25
(*Heinz* Home Style Fat Free) . . . . . . . . . . . . . . . . . . . . . . .10
**Turkey gravy mix** (*Lawry's*), 1 tbsp. . . . . . . . . . . . . . . . . . .25
**Turkey ham,** 2 oz., except as noted:
(*Healthy Deli*) . . . . . . . . . . . . . . . . . . . . . . . . . . . . . . . . .70
(*Jennie-O*), 1 oz. . . . . . . . . . . . . . . . . . . . . . . . . . . . . . .60
(*The Turkey Store*) . . . . . . . . . . . . . . . . . . . . . . . . . . . . .70
(*Wampler* Family Size Chunk) . . . . . . . . . . . . . . . . . . . . . .60
Black Forest (*Shady Brook Farms*) . . . . . . . . . . . . . . . . . . .70
Black Forest (*Wampler/Wampler Deli Roast Collection*) . . . . .60
honey-cured (*Jennie-O*), 1 oz. . . . . . . . . . . . . . . . . . . . . . .70
**Turkey ham salad** (*Wampler*), ⅓ cup . . . . . . . . . . . . . . . .150
**Turkey lunch meat** (see also "Turkey ham," etc.), breast,
2 oz., except as noted:
(*Alpine Lace* Fat Free) . . . . . . . . . . . . . . . . . . . . . . . . . . .45
(*Boar's Head* Premium/*Boar's Head Salsalito*) . . . . . . . . . . .60
(*Jennie-O/Jennie-O* Skinless) . . . . . . . . . . . . . . . . . . . . . . .50
(*Norbest* Gold Label Golden Browned) . . . . . . . . . . . . . . . .60
(*Shady Brook Farms* No Salt) . . . . . . . . . . . . . . . . . . . . . . .70
Cajun, garlic pesto, or honey Dijon (*The Turkey Store*) . . . . .50
cured (*Norbest* Gourmet) . . . . . . . . . . . . . . . . . . . . . . . . . .70
honey-roasted (*Healthy Deli*) . . . . . . . . . . . . . . . . . . . . . . .60
honey-roasted (*Perdue Carving*) . . . . . . . . . . . . . . . . . . . . .50
honey-roasted (*Shady Brook Farms*) . . . . . . . . . . . . . . . . . .60
lemon pepper (*The Turkey Store*) . . . . . . . . . . . . . . . . . . . .50
maple-glazed (*Boar's Head Honey Coat*) . . . . . . . . . . . . . . .70
oven-roasted (*Boar's Head Ovengold*) . . . . . . . . . . . . . . . . .60
oven-roasted (*Hebrew National* Thin), 5 slices, 2 oz. . . . . . . .50
oven-roasted (*Norbest* Bronze/Gold/Silver Label) . . . . . . . . .60
oven-roasted (*Perdue*) . . . . . . . . . . . . . . . . . . . . . . . . . . . .50
oven-roasted (*Perdue Carving*) . . . . . . . . . . . . . . . . . . . . . .70
oven-roasted (*Shady Brook Farms*) . . . . . . . . . . . . . . . . . . .60
oven-roasted (*The Turkey Store*) . . . . . . . . . . . . . . . . . . . . .50
oven-roasted (*Wampler* 3/2/1 Diamond) . . . . . . . . . . . . . . . .50
oven-roasted, glazed (*Healthy Deli* Gourmet) . . . . . . . . . . . .60
oven-roasted, Italian (*Healthy Deli*) . . . . . . . . . . . . . . . . . .70
pan-roasted (*Perdue Carving Classics*) . . . . . . . . . . . . . . . . .70
pan-roasted (*Perdue Carving Classics* Skinless) . . . . . . . . . .60

pan-roasted (*Wampler Deli Roast Collection*) . . . . . . . . . . . . .60
pan-roasted, cracked pepper (*Perdue Carving Classics*) . . . .50
pepper (*Healthy Choice*), 1-oz. slice . . . . . . . . . . . . . . . . . . .25
pepper (*Healthy Deli* Tutta Bella) . . . . . . . . . . . . . . . . . . . . . .60
pepper (*Wampler Deli Roast Collection*) . . . . . . . . . . . . . . . .40
pepper, cracked (*The Turkey Store*) . . . . . . . . . . . . . . . . . . . .50
pepper, hot red, garlic, or smoked (*Jennie-O*) . . . . . . . . . . . .60
rotisserie-seasoned (*Wampler Deli Roast Collection*) . . . . . .50
salsa-roasted (*Shady Brook Farms*) . . . . . . . . . . . . . . . . . . . .50
smoked (*Healthy Deli* Brick Oven) . . . . . . . . . . . . . . . . . . . . .60
smoked (*Norbest* Bronze/Gold Label) . . . . . . . . . . . . . . . . . . .60
smoked, all varieties (*Boar's Head*) . . . . . . . . . . . . . . . . . . . .60
smoked, cured, hickory or mesquite (*Jennie-O*) . . . . . . . . . .50
smoked, hardwood (*Sara Lee*) . . . . . . . . . . . . . . . . . . . . . . . .60
smoked, hickory (*Jennie-O*) . . . . . . . . . . . . . . . . . . . . . . . . . .60
smoked, hickory (*Perdue*) . . . . . . . . . . . . . . . . . . . . . . . . . . . .60
smoked, hickory (*Shady Brook Farms*) . . . . . . . . . . . . . . . . .50
smoked, hickory, honey-cured (*The Turkey Store*) . . . . . . . . .60
smoked, honey (*Healthy Choice*) . . . . . . . . . . . . . . . . . . . . . . .60
smoked, honey (*Perdue Carving*) . . . . . . . . . . . . . . . . . . . . . .50
smoked, honey-cured, hickory or mesquite (*Jennie-O*) . . . . .50
smoked, mesquite (*Perdue Carving*) . . . . . . . . . . . . . . . . . . . .50
smoked, mesquite (*Sara Lee*) . . . . . . . . . . . . . . . . . . . . . . . . .60
smoked, mesquite, honey-cured (*Wampler* 4 Diamond) . . . .50
smoked, picnic, dark (*Wampler* Family Size Chunk) . . . . . . .80
spiced (*Wampler Deli Roast Collection* Classic) . . . . . . . . . . .70
sun-dried tomato (*The Turkey Store*) . . . . . . . . . . . . . . . . . . .50
Tex-Mex (*Black Bear*) . . . . . . . . . . . . . . . . . . . . . . . . . . . . . . .60
**Turkey meatballs,** see "Meatballs"
**Turkey pastrami,** 2 oz.:
(*Boar's Head*) . . . . . . . . . . . . . . . . . . . . . . . . . . . . . . . . . . . .60
(*Jennie-O*) . . . . . . . . . . . . . . . . . . . . . . . . . . . . . . . . . . . . . .70
(*Shady Brook Farms*) . . . . . . . . . . . . . . . . . . . . . . . . . . . . . . .60
(*The Turkey Store*) . . . . . . . . . . . . . . . . . . . . . . . . . . . . . . . . .70
(*Wampler*) . . . . . . . . . . . . . . . . . . . . . . . . . . . . . . . . . . . . . . .80
hickory-smoked (*Perdue*) . . . . . . . . . . . . . . . . . . . . . . . . . . . .70
**Turkey pepperoni** (*Hormel Pillow Pack*), 1.1 oz. . . . . . . . . . . .80
**Turkey pie,** see "Turkey entree"
**Turkey pocket,** frozen, 4.5-oz. pc.:
broccoli and cheese (*Lean Pockets*) . . . . . . . . . . . . . . . . . .230

**Turkey pocket, frozen *(cont.)***
ham and cheddar (*Lean Pockets*) . . . . . . . . . . . . . . . . . . . . .290
ham and cheese (*Croissant Pockets*) . . . . . . . . . . . . . . . . . .320
ham and cheese (*Hot Pockets*) . . . . . . . . . . . . . . . . . . . . . . .310
**Turkey salami:**
(*Norbest*), 2 oz. . . . . . . . . . . . . . . . . . . . . . . . . . . . . . . .85
(*Wampler*), 2 oz. . . . . . . . . . . . . . . . . . . . . . . . . . . . . . .90
**Turkey sausage,** see "Sausage"
**Turkish salad** (*Sabra Salads*), 1 oz. . . . . . . . . . . . . . . . . . . .13
**Turmeric,** ground, 1 tsp. . . . . . . . . . . . . . . . . . . . . . . . . . .8
**Turnip,** fresh:
boiled, cubed, ½ cup . . . . . . . . . . . . . . . . . . . . . . . . . . . .14
boiled, mashed, ½ cup . . . . . . . . . . . . . . . . . . . . . . . . . . .18
**Turnip greens,** fresh:
raw, chopped, ½ cup . . . . . . . . . . . . . . . . . . . . . . . . . . . . .7
boiled, chopped, ½ cup . . . . . . . . . . . . . . . . . . . . . . . . . . .15
**Turnip greens, canned,** chopped, ½ cup:
(*Bush's Best*) . . . . . . . . . . . . . . . . . . . . . . . . . . . . . . . .25
(*Stubb's*) . . . . . . . . . . . . . . . . . . . . . . . . . . . . . . . . . . .25
w/diced turnips (*Bush's Best*) . . . . . . . . . . . . . . . . . . . . . .30
seasoned (*Glory Foods*) . . . . . . . . . . . . . . . . . . . . . . . . . .45
seasoned (*Sylvia's*) . . . . . . . . . . . . . . . . . . . . . . . . . . . . .40
**Turnip greens, frozen:**
chopped (*Birds Eye* Southern), 1 cup . . . . . . . . . . . . . . . . . .30
w/diced turnips (*Birds Eye* Southern), 1 cup . . . . . . . . . . . . .25
**Turnover,** frozen or refrigerated, 1 pc.:
apple or cherry (*Pillsbury*) . . . . . . . . . . . . . . . . . . . . . . . .170
raspberry (*Pepperidge Farm*) . . . . . . . . . . . . . . . . . . . . . . .290

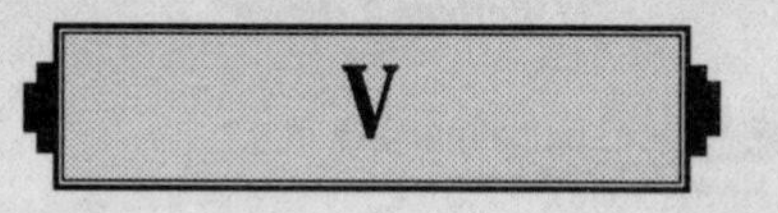

| FOOD AND MEASURE | CALORIES |
|---|---|
| **Vanilla syrup** (*Fox's U-Bet*), 2 tbsp. | 80 |
| **Veal,** meat only, 4 oz.: | |
| cubed, lean only, braised or stewed | 213 |
| ground, broiled | 195 |
| leg, braised, lean w/fat | 239 |
| leg, braised, lean only | 230 |
| leg, roasted, lean w/fat | 181 |
| leg, roasted, lean only | 170 |
| loin, braised, lean w/fat | 322 |
| loin, braised, lean only | 256 |
| loin, roasted, lean w/fat | 246 |
| loin, roasted, lean only | 198 |
| rib, braised, lean w/fat | 285 |
| rib, braised, lean only | 247 |
| rib, roasted, lean w/fat | 259 |
| rib, roasted, lean only | 201 |
| shoulder, whole, braised, lean w/fat | 259 |
| shoulder, whole, braised, lean only | 226 |
| shoulder, whole, roasted, lean w/fat | 209 |
| shoulder, whole, roasted, lean only | 193 |
| shoulder, arm, braised, lean w/fat | 268 |
| shoulder, arm, braised, lean only | 228 |
| shoulder, arm, roasted, lean w/fat | 208 |
| shoulder, arm, roasted, lean only | 186 |
| shoulder, blade, braised, lean w/fat | 255 |
| shoulder, blade, braised, lean only | 224 |
| shoulder, blade, roasted, lean w/fat | 211 |
| shoulder, blade, roasted, lean only | 194 |
| sirloin, braised, lean w/fat | 286 |
| sirloin, braised, lean only | 231 |
| sirloin, roasted, lean w/fat | 229 |
| sirloin, roasted, lean only | 191 |

**Veal dinner,** frozen, parmigiana, 1 pkg.:
(*Stouffer's* HomeStyle), 17.5 oz. . . . . . . . . . . . . . . . . . . . . . .530
(*Swanson Traditional Favorites*), 11.25 oz. . . . . . . . . . . . . .390
**Veal entree,** frozen, parmigiana, 1 pkg.:
(*Banquet*), 8.75 oz. . . . . . . . . . . . . . . . . . . . . . . . . . . .330
(*Freezer Queen* Meal), 9 oz. . . . . . . . . . . . . . . . . . . . . .330
(*Stouffer's* HomeStyle), 11⅝ oz. . . . . . . . . . . . . . . . . . . . .410
**Vegetable batter mix** (*McCormick Produce Partners*),
¼ cup . . . . . . . . . . . . . . . . . . . . . . . . . . . . . . . . . . . .120
**Vegetable burger,** see "Burger, vegetarian"
**Vegetable chips** (see also specific listings):
(*Snyder's Eat Smart* Crisps), 1 oz. . . . . . . . . . . . . . . . . . .160
(*Terra Chips*), 1 oz. . . . . . . . . . . . . . . . . . . . . . . . . . . .140
(*Terra Stix*), 1 oz. . . . . . . . . . . . . . . . . . . . . . . . . . . . .150
plain or wasabi (*Eden*), 1.1 oz. . . . . . . . . . . . . . . . . . . . .130
sea (*Eden*), 1.1 oz. . . . . . . . . . . . . . . . . . . . . . . . . . . . .140
**Vegetable dinner,** frozen, 1 pkg.:
(*Amy's* Country), 11 oz. . . . . . . . . . . . . . . . . . . . . . . . .380
veggie loaf (*Amy's*), 10 oz. . . . . . . . . . . . . . . . . . . . . . .260
**Vegetable dip mix,** garden (*McCormick*), 2 tbsp.* . . . . . . . .35
**Vegetable dish, can or jar,** ½ cup, except as noted:
curry, 1½ cups:
(*Patak's* Aloo Mattar Sabzi) . . . . . . . . . . . . . . . . . . . . .240
(*Patak's* Tikka Masala) . . . . . . . . . . . . . . . . . . . . . . . . .190
hot and spicy (*House of Tsang* Szechuan) . . . . . . . . . . . . . . .70
sweet and sour (*House of Tsang* Hong Kong) . . . . . . . . . . .160
teriyaki (*House of Tsang* Tokyo) . . . . . . . . . . . . . . . . . . . .100
**Vegetable dish, frozen** (see also "Vegetable entree,"
"Pasta dish," and specific listings):
Bavarian style (*Birds Eye*), ½ of 9-oz. pkg. . . . . . . . . . . . . .150
California style (*Birds Eye*), ½ cup . . . . . . . . . . . . . . . . . .100
French country style (*Birds Eye*), ⅔ cup . . . . . . . . . . . . . . .110
Italian style, and bow-tie pasta (*Birds Eye*), 1 cup . . . . . . . .150
Oriental or stir-fry style (*Birds Eye*), ½ cup . . . . . . . . . . . . . .60
New England style and shells (*Birds Eye*), 9-oz. pkg. . . . . . .260
pancake (*King Kold*), 2 cakes, 2 oz. . . . . . . . . . . . . . . . . . .120
**Vegetable entree, can or jar,** see "Vegetable dish, can or jar"
**Vegetable entree, frozen** (see also "Vegetable entree mix,
frozen" and "Vegetarian entree"), 1 pkg.:
au gratin (*Cascadian Farm Veggie Bowl*), 9 oz. . . . . . . . . . .170

and chicken, see "Chicken entree, frozen"
Caribbean (*Cascadian Farm Veggie Bowl*), 9 oz. . . . . . . . . . .280
casserole, fiesta (*Cascadian Farm Veggie Bowl*), 9 oz. . . . .340
Chinese or Italian style, and white chicken, w/rice
(*Budget Gourmet*), 8 oz. . . . . . . . . . . . . . . . . . . . . . . .250
pie (*Amy's*), 7.5 oz. . . . . . . . . . . . . . . . . . . . . . . . . . . .420
pie (*Amy's* Country), 7.5 oz. . . . . . . . . . . . . . . . . . . . . .370
pie (*Amy's* Nondairy), 7.5 oz. . . . . . . . . . . . . . . . . . . . .320
pie (*Cedarlane* Less Fat), 7.4 oz. . . . . . . . . . . . . . . . . . .390
pie, w/beef (*Morton*), 7 oz. . . . . . . . . . . . . . . . . . . . . . .190
pie, w/chicken (*Morton*), 7 oz. . . . . . . . . . . . . . . . . . . .320
pie, Mediterranean or Santa Fe (*Cedarlane*), 7.5 oz. . . . . . . .490
pie, w/turkey (*Morton*), 7 oz. . . . . . . . . . . . . . . . . . . . . .310
shepherd's pie (*Amy's*), 8 oz. . . . . . . . . . . . . . . . . . . . . .160
spicy Szechuan style, and white chicken, w/pasta
(*Budget Gourmet*), 8 oz. . . . . . . . . . . . . . . . . . . . . . . .280
stir-fry, w/rice (*Michelina's*), 8 oz. . . . . . . . . . . . . . . . . .240
**Vegetable entree mix*, frozen,** 1¼ cups, except as noted:
beef broccoli stir-fry (*Green Giant Create a Meal!*),
1⅓ cups . . . . . . . . . . . . . . . . . . . . . . . . . . . . . . . . .290
beefy noodle (*Green Giant Create a Meal!*) . . . . . . . . . . . .350
cheesy pasta–vegetable (*Green Giant Create a Meal!*) . . . . .420
chicken Alfredo (*Green Giant Create a Meal!*) . . . . . . . . . . .400
curry, South Indian (*Cascadian Farm Quickstart*),
2¼ cups . . . . . . . . . . . . . . . . . . . . . . . . . . . . . . . . .300
garlic ginger stir-fry (*Green Giant Create a Meal!*),
1½ cups . . . . . . . . . . . . . . . . . . . . . . . . . . . . . . . . .270
garlic herb (*Green Giant Create a Meal!* Oven Roasted),
1¾ cups . . . . . . . . . . . . . . . . . . . . . . . . . . . . . . . . .350
garlic herb pasta (*Green Giant Create a Meal!*), . . . . . . . . .380
lemon pepper chicken (*Green Giant Create a Meal!*
Oven Roasted), 1⅔ cups . . . . . . . . . . . . . . . . . . . . . .310
lo mein stir-fry (*Green Giant Create a Meal!*) . . . . . . . . . . .320
Parmesan herb (*Green Giant Create a Meal!*
Oven Roasted), 1¾ cups . . . . . . . . . . . . . . . . . . . . . . .340
Southwest skillet (*Cascadian Farm Quickstart*),
2¼ cups . . . . . . . . . . . . . . . . . . . . . . . . . . . . . . . . .290
stew, homestyle (*Green Giant Create a Meal!*), 1 cup . . . . .340
sweet and sour stir-fry (*Green Giant Create a Meal!*) . . . . .340
Szechuan stir-fry (*Green Giant Create a Meal!*) . . . . . . . . . .310

**Vegetable entree mix*, frozen *(cont.)***
teriyaki stir-fry (*Green Giant Create a Meal!*) . . . . . . . . . . . .230
teriyaki stir-fry (*Tree of Life EasyMeal*), 1 pkg. . . . . . . . . . . .270
teriyaki veggies/rice (*Cascadian Farm Quickstart*), 2¼ cups . . . . . . . . . . . . . . . . . . . . . . . . . . . . . . . . . . .330
Thai stir-fry (*Tree of Life EasyMeal*), 1 pkg. . . . . . . . . . . . .270
Thai veggies/rice (*Cascadian Farm Quickstart*), 2¼ cups . . . . . . . . . . . . . . . . . . . . . . . . . . . . . . . . . . .310
**Vegetable juice,** 8 fl. oz.:
(*Red Gold*) . . . . . . . . . . . . . . . . . . . . . . . . . . . . . . . . . .50
all varieties (*V8*) . . . . . . . . . . . . . . . . . . . . . . . . . . . . .50
**Vegetable oyster,** see "Salsify"
**Vegetable pie,** see "Vegetable entree, frozen"
**Vegetable pocket** (see also specific listings), 1 pc.:
Mediterranean (*Amy's*), 4.5 oz. . . . . . . . . . . . . . . . . . . . . . .220
pie (*Amy's*), 5 oz. . . . . . . . . . . . . . . . . . . . . . . . . . . . . .300
roasted vegetables (*Amy's*), 4.5 oz. . . . . . . . . . . . . . . . . . .220
**Vegetables,** see specific listings
**Vegetables, mixed,** fresh:
(*Mann's* Medley), 4 oz. . . . . . . . . . . . . . . . . . . . . . . . . . . .35
Oriental stir-fry (*Frieda's*), 3 oz. . . . . . . . . . . . . . . . . . . . .15
**Vegetables, mixed, can or jar,** ½ cup, except as noted:
(*Del Monte*) . . . . . . . . . . . . . . . . . . . . . . . . . . . . . . . . . .40
(*Libby's*) . . . . . . . . . . . . . . . . . . . . . . . . . . . . . . . . . . .45
(*Veg-All* Original/Homestyle Large Cut/Hot/Spicy) . . . . . . . . .40
Cajun (*Veg-All*) . . . . . . . . . . . . . . . . . . . . . . . . . . . . . . .50
Chinese, mixed (*La Choy*) . . . . . . . . . . . . . . . . . . . . . . . . .10
chop suey (*La Choy*), ⅔ cup . . . . . . . . . . . . . . . . . . . . . . . .15
**Vegetables, mixed, frozen** (see also "Vegetable dish, frozen" and specific listings):
(*Birds Eye*), ⅓ cup . . . . . . . . . . . . . . . . . . . . . . . . . . . . .50
(*Green Giant*), ¾ cup . . . . . . . . . . . . . . . . . . . . . . . . . . . .50
(*John Cope's* 4/5-Way), ⅔ cup . . . . . . . . . . . . . . . . . . . . . .60
(*Seabrook Farms*), ⅔ cup . . . . . . . . . . . . . . . . . . . . . . . . .70
(*Tree of Life* Organic), ½ cup . . . . . . . . . . . . . . . . . . . . . .65
Alfredo (*Green Giant*), ¾ cup . . . . . . . . . . . . . . . . . . . . . . .70
California blend (*Cascadian Farm*), ⅔ cup . . . . . . . . . . . . . .20
California blend (*John Cope's*), ¾ cup . . . . . . . . . . . . . . . . .30
in cheddar cheese sauce (*Cascadian Farm*), ⅔ cup . . . . . . . .80
Chinese stir-fry (*Cascadian Farm*), 1 cup . . . . . . . . . . . . . .25

gumbo blend (*Birds Eye*), ¾ cup . . . . . . . . . . . . . . . . . . . . . .40
gumbo blend (*McKenzie's*), ⅔ cup . . . . . . . . . . . . . . . . . . . .35
Santa Fe blend (*Cascadian Farm*), 3 oz. . . . . . . . . . . . . . . . . .60
seasoning blend (*Birds Eye*), ¾ cup . . . . . . . . . . . . . . . . . . .20
seasoning blend (*McKenzie's*), 1.1 oz. . . . . . . . . . . . . . . . . .10
soup mix (*Birds Eye*), ⅔ cup . . . . . . . . . . . . . . . . . . . . . . . .45
soup mix (*McKenzie's*), ⅔ cup . . . . . . . . . . . . . . . . . . . . . .40
stew mix (*Birds Eye* Southern), ⅔ cup . . . . . . . . . . . . . . . . .40
teriyaki (*Green Giant*), 1¼ cup . . . . . . . . . . . . . . . . . . . . . .80
Thai stir-fry (*Cascadian Farm*), ¾ cup . . . . . . . . . . . . . . . . .25
winter blend (*John Cope's*), 1 cup . . . . . . . . . . . . . . . . . . . .25
**Vegetarian burger,** see "Burger, vegetarian"
**Vegetarian dish** (see also specific listings), frozen:
(*Worthington* Dinner Roast), ¾" slice, 3 oz. . . . . . . . . . . . . .180
(*Worthington FriPats*), 1 patty . . . . . . . . . . . . . . . . . . . . . .130
(*Worthington Stakelets*), 1 pc. . . . . . . . . . . . . . . . . . . . . . .140
black pepper steak (*Veggie Master* Vege), ¼ pkg. . . . . . . . . .97
croquettes (*Worthington* Golden), 4 pcs. . . . . . . . . . . . . . . .210
ground, original or Italian (*Yves* Ground Round), ⅓ cup . . . .60
**Vegetarian entree, frozen** (see also "Vegetable entree" and specific listings), 3½ cups, except as noted:
Aztec or Cajun (*Cascadian Farm Meals for a Small Planet*) . . . . . . . . . . . . . . . . . . . . . . . . . . . . . . .290
Indian (*Cascadian Farm Meals for a Small Planet*) . . . . . . .340
Mediterranean (*Cascadian Farm Meals for a Small Planet*), 3¼ cups . . . . . . . . . . . . . . . . . . . . . . . . . . . . . . . . .230
Moroccan (*Cascadian Farm Meals for a Small Planet*) . . . .310
pot pie, see "Vegetable entree, frozen"
stew, country, w/"meatballs" (*Yves*), 10.5-oz. pkg. . . . . . . .170
Szechuan (*Cascadian Farm Meals for a Small Planet*) . . . . .340
Szechuan (*Cedarlane* Veggie Chick'n), ½ of 10-oz. pkg. . . .220
teriyaki (*Cedarlane* Veggie Chick'n), ½ of 10-oz. pkg. . . . . .220
**Venison,** meat only, roasted, 4 oz. . . . . . . . . . . . . . . . . . .179
**Vermicelli pasta dish, mix,** roast garlic and olive oil:
(*Near East*), 1 cup* . . . . . . . . . . . . . . . . . . . . . . . . . . . . . .310
(*Pasta Roni*), 1 cup* . . . . . . . . . . . . . . . . . . . . . . . . . . . . .360
**Vienna sausage,** see "Sausage, canned"
**Vindaloo sauce,** see "Curry sauce"
**Vinegar,** 1 tbsp.:
all varieties, except balsamic (*Progresso*) . . . . . . . . . . . . . . .0

**Vinegar *(cont.)***
balsamic (*Pompeian*) . . . . . . . . . . . . . . . . . . . . . . . . . . . . .5
balsamic (*Progresso*) . . . . . . . . . . . . . . . . . . . . . . . . . . . .10
balsamic (*Regina*) . . . . . . . . . . . . . . . . . . . . . . . . . . . . . . .5
plum or brown rice (*Eden* Organic) . . . . . . . . . . . . . . . . . . .2
red wine (*Pompeian*) . . . . . . . . . . . . . . . . . . . . . . . . . . . . .2
red or white wine (*Regina*) . . . . . . . . . . . . . . . . . . . . . . . .0
sushi (*Sushi Chef*) . . . . . . . . . . . . . . . . . . . . . . . . . . . . .20

# W

**FOOD AND MEASURE** **CALORIES**

**Waffle,** 1 pc.:
blueberry or homestyle (*Thomas'*) . . . . . . . . . . . . . . . . . . .140
buttermilk (*Thomas'*) . . . . . . . . . . . . . . . . . . . . . . . . . .130
**Waffle, frozen,** 2 pcs., except as noted:
(*Aunt Jemima* Homestyle) . . . . . . . . . . . . . . . . . . . . .200
(*Aunt Jemima* Lowfat) . . . . . . . . . . . . . . . . . . . . . . . .170
(*Belgian Chef*) . . . . . . . . . . . . . . . . . . . . . . . . . . . . .180
(*Eggo* Homestyle) . . . . . . . . . . . . . . . . . . . . . . . . . . .190
(*Eggo Minis* Homestyle), 3 sets of 4 pcs. . . . . . . . . . . . . .260
(*Eggo Nutri-Grain*) . . . . . . . . . . . . . . . . . . . . . . . . . .170
(*Eggo Special K*) . . . . . . . . . . . . . . . . . . . . . . . . . . .120
(*Hungry Jack* Homestyle) . . . . . . . . . . . . . . . . . . . . . .180
(*Hungry Jack* Homestyle Low Fat) . . . . . . . . . . . . . . . . .170
apple cinnamon, blueberry, or chocolate chip (*Eggo*) . . . . .200
apple cinnamon or wildberry (*Hungry Jack*) . . . . . . . . . . .200
banana bread (*Eggo*) . . . . . . . . . . . . . . . . . . . . . . . . .190
blueberry (*Aunt Jemima*) . . . . . . . . . . . . . . . . . . . . . . .210
blueberry (*Eggo Nutri-Grain* Low Fat) . . . . . . . . . . . . . . .150
blueberry (*Hungry Jack*) . . . . . . . . . . . . . . . . . . . . . . .210
buttermilk (*Aunt Jemima*) . . . . . . . . . . . . . . . . . . . . . .200
buttermilk (*Eggo*) . . . . . . . . . . . . . . . . . . . . . . . . . . .190
buttermilk (*Hungry Jack*) . . . . . . . . . . . . . . . . . . . . . .190
cinnamon toast (*Eggo*), 3 sets of 4 . . . . . . . . . . . . . . . . .290
cinnamon toast (*Hungry Jack*), 3 sets of 4 . . . . . . . . . . . .270
multibran (*Eggo Nutri-Grain*) . . . . . . . . . . . . . . . . . . . .160
nut and honey (*Eggo*) . . . . . . . . . . . . . . . . . . . . . . . . .220
oat, golden (*Eggo*) . . . . . . . . . . . . . . . . . . . . . . . . . .140
strawberry (*Eggo*) . . . . . . . . . . . . . . . . . . . . . . . . . . .200
**Waffle mix,** see "Pancake mix"
**Waffle sticks,** frozen, 3 pcs.:
(*Aunt Jemima* Homestyle) . . . . . . . . . . . . . . . . . . . . .310
chocolate chip (*Aunt Jemima*) . . . . . . . . . . . . . . . . . . .330
cinnamon sugar (*Aunt Jemima*) . . . . . . . . . . . . . . . . . .320

**Walnut,** dried, shelled:
(*Blue Diamond* Halves and Pieces), ⅓ cup . . . . . . . . . . . . .210
(*Fisher*), 1 oz. . . . . . . . . . . . . . . . . . . . . . . . . . . . . . .200
black, 1 oz. . . . . . . . . . . . . . . . . . . . . . . . . . . . . . . . .172
black, chopped, ¼ cup . . . . . . . . . . . . . . . . . . . . . . . . .190
English or Persian, pieces, ¼ cup . . . . . . . . . . . . . . . . . .193
English or Persian, halves, ¼ cup . . . . . . . . . . . . . . . . . .160
sesame-glazed (*Diamond*), ¼ cup . . . . . . . . . . . . . . . . . .190
**Walnut topping,** in syrup (*Smucker's*), 2 tbsp. . . . . . . . . . .170
**Water chestnuts,** Chinese, fresh:
(*Frieda's*), 1 tbsp., 1.1 oz. . . . . . . . . . . . . . . . . . . . . . . .30
sliced, ½ cup . . . . . . . . . . . . . . . . . . . . . . . . . . . . . . . .60
**Water chestnuts, canned:**
whole, 4 pcs., 1 oz. . . . . . . . . . . . . . . . . . . . . . . . . . . .14
sliced (*La Choy*), ½ cup . . . . . . . . . . . . . . . . . . . . . . . . .25
**Watercress:**
(*Frieda's*), 1 cup, 3 oz. . . . . . . . . . . . . . . . . . . . . . . . . .10
10 sprigs, 1¼" . . . . . . . . . . . . . . . . . . . . . . . . . . . . . . . .3
**Watermelon,** fresh:
1" slice, 10" diam. . . . . . . . . . . . . . . . . . . . . . . . . . . . .152
balls or diced, ½ cup . . . . . . . . . . . . . . . . . . . . . . . . . . .25
yellow, seedless (*Frieda's*), ½ cup, 3 oz. . . . . . . . . . . . . . . .25
**Watermelon seed,** dried, 1 oz. . . . . . . . . . . . . . . . . . . . . .158
**Wax beans,** fresh, see "Green bean"
**Wax beans, can or jar,** ½ cup:
cut (*Del Monte* Golden) . . . . . . . . . . . . . . . . . . . . . . . . .20
cut (*Libby's*) . . . . . . . . . . . . . . . . . . . . . . . . . . . . . . . .25
cut or French sliced (*Blue Boy*) . . . . . . . . . . . . . . . . . . . .25
**Wax gourd,** boiled, cubed, ½ cup . . . . . . . . . . . . . . . . . . .11
**Welsh rarebit,** frozen (*Stouffer's* Side Dish),
¼ cup . . . . . . . . . . . . . . . . . . . . . . . . . . . . . . . . . . .120
***Wendy's,*** 1 serving:
sandwiches:
bacon cheeseburger, jr. . . . . . . . . . . . . . . . . . . . . . . . .360
*Big Bacon Classic* . . . . . . . . . . . . . . . . . . . . . . . . . . .580
cheeseburger, jr. . . . . . . . . . . . . . . . . . . . . . . . . . . . .320
cheeseburger, jr., deluxe . . . . . . . . . . . . . . . . . . . . . . .360
cheeseburger Kid's Meal . . . . . . . . . . . . . . . . . . . . . . . .320
chicken, breaded fillet . . . . . . . . . . . . . . . . . . . . . . . . .440
chicken, club . . . . . . . . . . . . . . . . . . . . . . . . . . . . . . .480

chicken, grilled .....300
chicken, spicy .....410
*Classic Single* .....360
*Classic Single* w/everything .....420
hamburger, jr. .....280
hamburger Kid's Meal .....270

components/condiments:
American cheese .....70
American cheese, jr. .....45
bacon, 1 slice .....20
honey mustard, reduced cal., 1 tsp. .....25
ketchup, 1 tsp. .....10
mayonnaise, ½ tsp. .....30
mustard, ½ tsp. .....0
onion, 4 rings .....5
pickles, 4 slices .....0
tomato, 1 slice .....5

*Fresh Stuffed Pitas:*
chicken, Caesar, or garden ranch .....480
classic Greek .....440
garden veggie .....400

pita sauce, 1 tbsp.:
Caesar vinaigrette, reduced fat/cal. .....70
garden ranch, reduced fat/cal. .....50

chicken nuggets, 5 pcs. .....230
chicken nuggets, 4 pc. Kid's Meal .....190

chicken nuggets' sauce, 1 pkt.:
barbecue .....45
honey .....90
honey mustard .....130
sweet and sour .....50

chili:
small, 8 oz. .....210
large, 12 oz. .....310
cheddar, shredded, 2 tbsp. .....70
saltines, 1 pkt. .....25

baked potato:
plain, 10 oz. .....310
bacon and cheese .....530
broccoli and cheese .....470

***Wendy's*, baked potato *(cont.)***
cheese . . . . . . . . . . . . . . . . . . . . . . . . . . . . . . . . .570
chili and cheese . . . . . . . . . . . . . . . . . . . . . . . . . .620
sour cream and chive . . . . . . . . . . . . . . . . . . . . . .370
sour cream pkt. . . . . . . . . . . . . . . . . . . . . . . . . . . . .60
whipped margarine pkt. . . . . . . . . . . . . . . . . . . . . .100
french fries, *Biggie* . . . . . . . . . . . . . . . . . . . . . . . . . . .470
french fries, *Great Biggie* . . . . . . . . . . . . . . . . . . . . . .570
french fries, small . . . . . . . . . . . . . . . . . . . . . . . . . . .270
salad, w/out dressing:
deluxe garden or side Caesar . . . . . . . . . . . . . . . . . .110
grilled chicken . . . . . . . . . . . . . . . . . . . . . . . . . . .190
side salad . . . . . . . . . . . . . . . . . . . . . . . . . . . . . . . .60
taco salad . . . . . . . . . . . . . . . . . . . . . . . . . . . . . .380
taco chips, 15 pcs. . . . . . . . . . . . . . . . . . . . . . . . .200
soft bread stick, 1 pc. . . . . . . . . . . . . . . . . . . . . . .130
dressing, 2 tbsp.:
blue cheese . . . . . . . . . . . . . . . . . . . . . . . . . . . . .180
French . . . . . . . . . . . . . . . . . . . . . . . . . . . . . . . . .120
French, fat free . . . . . . . . . . . . . . . . . . . . . . . . . . . .30
Italian, reduced fat/cal. . . . . . . . . . . . . . . . . . . . . . .40
Italian Caesar . . . . . . . . . . . . . . . . . . . . . . . . . . . .150
ranch, *Hidden Valley* . . . . . . . . . . . . . . . . . . . . . . .100
ranch, *Hidden Valley,* reduced fat/cal. . . . . . . . . . . . . . .60
Thousand Island . . . . . . . . . . . . . . . . . . . . . . . . . .130
*Frosty,* large . . . . . . . . . . . . . . . . . . . . . . . . . . . . . . .540
*Frosty,* medium . . . . . . . . . . . . . . . . . . . . . . . . . . . . .440
*Frosty,* small . . . . . . . . . . . . . . . . . . . . . . . . . . . . . . .330
**Wheat,** whole-grain, 1 cup:
durum . . . . . . . . . . . . . . . . . . . . . . . . . . . . . . . . . . . . .651
hard red spring . . . . . . . . . . . . . . . . . . . . . . . . . . . . .632
hard red winter . . . . . . . . . . . . . . . . . . . . . . . . . . . . .628
soft red winter . . . . . . . . . . . . . . . . . . . . . . . . . . . . . .556
hard white . . . . . . . . . . . . . . . . . . . . . . . . . . . . . . . . .657
soft white . . . . . . . . . . . . . . . . . . . . . . . . . . . . . . . . .571
**Wheat, parboiled,** see "Bulgur"
**Wheat, sprouted,** 1 cup . . . . . . . . . . . . . . . . . . . . . . .214
**Wheat bran** (see also "Cereal"):
crude, 2 tbsp. . . . . . . . . . . . . . . . . . . . . . . . . . . . . . . . .15

toasted (*Kretschmer*), ¼ cup . . . . . . . . . . . . . . . . . . . . . .30
unprocessed (*Quaker*), ⅓ cup . . . . . . . . . . . . . . . . . . . . .30
untoasted (*Hodgson Mill*), 2 tbsp. . . . . . . . . . . . . . . . . . .55
**Wheat dish mix** (see also "Tabouli"), 1 cup*:
pilaf (*Near East*) . . . . . . . . . . . . . . . . . . . . . . . . . . . .220
w/rice, creamy Parmesan (*Near East* Creative Grains) . . . . .280
w/rice, roasted pecan and garlic (*Near East* Creative
Grains) . . . . . . . . . . . . . . . . . . . . . . . . . . . . . . . . .240
w/rice and barley, chicken and herbs (*Near East* Creative
Grains) . . . . . . . . . . . . . . . . . . . . . . . . . . . . . . . . .270
roasted garlic (*Near East* Creative Grains) . . . . . . . . . . . . .220
**Wheat flakes,** rolled (*Arrowhead Mills*), ⅓ cup . . . . . . . . . .110
**Wheat flour,** ¼ cup, except as noted:
(*Hodgson Mill* 50/50 Wheat) . . . . . . . . . . . . . . . . . . . . .100
(*La Piña*) . . . . . . . . . . . . . . . . . . . . . . . . . . . . . . . . .100
all varieties, except whole wheat (*Gold Medal*) . . . . . . . . . .100
all-purpose, white, unbleached (*Pillsbury*) . . . . . . . . . . . .100
bread (*Eagle Mills* Bread Machine) . . . . . . . . . . . . . . . . .100
bread (*Hodgson Mill* Best for Bread) . . . . . . . . . . . . . . . .100
cake, white (*Betty Crocker Softasilk*) . . . . . . . . . . . . . . .100
mix, self-rising (*Aunt Jemima*), 3 tbsp. . . . . . . . . . . . . . . .90
pasta, see "Semolina flour"
pastry, whole wheat (*Hodgson Mill*) . . . . . . . . . . . . . . . .110
presifted (*Pillsbury* Shake & Blend) . . . . . . . . . . . . . . . .100
presifted (*Wondra*) . . . . . . . . . . . . . . . . . . . . . . . . . .100
seasoned (*Kentucky Kernel*) . . . . . . . . . . . . . . . . . . . . . .90
self-rising, white (*Pillsbury*) . . . . . . . . . . . . . . . . . . . .100
whole wheat (*Gold Medal*) . . . . . . . . . . . . . . . . . . . . . . .90
whole wheat, white (*Hodgson Mill*) . . . . . . . . . . . . . . . . .100
**Wheat germ:**
(*Kretschmer* Original), 2 tbsp. . . . . . . . . . . . . . . . . . . . .50
crude, 1 oz. . . . . . . . . . . . . . . . . . . . . . . . . . . . . . . .102
honey crunch (*Kretschmer*), 1⅔ tbsp. . . . . . . . . . . . . . . . .50
toasted, 1 oz. . . . . . . . . . . . . . . . . . . . . . . . . . . . . . .108
**Wheat gluten:**
(*Arrowhead Mills* Vital), 3 tbsp. . . . . . . . . . . . . . . . . . . .35
(*General Mills* Supreme Hygluten), ¼ cup . . . . . . . . . . . . .100
**Wheat kernels** (*Purity Foods* Berries), ¼ cup . . . . . . . . . . .160
**Whelk,** meat only, raw, 4 oz. . . . . . . . . . . . . . . . . . . . . .156

**Whipped topping,** see "Cream topping"
**Whiskey,** see "Liquor"
**Whiskey sour drink mixer** (*Mr & Mrs T*), 4 fl. oz. . . . . . . .100
**White bean,** mature:
boiled, ½ cup . . . . . . . . . . . . . . . . . . . . . . . . . . . . .125
small, dry (*Jack Rabbit*), ¼ cup . . . . . . . . . . . . . . . . . . .70
small, boiled, ½ cup . . . . . . . . . . . . . . . . . . . . . . . . .127
**White bean, canned,** Spanish style (*Goya*), 7.5 oz. . . . . . .130
***White Castle:***
sandwiches, 1 pc.:
  breakfast . . . . . . . . . . . . . . . . . . . . . . . . . . . . .340
  cheeseburger . . . . . . . . . . . . . . . . . . . . . . . . . . .160
  cheeseburger, bacon . . . . . . . . . . . . . . . . . . . . . . .200
  cheeseburger, double . . . . . . . . . . . . . . . . . . . . . .290
  chicken ring . . . . . . . . . . . . . . . . . . . . . . . . . . .200
  fish . . . . . . . . . . . . . . . . . . . . . . . . . . . . . . . .180
  hamburger . . . . . . . . . . . . . . . . . . . . . . . . . . . .140
  hamburger, double . . . . . . . . . . . . . . . . . . . . . . . .240
chicken rings, 6 pcs. . . . . . . . . . . . . . . . . . . . . . . . .210
sides:
  cheese sticks, 5 pcs. . . . . . . . . . . . . . . . . . . . . . .420
  french fries, small . . . . . . . . . . . . . . . . . . . . . . .115
  onion rings, 8 pcs. . . . . . . . . . . . . . . . . . . . . . . .290
shake, chocolate, 16 oz. . . . . . . . . . . . . . . . . . . . . . .250
shake, vanilla, 16 oz. . . . . . . . . . . . . . . . . . . . . . . .260
**White sauce mix** (*Knorr* Classic), 2 tsp. . . . . . . . . . . . . . .25
**Whitefish,** meat only:
raw, 4 oz. . . . . . . . . . . . . . . . . . . . . . . . . . . . . . .153
baked, broiled, or microwaved, 4 oz. . . . . . . . . . . . . . . . .195
**Whitefish, smoked** (*Ducktrap River*), 2 oz. . . . . . . . . . . . .70
**Whiting,** meat only:
raw, 4 oz. . . . . . . . . . . . . . . . . . . . . . . . . . . . . . .102
baked, broiled, or microwaved, 4 oz. . . . . . . . . . . . . . . . .130
**Wiener,** see "Frankfurter"
**Wild rice:**
raw (*Gourmet House/Gourmet House* Quick), ¼ cup . . . . . .170
raw (*Lundberg* Organic), ¼ cup . . . . . . . . . . . . . . . . . .160
cooked, 1 cup . . . . . . . . . . . . . . . . . . . . . . . . . . . .166
blends, see "Rice"

**Wild rice dishes,** see "Rice dishes"
**Wine,** 1 fl. oz.:
dessert or apertif[1] .45
dry or table[2] .21
**Wine, cooking,** 2 tbsp., except as noted:
Burgundy (*Regina*) .25
Marsala (*Holland House*) .45
red or white (*Holland House*) .20
rice (*Sun Luck* Mirin), 1 tbsp. .20
Sauterne (*Regina*) .20
sherry (*Holland House*) .45
sherry (*Regina*) .35
**Winged bean,** fresh:
raw, sliced, ½ cup .11
boiled, drained, ½ cup .12
**Winged bean, mature,** boiled, ½ cup 126
**Wolf fish,** Atlantic, meat only:
raw, 4 oz. 109
baked, broiled, or microwaved, 4 oz. 139
**Wonton wrapper:**
(*Frieda's*), 4 pcs., 1 oz. .80
(*Nasoya*), 8 pcs., 2.1 oz. 260
**Worcestershire sauce** (*Lea & Perrins*), 1 tsp. .5
**Wraps** (see also "Tortilla"), 2-oz. pc., except as noted:
plain (*Aladdin Bread*) 190
garlic pesto (*Aladdin Bread*) 180
garlic pesto (*Cedar's*), 2.5 oz. 190
multigrain, 6 (*Cedar's* Mountain Bread) 200
jalapeño (*Aladdin Bread*) 190
Southwestern (*Aladdin Bread*) 190
Southwestern (*Cedar's*), 2.5 oz. 185
spinach (*Cedar's*), 2.5 oz. 180
tomato basil (*Cedar's*), 2.5 oz. 185
wheat (*Cedar's* Mountain Bread) 180

[1]Includes fortified wines containing more than 15% alcohol, such as port, sherry, vermouth, etc.
[2]Includes wines containing less than 15% alcohol, such as burgundy, Chablis, champagne, etc.

**Wraps** ***(cont.)***
wheat, whole (*Aladdin Bread*) . . . . . . . . . . . . . . . . . . . . . . .180
white (*Cedar's* Mountain Bread) . . . . . . . . . . . . . . . . . . . . .180
**Wraps, filled,** frozen, 6-oz. pc., except as noted:
couscous/vegetable (*Cedarlane* Veggie Wrap) . . . . . . . . . . .220
pasta (*Wolfgang Puck's*), 12-oz. pc. . . . . . . . . . . . . . . . . . .340
rice/vegetable teriyaki (*Cedarlane* Veggie Wrap) . . . . . . . . .280
vegetarian pizza (*Cedarlane* Veggie Wrap) . . . . . . . . . . . . . .220

# Y-Z

| FOOD AND MEASURE | CALORIES |
|---|---|
| **Yam,** fresh, baked, or boiled, ½ cup | 79 |
| **Yam, canned or frozen,** see "Sweet potato" | |
| **Yam, mountain,** Hawaiian, ½ cup: | |
| raw, cubed | 46 |
| steamed, cubed | 59 |
| **Yam bean tuber,** fresh: | |
| raw (*Frieda's* Jicama), ¾ cup, 3 oz. | 35 |
| raw, sliced, ½ cup | 23 |
| boiled, drained, 4 oz. | 43 |
| **Yard-long bean,** fresh, ½ cup, except as noted: | |
| (*Frieda's* Long Bean), ¾ cup, 3 oz. | 40 |
| sliced, raw | 22 |
| sliced, boiled, drained | 25 |
| **Yard-long bean, mature,** boiled, ½ cup | 102 |
| **Yellow beans,** mature, boiled, ½ cup | 126 |
| **Yellow-eye beans,** dry (*Frieda's*), ½ cup | 120 |
| **Yellow squash,** fresh, see "Crookneck squash" | |
| **Yellow squash, canned** (*Sunshine*), ½ cup | 25 |
| **Yellow squash, frozen,** sliced (*Birds Eye*), ⅔ cup | 15 |
| **Yellowtail,** meat only: | |
| raw, 4 oz. | 166 |
| baked, broiled, or microwaved, 4 oz. | 212 |
| **Yogurt,** 8 oz., except as noted: | |
| plain (*Colombo* Fat Free) | 100 |
| plain (*Colombo* Lowfat) | 130 |
| plain (*Crowley* Nonfat) | 100 |
| plain (*Dannon* Lowfat) | 150 |
| plain (*Dannon* Nonfat) | 130 |
| plain (*Darigold* Lowfat) | 160 |
| plain (*Friendship*) | 150 |
| plain (*Stonyfield Farm*), 1 cup | 180 |
| plain (*Stonyfield Farm* Lowfat), 6 oz. | 80 |
| plain (*Stonyfield Farm* Nonfat) | 100 |
| plain (*Yoplait* Fat Free), 6 oz. | 80 |

**Yogurt *(cont.)***

all flavors (*Colombo* Light) . . . . . . . . . . . . . . . . . . . . . . . . .120
all flavors (*Dannon La Crème*), 4 oz. . . . . . . . . . . . . . . . . . . . .140
all flavors (*Dannon Light 'n Fit*) . . . . . . . . . . . . . . . . . . . . . .120
all flavors (*Dannon Sprinkl'ins*), 4.1 oz. . . . . . . . . . . . . . . . .120
all flavors (*Darigold* Light), 6 oz. . . . . . . . . . . . . . . . . . . . . .100
all flavors (*Darigold* Lowfat) . . . . . . . . . . . . . . . . . . . . . . . .240
all flavors (*Yoplait* Light), 6 oz. . . . . . . . . . . . . . . . . . . . . . .100
all flavors (*Yoplait Custard Style*), 6 oz. . . . . . . . . . . . . . . . .190
all fruit flavors (*Crowley* Swiss Style) . . . . . . . . . . . . . . . . . .240
all fruit flavors (*Yoplait* 99% Fat Free), 6 oz. . . . . . . . . . . . .170
all fruit flavors (*Yoplait Custard Style*), 4 oz. . . . . . . . . . . . .120
all fruit flavors (*Yoplait Exprésse/Go-Gurt*), 2.25 oz. . . . . . . .70
all fruit flavors (*Yoplait Trix/Yumsters*), 4 oz. . . . . . . . . . . . .120
all fruit flavors, except banana/strawberry
(*Colombo* Classic) . . . . . . . . . . . . . . . . . . . . . . . . . . . . . . .220
apple cinnamon (*Dannon* Fruit on the Bottom) . . . . . . . . . . .210
apricot mango (*Stonyfield Farm* Nonfat) . . . . . . . . . . . . . . . .160
banana (*Stonyfield Farm* Blended), 6 oz. . . . . . . . . . . . . . . . .170
banana/strawberry (*Colombo* Classic) . . . . . . . . . . . . . . . . . .230
berries, mixed (*Dannon* Fruit on the Bottom) . . . . . . . . . . . .210
blueberry (*Dannon* Fruit on the Bottom) . . . . . . . . . . . . . . . .210
blueberry (*Stonyfield Farm* Lowfat), 6 oz. . . . . . . . . . . . . . . .130
blueberry (*Stonyfield Farm* Nonfat) . . . . . . . . . . . . . . . . . . . .160
blueberry, wild (*Stonyfield Farm*), 6 oz. . . . . . . . . . . . . . . . .160
blueberry peach (*Dannon* Fruit on the Bottom), 4 oz. . . . . .100
blueberry vanilla cream (*Dannon Double Delights*), 6 oz. . . .180
boysenberry (*Dannon* Fruit on the Bottom) . . . . . . . . . . . . .210
cappuccino (*Stonyfield Farm* Underground Nonfat) . . . . . . .160
caramel (*Stonyfield Farm* Lowfat), 6 oz. . . . . . . . . . . . . . . . .170
caramel (*Stonyfield Farm* Nonfat) . . . . . . . . . . . . . . . . . . . . .220
caramel chocolate (*Stonyfield Farm*), 4 oz. . . . . . . . . . . . . .110
cherry (*Dannon* Fruit on the Bottom) . . . . . . . . . . . . . . . . . .210
cherry (*Stonyfield Farm* Nonfat) . . . . . . . . . . . . . . . . . . . . . .160
cherry (*Stonyfield Farm* Underground Nonfat) . . . . . . . . . . .200
chocolate (*Stonyfield Farm* Underground Nonfat) . . . . . . . .200
coconut cream pie (*Yoplait*), 6 oz. . . . . . . . . . . . . . . . . . . . .190
coffee or cranberry raspberry (*Dannon*) . . . . . . . . . . . . . . . .220
lemon (*Colombo* Classic) . . . . . . . . . . . . . . . . . . . . . . . . . . . .180
lemon (*Dannon*) . . . . . . . . . . . . . . . . . . . . . . . . . . . . . . . . . . .220

lemon (*Stonyfield Farm* Lotsa Nonfat) . . . . . . . . . . . . . . . . .160
lemon (*Stonyfield Farm* Luscious Lowfat), 6 oz. . . . . . . . . . .130
lemon (*Yoplait*), 6 oz. . . . . . . . . . . . . . . . . . . . . . . . . . . . . . .180
lemon meringue pie (*Dannon Double Delights*), 6 oz. . . . . .180
maple, creamy (*Stonyfield Farm*), 6 oz. . . . . . . . . . . . . . . . . .160
maple vanilla (*Stonyfield Farm* Lowfat), 6 oz. . . . . . . . . . . .120
mocha (*Stonyfield Farm* Mocha-ccino), 6 oz. . . . . . . . . . . .170
mocha latte (*Stonyfield Farm* Lowfat), 6 oz. . . . . . . . . . . . .120
peach (*Dannon* Fruit on the Bottom) . . . . . . . . . . . . . . . . . .210
peach (*Stonyfield Farm* Blended), 6 oz. . . . . . . . . . . . . . . . .170
peach (*Stonyfield Farm* Just Peachy Lowfat), 6 oz. . . . . . . .130
peach (*Stonyfield Farm* Nonfat) . . . . . . . . . . . . . . . . . . . . .150
piña colada (*Yoplait*), 6 oz. . . . . . . . . . . . . . . . . . . . . . . . .170
strawberries and cream (*Stonyfield Farm*), 6 oz. . . . . . . . . .160
raspberry Bavarian creme (*Dannon Double Delights*),
 6 oz. . . . . . . . . . . . . . . . . . . . . . . . . . . . . . . . . . . . . . . . .170
raspberry or strawberry (*Dannon* Fruit on the Bottom) . . . .210
raspberry or strawberry (*Stonyfield Farm* Lowfat), 6 oz. . . .130
raspberry or strawberry (*Stonyfield Farm* Nonfat) . . . . . . . .160
strawberry (*Colombo* Lowfat) . . . . . . . . . . . . . . . . . . . . . . .190
strawberry (*Stonyfield Farm* Blended), 6 oz. . . . . . . . . . . . .170
strawberry banana (*Dannon* Fruit on the Bottom) . . . . . . . .210
strawberry banana (*Stonyfield Farm*), 4 oz. . . . . . . . . . . . . .100
strawberry banana, blueberry, cherry, or raspberry
 (*Dannon* Blended Nonfat), 4 oz. . . . . . . . . . . . . . . . . . . .100
strawberry peach (*Dannon* Blended Nonfat), 4 oz. . . . . . . . .100
tropical w/peaches (*Dannon* Fruit on the Bottom) . . . . . . . .240
vanilla (*Colombo* Classic) . . . . . . . . . . . . . . . . . . . . . . . . . .180
vanilla (*Colombo* Fat Free) . . . . . . . . . . . . . . . . . . . . . . . . .160
vanilla (*Dannon*) . . . . . . . . . . . . . . . . . . . . . . . . . . . . . . . . .230
vanilla (*Stonyfield Farm*), 1 cup . . . . . . . . . . . . . . . . . . . .230
vanilla (*Stonyfield Farm* Lowfat), 6 oz. . . . . . . . . . . . . . . .120
vanilla, French (*Colombo* Lowfat) . . . . . . . . . . . . . . . . . . . .180
vanilla, French (*Stonyfield Farm*), 6 oz. . . . . . . . . . . . . . . .170
vanilla, French (*Stonyfield Farm* Nonfat) . . . . . . . . . . . . . .160
vanilla truffle (*Stonyfield Farm*), 6 oz. . . . . . . . . . . . . . . . .220
vanilla raspberry or strawberry, French (*Dannon* Fruit
 on the Bottom) . . . . . . . . . . . . . . . . . . . . . . . . . . . . . . . . .240

**Yogurt, frozen,** ½ cup:
apple pie (*Häagen-Dazs*) . . . . . . . . . . . . . . . . . . . . . . . . . .230

**Yogurt, frozen *(cont.)***

(*Ben & Jerry's Phish Food*) . . . . . . . . . . . . . . . . . . . . . . . . .230
(*Ben & Jerry's Raspberry Gone Coconuts*) . . . . . . . . . . . . . .210
caramel w/cake (*Ben & Jerry's Ooey Gooey Cake*) . . . . . . . . .190
caramel fudge (*Dreyer's/Edy's Caramel Fudge Cosmo*) . . . .140
cherry fudge chip (*Ben & Jerry's Cherry Garcia*) . . . . . . . . . .170
chocolate (*Breyers*) . . . . . . . . . . . . . . . . . . . . . . . . . . . . . . . .130
chocolate (*Cascadian Farm*) . . . . . . . . . . . . . . . . . . . . . . . . .130
chocolate (*Dreyer's/Edy's* Decadence) . . . . . . . . . . . . . . . . .120
chocolate (*Stonyfield Farm*) . . . . . . . . . . . . . . . . . . . . . . . . .100
chocolate cherry cordial (*Turkey Hill* Fat Free) . . . . . . . . . . .110
chocolate chip (*Dreyer's/Edy's Chips Supreme*) . . . . . . . . . . .120
chocolate chip, chocolate (*Häagen-Dazs*) . . . . . . . . . . . . . . .230
chocolate chip cookie dough (*Ben & Jerry's*) . . . . . . . . . . . .200
chocolate chip cookie dough (*Turkey Hill*) . . . . . . . . . . . . . .140
chocolate fudge (*Dreyer's/Edy's* Fat Free) . . . . . . . . . . . . . .100
chocolate fudge brownie (*Ben & Jerry's*) . . . . . . . . . . . . . . .190
chocolate marshmallow (*Turkey Hill* Fat Free) . . . . . . . . . . .130
coffee (*Häagen-Dazs*) . . . . . . . . . . . . . . . . . . . . . . . . . . . . .200
coffee (*Stonyfield Farm* Decaf/Soft Gourmet) . . . . . . . . . . . .90
coffee fudge sundae (*Edy's* Fat Free) . . . . . . . . . . . . . . . . . .100
cookies and cream (*Dreyer's/Edy's*) . . . . . . . . . . . . . . . . . . .110
cookies and cream, mint (*Turkey Hill* Fat Free) . . . . . . . . . .110
creme caramel (*Stonyfield Farm*) . . . . . . . . . . . . . . . . . . . . .120
dulce de leche (*Häagen-Dazs*) . . . . . . . . . . . . . . . . . . . . . . .190
lemon chiffon (*Cascadian Farm*) . . . . . . . . . . . . . . . . . . . . . .120
mint chocolate chip or mocha almond
(*Stonyfield Farm*) . . . . . . . . . . . . . . . . . . . . . . . . . . . . .130
mocha fudge (*Cascadian Farm*) . . . . . . . . . . . . . . . . . . . . . .120
Neapolitan (*Turkey Hill* Fat Free) . . . . . . . . . . . . . . . . . . . . .100
peach raspberry (*Turkey Hill*) . . . . . . . . . . . . . . . . . . . . . . .110
raspberry (*Stonyfield Farm*) . . . . . . . . . . . . . . . . . . . . . . . . .100
raspberry (*Stonyfield Farm* Soft) . . . . . . . . . . . . . . . . . . . . . .90
raspberry, black (*Turkey Hill*) . . . . . . . . . . . . . . . . . . . . . . .110
raspberry chocolate swirl (*Cascadian Farm*) . . . . . . . . . . . .110
strawberry (*Breyers*) . . . . . . . . . . . . . . . . . . . . . . . . . . . . . .120
strawberry (*Häagen-Dazs* Nonfat) . . . . . . . . . . . . . . . . . . . .140
tin roof sundae (*Dreyer's/Edy's* Ultimate) . . . . . . . . . . . . . .130
tin roof sundae (*Turkey Hill*) . . . . . . . . . . . . . . . . . . . . . . . .140
toffee crunch (*Dreyer's/Edy's Heath*) . . . . . . . . . . . . . . . . . .120

vanilla (*Breyers*) . . . . . . . . . . . . . . . . . . . . . . . . . . . . 120
vanilla (*Cascadian Farm*) . . . . . . . . . . . . . . . . . . . . . . 130
vanilla (*Dreyer's/Edy's*) . . . . . . . . . . . . . . . . . . . . . . . . 100
vanilla (*Häagen-Dazs*) . . . . . . . . . . . . . . . . . . . . . . . . . 200
vanilla (*Stonyfield Farm*) . . . . . . . . . . . . . . . . . . . . . . . 90
vanilla, French or simply (*Stonyfield Farm* Soft) . . . . . . . . . . 90
vanilla bean (*Turkey Hill*) . . . . . . . . . . . . . . . . . . . . . . . 110
vanilla–chocolate (*Turkey Hill*) . . . . . . . . . . . . . . . . . . . 110
vanilla–chocolate swirl (*Dreyer's/Edy's* Fat Free) . . . . . . . . . . 90
vanilla–chocolate–strawberry (*Breyers*) . . . . . . . . . . . . . . 120
vanilla fudge (*Häagen-Dazs*) . . . . . . . . . . . . . . . . . . . . . 220
vanilla fudge (*Turkey Hill* Fat Free) . . . . . . . . . . . . . . . . 110
vanilla fudge swirl (*Stonyfield Farm*) . . . . . . . . . . . . . . . . 110
vanilla raspberry swirl (*Häagen-Dazs*) . . . . . . . . . . . . . . . 170
**"Yogurt," soy:**
plain (*Silk*), 8 oz. . . . . . . . . . . . . . . . . . . . . . . . . . . . 150
all fruit flavors (*Stonyfield Farm O'Soy*), 4 oz. . . . . . . . . . . . 90
all fruit flavors, except black cherry (*Silk*) . . . . . . . . . . . . . 170
cherry, black (*Silk*), 6 oz. . . . . . . . . . . . . . . . . . . . . . . 160
vanilla (*Silk*), 6 oz. . . . . . . . . . . . . . . . . . . . . . . . . . . 110
vanilla (*Silk*), 8 oz. . . . . . . . . . . . . . . . . . . . . . . . . . . 150
**Yogurt bar,** frozen, 1 pc.:
blackberry (*Cascadian Farm*) . . . . . . . . . . . . . . . . . . . . . . 80
cherry fudge chip (*Ben & Jerry's Cherry Garcia*) . . . . . . . . . 250
chocolate or vanilla (*Cascadian Farm*) . . . . . . . . . . . . . . . 100
**Yogurt drink,** all flavors:
(*Dannon Actimel*), 3.3 fl. oz. . . . . . . . . . . . . . . . . . . . . . 90
(*Dannon Frusion* Smoothie), 1 bottle . . . . . . . . . . . . . . . . 270
**Youngberry juice,** blend (*Ceres*), 5.25 fl. oz. . . . . . . . . . . . 87
**Yu choy sum** (*Frieda's*), 1 cup, 3 oz. . . . . . . . . . . . . . . . . 20
**Yuca root** (*Frieda's*), ⅔ cup, 3 oz. . . . . . . . . . . . . . . . . 100
**Ziti entree,** frozen:
baked (*Celentano*), 9 oz., ⅛ pkg. . . . . . . . . . . . . . . . . . . 250
Parmesano (*Budget Gourmet*), 8-oz. pkg. . . . . . . . . . . . . . 260
**Zucchini,** fresh, ½ cup, except as noted:
raw, sliced . . . . . . . . . . . . . . . . . . . . . . . . . . . . . . . . . 9
raw, baby (*Frieda's*), ⅔ cup, 3 oz. . . . . . . . . . . . . . . . . . . 20
raw, baby, 1 large, 3⅛" . . . . . . . . . . . . . . . . . . . . . . . . . . 3
boiled, drained, sliced . . . . . . . . . . . . . . . . . . . . . . . . . . 14
boiled, drained, mashed . . . . . . . . . . . . . . . . . . . . . . . . . 19

**Zucchini, canned,** Italian style:
(*Del Monte*), ½ cup . . . . . . . . . . . . . . . . . . . . . . . . . . .30
w/tomato juice, ½ cup . . . . . . . . . . . . . . . . . . . . . . . . .33
**Zucchini, marinated,** sun-dried, in jars (*Antica Italia*), 1 oz. . . . . . . . . . . . . . . . . . . . . . . . . . . . . . . . . . . . .160
**Zucchini soufflé,** frozen (*Melrose*), ½ cup . . . . . . . . . . . . . .90